EPIDEMIOLOGY

Yevhen Tarasov

ALLIED HEALTH PRESS

Epidemiology

Author: **Yevhen Tarasov**

Allied Health Press
4164 Lakeshore Road
Burlington ON L7L 1A4
Canada
www.alliedhealthpress.com
Email: orders@arclereducation.com

ISBN: 978-1-77956-251-7

ABOUT THE AUTHOR

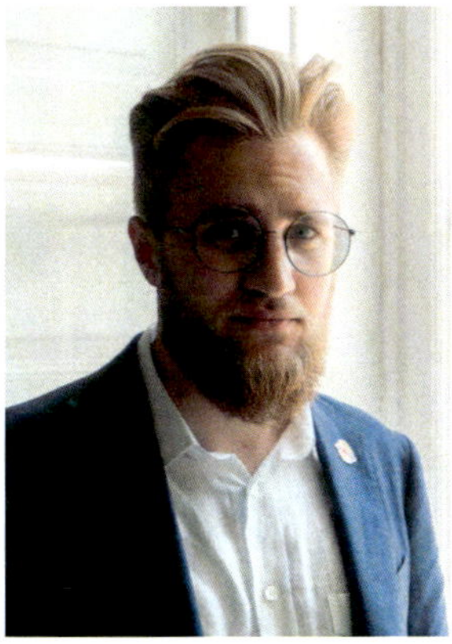

Yevhen Tarasov, MD, EuSpLM is an assistant professor at the Department of General and Clinical Epidemiology and Biosafety with course on Microbiology and Virology at Odesa National Medical University. Yevhen Tarasov received his MD in 2018 and got specialization in Medical Laboratory Science in 2019 with residency at The Filatov Institute of Eye Diseases and Tissue Therapy of the National Academy if Medical Science of Ukraine. He then joined the at the Department of General and Clinical Epidemiology and Biosafety with course on Microbiology and Virology at Odesa National Medical University, Odesa, Ukraine as an assistant professor. His research interests include epidemiology and diagnostics of autoimmune diseases and allergy. He is a group leader of work group on Ukrainian adaptation of the the International Consensus on Antinuclear Antibody (ANA) Patterns (ICAP).

Word Roots, Prefixes, and Suffixes by Chapter

Chapter 1 Introduction to Epidemiology

Epidemio-: Populations or epidemics.

-logy: (study of) astrology, biology, ecology, zoology

Epi-: pidemic, epidermis, epiphenomenon, episode

-demic: Pertaining to a population or geographic area affected by a disease.

-emia: blood (used in epidemiology to denote the presence of a substance in the blood).

Endo-: (inside) endocrine, endoskeleton, endothermic

-idemiology: Study and analysis of the patterns, causes, and effects of health and disease conditions in defined populations.

Patho-: Disease, suffering (used in epidemiology to denote the study of the origin and development of a disease).

-genic: (creating) carcinogenic, eugenic, mutagenic, photogenic

Chapter 2 Measuring Health and Disease

Patho-: Disease

Dys-: Abnormal, difficult, or painful

-itis: Inflammation

-logy: Study or science of

Hyper-: Excessive or above normal

-emia: Condition of the blood

-genic: Produced by or related to

-osis: Condition, usually abnormal

Chapter 3 Study Designs in Epidemiology

-graphic: Pertaining to writing or recording

Prevalence-: The proportion of a population found to have a condition

-Demics: Pertaining to populations or people.

Pandemics (widespread outbreak of disease affecting many people).

Prevent-: Before or in advance.

Co-: together, -study: the act of studying.

-sectional: relating to a section or segment.

Chapter 4 Infectious Disease Epidemiology

Infect-: To infect, to contaminate

Patho-: Disease

Micro-: Small, minute

-osis: Condition, usually abnormal

-emia: Condition of the blood

Zoono-: Animal

-viridae: Family of viruses

Immuno-: Immune system

Chapter 5 Descriptive Epidemiology

Descriptive-: To describe or characterize

Geo-: Earth, geography

-incidence: The rate of occurrence of new cases of a disease

Morb-: Disease or sickness

Mortal-: Death

Chapter 6 Clinical Epidemiology and Its Relevance for Public Health

Public-: Pertaining to the community or general population.

-Health: State of being whole or free from illness.

Clinical-: Pertaining to or based on observation and treatment of patients.

-Iatry: Medical treatment or healing.

Eco-: Environment or ecological system.

-Pathy: Disease or suffering.

Chapter 7 Social Epidemiology: Past, Present, and Future

Socio-: Pertaining to society or social conditions.

-Metrics: Measurement or study of measurement.

Anthropo-: Human or relating to humans.

-Pandemic: Affecting a whole people or region.

Cultural-: Pertaining to culture or customs.

Chapter 8 Epidemiological Burden of Tuberculosis in Developing Countries

Tuberculo-: Relating to a small swelling or nodule.

Mycobacterium: A genus of bacteria.

-Bacterium: Bacterium (plural: bacteria).

Pulmo-: Relating to the lungs.

-ary: Relating to or pertaining to.

Anti-: Against or opposing.

-cidal: Killing or destroying.

Multi-: Many or multiple.

-therapy: Treatment or therapy.

Chapter 9 Environmental and Occupational Epidemiology

Environment-: Surroundings or external conditions.

Occupational-: Pertaining to work or employment.

-al: Pertaining to or relating to.

Toxico-: Poisonous or toxic.

-ic: Pertaining to or characterized by.

Expo-: Exposure or contact with.

-ure: Result of an action or process.

-opathy: Disease or disorder.

Chapter 10 Epidemiology to Evaluation and Policy

Evalua-: To determine the significance, worth, or condition of something.

-ation: Action or process.

Policy-: A principle or rule to guide decisions and achieve rational outcomes.

-ician: Practitioner or specialist.

-Eval: Shortened form of evaluation.

Stat-: To stand or determine.

-oid: Resembling or like.

Quan-: Quantify.

Table of Contents

3 Study Designs in Epidemiology 59

4 Infectious Disease Epidemiology 119

LIST OF FIGURES

LIST OF TABLES

PREFACE

Epidemiology is the scientific discipline that focuses on understanding the prevalence and distribution of diseases across different population groups, and the factors that influence these patterns. It plays a crucial role in public health by providing data that helps in designing and assessing preventive measures, as well as in managing diseases in populations where they have already emerged. The discipline uses specialized methods for collecting and analyzing data, along with a specific set of technical terminology that is essential for effective communication within the field.

As a fundamental component of medical research, the epidemiology of a disease is as critical as its clinical symptoms and pathological features in describing its overall nature. The process often involves identifying a specific population to study, termed the 'target population,' which forms the basis for drawing broader conclusions about the disease. In some instances, such as in the evaluation of dust control measures in British coal mines, epidemiologists have access to data encompassing the entire target population, enabling comprehensive analysis of all new cases of diseases like coal workers' pneumoconiosis across a defined area.

However, it is more common for epidemiologists to work with a subset of the target population, known as a study sample, due to practical limitations. This approach can be seen in scenarios where a specialist, such as a gastroenterologist, may use data from their clinical practice to make generalizations about the long-term outcomes of diseases like Crohn's disease. The validity and reliability of the conclusions drawn from such samples are heavily dependent on the size of the sample and the method of selection. Small sample sizes are particularly vulnerable to random variations that may skew the results, and these potential errors can be assessed statistically.

A more challenging issue arises from the method of sample selection, which can introduce systematic biases. For example, a specialist dealing with a high number of complex or severe cases may have a patient pool that does not accurately represent the typical progression and complications of a disease. Such biases are difficult to quantify and often require subjective judgment to evaluate.

To mitigate these issues, epidemiologists can employ random sampling techniques where each individual in the target population has a known and equal chance of being selected. This strategy, however, presupposes the ability to identify and enumerate every individual within the target population, a task that is not always feasible due to various logistical constraints. Therefore, while epidemiology provides invaluable insights into disease patterns and their determinants, researchers must carefully consider the limitations and potential biases inherent in their study designs.

The primary objective of the textbook "Epidemiology" is to furnish students, academicians, and professionals in the field of public health with a comprehensive, detailed, and accessible resource on the principles and practices of epidemiology. This textbook aims to enhance the understanding of the patterns, causes, and effects of health and disease conditions in defined populations. It serves as both an introductory guide for newcomers and a thorough reference for seasoned professionals.

This textbook is designed to provide a foundational understanding of the various methods and techniques used in the study of epidemiology, integrating both classical concepts and contemporary developments. It covers a broad spectrum of topics, including the distribution of diseases, the dynamics of transmission, and the effectiveness of health interventions, policies, and public health practices. The goal is to equip readers with the skills necessary to conduct epidemiological research and to apply epidemiological knowledge to the solving of real-world health problems.

Structured to cater to an audience that ranges from undergraduate and graduate students in public health and related fields to healthcare providers, policy makers, and researchers in epidemiology, the book ensures that its content is accessible without sacrificing depth or scientific rigor. Each chapter includes detailed explanations and illustrative examples that provide practical insights into the application of epidemiological principles.

The textbook also emphasizes the critical role of epidemiology in informing public health decisions, guiding preventive healthcare, and advancing medical research. It addresses the ethical considerations inherent in epidemiological studies and the importance of statistical methods in analyzing epidemiological data. Special attention is given to emerging challenges in global health, including the management of pandemics and the impact of environmental and social factors on health.

In addition to theoretical content, this book incorporates interactive components such as data sets for analysis, questions for reflection, and tasks designed to enhance analytical skills. These interactive elements encourage active learning and help students develop practical skills in data interpretation and critical thinking relevant to epidemiological contexts.

The textbook aims to foster a thorough and nuanced understanding of epidemiology as a discipline pivotal to public health, enhancing the capacity of readers to contribute effectively to health surveillance, disease prevention, and health promotion initiatives. Providing comprehensive coverage of both the foundational elements and the cutting-edge issues in epidemiology, the textbook strives to prepare its readers to address the complex health challenges of today and tomorrow.

Chapter

INTRODUCTION TO EPIDEMIOLOGY

1

Contents

Introduction

Epidemiology serves as a cornerstone in understanding the distribution and determinants of health-related states or events within populations, along with the application of this knowledge to control health problems. At its essence, epidemiology delves into patterns of disease occurrence and explores the factors influencing these patterns. It plays a crucial role in public health by providing insights into the causes and spread of diseases, informing preventive measures, and guiding health policies and interventions.

One fundamental aspect of epidemiology is its focus on populations rather than individuals. By studying groups of people, epidemiologists can identify commonalities and trends that may not be apparent at the individual level. Through various study designs, such as observational studies and clinical trials, epidemiologists gather data to examine the relationships between exposures (such as lifestyle factors, environmental conditions, or genetic predispositions) and health outcomes (such as diseases, injuries, or deaths). Epidemiological research employs rigorous methods to collect, analyze, and interpret data. This involves establishing clear study objectives, designing appropriate study protocols, and employing statistical techniques to draw valid conclusions. Epidemiologists also assess the validity and reliability of their findings, considering factors such as bias, confounding variables, and chance.

Moreover, epidemiology is interdisciplinary in nature, drawing on knowledge and methodologies from fields such as biology, statistics, sociology, and environmental science. This interdisciplinary approach allows epidemiologists to investigate complex health issues from multiple perspectives, facilitating a more comprehensive understanding of disease dynamics and risk factors.

Ultimately, the insights gained from epidemiological studies contribute to the development of evidence-based strategies for disease prevention, health promotion, and healthcare planning. By identifying high-risk populations, elucidating causal pathways, and evaluating the effectiveness of interventions, epidemiology plays a vital role in improving public health outcomes and reducing the burden of diseases worldwide.

Orientation and Directional Terms

Term	Definition	Illustration
Clinical Trials	Clinical trials are research studies that test a medical, surgical, or behavioral intervention in people. These trials are the primary way that researchers determine if a new form of treatment or prevention, such as a new drug, diet, or medical device (for example, a pacemaker), is safe and effective in people.	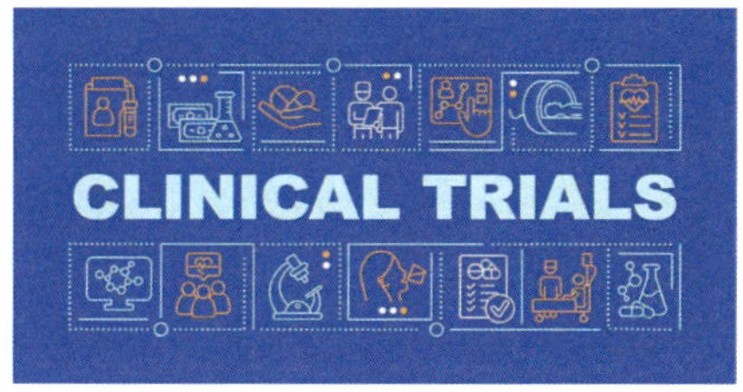
Lung Cancer	Lung cancer is cancer that forms in tissues of the lung, usually in the cells that line the air passages. It is the leading cause of cancer death in both men and women.	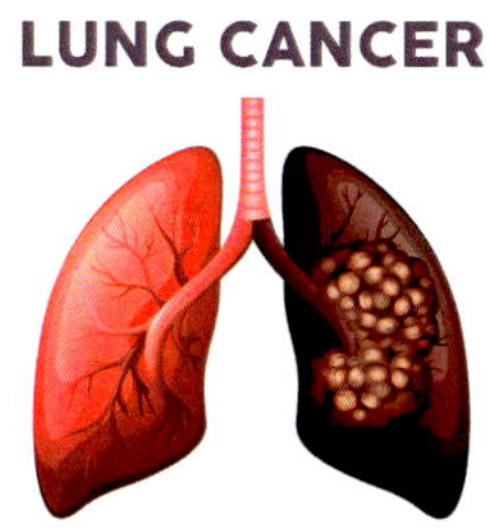
Morbidity	Morbidity” refers to the state of being diseased or unhealthy within a population. It is often used in epidemiology and public health to describe the prevalence of diseases, illnesses, or other health-related conditions within a specific group or population over a certain period of time.	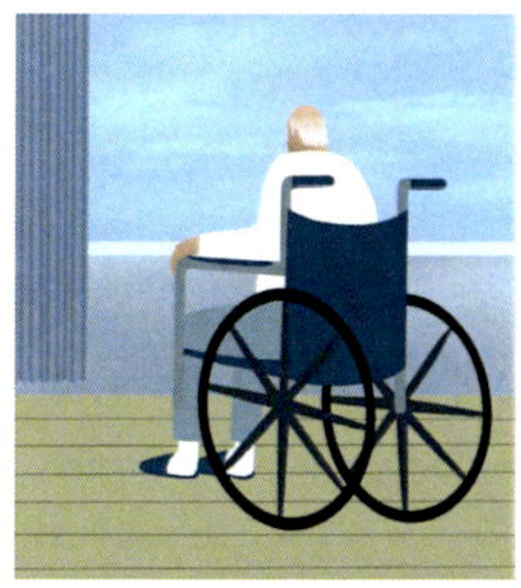
Mortality	Mortality” refers to the state of being subject to death, or the incidence of death within a population. It is a crucial measure in epidemiology, demography, and public health, providing insights into the overall health and well-being of a population.	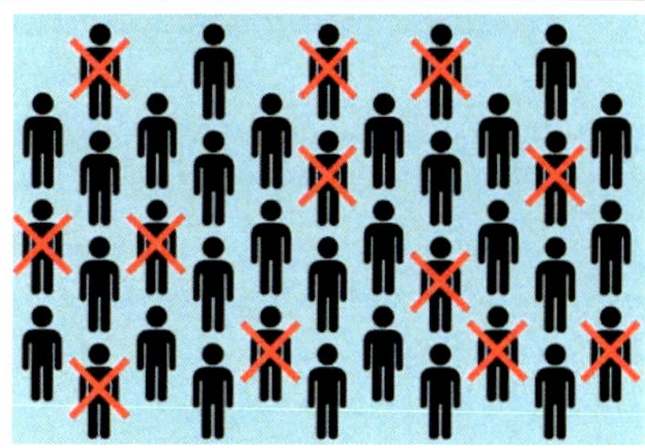
Prostate-specific antigen (PSA)	Prostate-specific antigen (PSA) test is a blood test used primarily to screen for prostate cancer. The test measures the amount of prostate-specific antigen (PSA) in your blood.	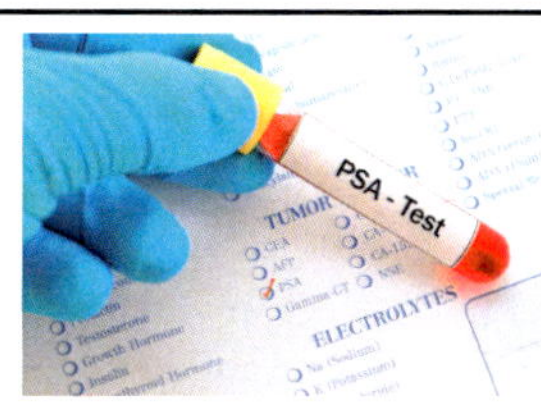

1.1. Basics of Epidemiology

The study of disease frequency, distribution, and determinants in human populations, as well as the application of this knowledge to health promotion, disease prevention, and disease control, is known as epidemiology.

1. Major Components of the Definition
   - **Population:** Epidemiology primarily examines the impact of diseases on populations rather than on individuals. For instance, while malaria is widespread in Ethiopia, cases of lung cancer are uncommon. When an individual does develop lung cancer, the likelihood of death is higher. Despite lung cancer being a more deadly condition, epidemiology places greater importance on diseases like malaria that affect larger numbers of people.
   - **Frequency:** This demonstrates that the science of epidemiology is primarily quantitative. The frequency (occurrence) of diseases and other health-related conditions is the focus of epidemiology. Morbidity and mortality rates are used to quantify the frequency of diseases.
   - **Health Related Conditions:** Because everything around us and everything we do has an impact on our health, epidemiology is concerned not only with disease but also with other conditions related to health. Conditions that impact or affect health, either directly or indirectly, are referred to as health-related conditions. These could include births, injuries, and health-related behaviors like smoking, being unemployed, being poor, etc.
   - **Distribution:** Distribution refers to the geographical distribution of diseases, the distribution in time, and the distribution by type of persons affected.
   - **Determinants:** Determinants are factors that determine whether or not a person will get a disease.
   - Application of the research to the prevention and management of health issues as well as the promotion of health. This means that finding efficient methods for disease prevention and control is the main goal of research on the frequency, distribution, and determinants of disease.

1.1.1. The Objectives of Epidemiology

What are the particular goals of epidemiology? The first is to determine the cause or etiology of an illness as well as any associated risk factors, or variables that raise an individual's risk of contracting an illness. How the illness spreads from one individual to another or from a nonhuman reservoir to a human population is what we are interested in learning. Intervention to lower disease-related morbidity and mortality is our ultimate goal. Creating a logical foundation for preventative initiatives is our goal. The foundation for disease prevention initiatives can be established if the etiologic or causative factors are identified and exposure to them is minimized or eliminated. Furthermore, we can create effective immunizations and therapies that stop the disease from spreading to other people.

Second, to assess the level of illness present in the neighborhood. To plan health services and facilities and to train future healthcare providers, it is imperative to know the burden of disease in the community.

Third, research disease prognosis and natural history. It is obvious that some diseases are more serious than others; some may present with a shorter time to death, while others may not. Others are not lethal. In order to compare the outcomes of using new modalities with the baseline data and assess whether our new strategies have been truly effective, we want to quantitatively define the baseline natural history of a disease. This will allow us to develop new modes of intervention, such as treatments or new ways to prevent complications.

The fourth step is to assess treatment and prevention strategies as well as new and current delivery methods. For example, does the prostate-specific antigen (PSA) test, which is used to screen men for prostate cancer, improve survival for those who are diagnosed with the disease? Has the rise of managed care and other innovative healthcare delivery and insurance systems affected the health outcomes and quality of life of the patients involved? If so, how has this impact been defined and quantified?

Fifth, to serve as the basis for creating public policy concerning genetic issues, environmental concerns, and other aspects of illness prevention and health promotion. For instance, is there a risk to human health from electromagnetic radiation emitted by heating pads, electric blankets, and other home appliances? Are there negative short- or long-term health effects in human populations caused by high atmospheric ozone or particulate matter levels? Is there a significant risk to human health from radon in homes? Which jobs are linked to a higher risk of illness among employees, and what kinds of regulations are necessary?

1.1.2. History of Epidemiology

The history of epidemiology stretches from 400 B.C. to the present day (Table 1.1).

Table 1.1. Historical Milestones are Described Against Each Period/Year

Period/Year	Milestone
400 B.C.	Hippocrates a Greek physician described the influence of the environment on diseases. Defined the words "epidemic" and "endemic."
1334	Clinical trial concept was proposed by Petrach.
1543	Girolamo Fracastoro, a physician from Italy proposed that disease is caused by live unseen small particles.
1546	The germ theory of disease was presented in the book titled "De Contagiosis Morbis" authored by Girolamo Fracastoro.
1646	Rene Descartes, A French scientist, proposed reductionism that is studying one factor at a time and depending on the evidence rather than imagination.
1662	Individual deaths and their causes in London were discussed. by Johan Grant in his book entitled "His Natural and Political Observations Upon the Bills of Mortality." He also used a quantitative approach on the patterns of birth, death and disease prevalence and proposed Life tables.
1668	Thomas Sydenham from England described the concept of generic diseases.

1675	By developing a microscope, Antonie von Leeuwenhoek, a Dutch scientist showed a shred of evidence for the germ theory of disease.
1700	Bernardino Ramazzini, an Italian physician wrote an account of the occurrence of similar cases in workers sharing the same space in his book titled "De Morbis Artificum Diatriba."
1706–1777	François Bossier de Lacroix first attempted to classify the diseases.
1707	Pathological investigations of a series of sudden deaths in the city of Rome, Italy were delineated in the book entitled "De Subitaneis Mortibus" authored by Giovanni Maria Lancisi.
1713	Bernardino Ramazzini reported a higher rate of breast cancer in nuns than married women.
1747	James Lind a Scottish physician in the first clinical trial proved that consuming citrus fruits cure the Scurvy disease.
1775	A causal association of exposure to suit with a higher incidence of scrotal cancer was proposed by Percivall Pott, an English surgeon.
1780	First dengue-like illness was reported in India from Chennai.
1798	Cow pox conferring protection on smallpox was proposed by Edward Jenner, a physician from England.
1801	Registration of deaths was introduced in England.
1802	Vaccination for smallpox was introduced in India.
1838	William Farr initiated the national system of death causes in England.
1842	A report on the Sanitary conditions of the Laboring population of Great Britain authored by Edwin Chadwick was published.
1842	Massachusetts system for registration of births, deaths and marriages was introduced in Massachusetts, United States.
1847	Ignaz Philipp Semmelweis, a Hungarian physician, proved that using of disinfected hands while treating pregnant women in obstetric clinics will prevent the occurrence of Puerperal fever.
1850	Report of Sanitary Commission of the State of Massachusetts was published by Lemuel Shattuck in the United States in 1853 John Snow, an English physician presented a paper on communicable diseases.
1854	John Snow reported the source of the Cholera outbreak in London.
1893	The First International Classification of diseases was adopted by the International statistical institute.
1894	*Yersinia pestis* was discovered by Alexander Yersin, a Swiss/French bacteriologist.
1897	The first vaccine in India was developed for plague by Dr. Waldemar Mordecai Haffkine.
1911	Indian Council of Medical Research was established.
1915	The application of Iodized salt for the eradication of goiter was proposed in Switzerland.
1924	Iodine salt was introduced at the community level in several countries

1939	AB Hill in England published a textbook entitled "Principles of Medical Statistics."
1948	World Health Organization was established.
1948	Framingham heart study was initiated in Framingham, Massachusetts, United States with a cohort of 5209 men and women aged 30–62 years to identify risk factors for cardiovascular diseases.
1950	Three case-control studies on the association of smoking and lung cancers were published by Morton L. Levin and co-workers, Ernest Ludwig Wynder and Evarts Ambrose Graham and Richard Shaboe Doll and Austin Bradford Hill.
1950	Methyl mercury poisoning of fish known as Minamata Disease was reported in Japan.
1950	Dengue was first discovered in the Philippines and Thailand.
1951	British Doctors Cohort study was initiated by Richard Doll and Austin Broad Ford- Hill in England.
1952	Zika virus disease in humans was first reported in Uganda and the United Republic of Tanzania.
1952	Primary Health Centers were started in India.
1953	United States Veteran's study on a cohort of 220000 males was commissioned by Harold Dorn.
1953	A national malaria control program was started in India.
1954	E. Culer Hammond and Daniel Horner initiated a study on the relationship between smoking and lung cancer in New York.
1954	The Salk vaccine trial was initiated in the United States to test the efficacy of Salk's killed virus to prevent poliomyelitis.
1955	The National Leprosy Control Program was launched in India.
1957	Jerry Morris, a Scottish epidemiologist published the first textbook on Non-communicable disease epidemiology textbook entitled "Uses of Epidemiology."
1957	Ancel Keys initiated the Seven Countries Study to study the relationship between diet and coronary artery disease.
1962	The National Tuberculosis Control Program was initiated in India.
1963–1964	The first clinically proved dengue case was reported in Kolkata, India.
1964	United States Surgeon General's report on smoking and health was submitted.
1965	A. Bradford-Hill in England proposed nine points to establish the casual association of disease.
1966	The last human plague case was reported in India.
1975	Eradication of smallpox was announced in India
1976	Ebola virus disease was reported in Sudan and the Democratic Republic of Congo.
1980	The eradication of smallpox was announced by World Health Organization.

1981	The first case of human immune deficiency was reported in the United States.
1983	The First National Health Policy was proposed in India.
1984	The Guinea worm eradication program was initiated in India.
1985	The Universal Immunization Program was started in India.
1986	HIV was first reported in India.
1992	Centre for Disease Control and Prevention, United States was Established.
1992–93	The first national health family survey was conducted in India.
1993	A revised national tuberculosis control program was launched in India.
1997	The national polio surveillance program was initiated in India.
1999	The National Institute of Epidemiology was established in India.
2002	Severe acute respiratory syndrome was reported in two patients in South China.
2002	The second National Health Policy was proposed in India.
2005	National Rural Health Mission was initiated in India.
2010	National program on the prevention and control of cancer, diabetes, CVD and stroke were initiated in India.
2017	The Third National Health Policy was presented in India.
2017	The first outbreak of Zika virus disease was reported in India from Gujarat and the second outbreak was in Tamil Nadu.
2018	International classification diseases version 11 was released.
2018	Ayushman Bharat, a national health protection scheme was launched.
2019	SARS Corona virus-2 was discovered in Wuhan of Hubei Province.

Source: https://egyankosh.ac.in/bitstream/123456789/71439/1/Unit-1.pdf.

1.2. Foundations of Epidemiology

Epidemiology Is Interdisciplinary

See Figure 1.1 for a description of the multidisciplinary roots of epidemiology. As a multidisciplinary field, epidemiology incorporates elements from the medical sciences, social and behavioral sciences, toxicology, pathology, virology, genetics, microbiology, and clinical medicine. Terris emphasized that epidemiology is a very sophisticated and rich science that draws methods and strategies from numerous fields. According to what he wrote, epidemiology "must synthesize and draw upon knowledge from the various sciences of the physical environment, from the sciences concerned with human society, and from the biological sciences of man and his parasites."

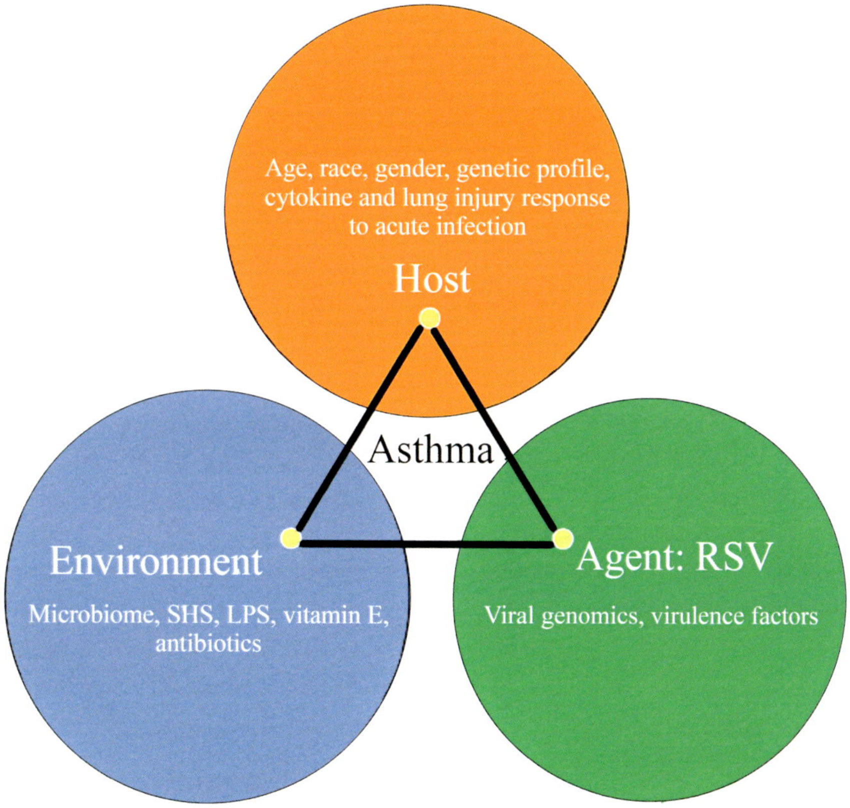

Figure 1.1. *The interdisciplinary foundations of epidemiology.*

Source: https://courses.lumenlearning.com/suny-buffalo-environmentalhealth/chapter/application-to-chronic-disease/.

These are a few examples of how other fields have influenced epidemiology. The study of microorganisms, or microbiology, provides details on the morphology and modes of transmission of particular disease agents. The fields of virology and bacteriology are related. Microbiologic techniques were employed in the previously discussed investigations of TSS, Legionnaires' disease, and anthrax to identify potential infectious agents. Epidemiologic studies of foodborne illnesses are another example (e.g., *E. coli*); these investigations use microbiologic techniques to identify the similarities among the bacteria causing an outbreak so as to determine whether a shared source was responsible.

When determining whether a patient has a particular disease or condition, clinical medicine plays a crucial role in the diagnosis process. The ability to distinguish between healthy and sick tissue may be aided by a pathologist's experience. Clinical medicine identified the symptoms or indicators of illness in the individuals from our earlier examples. Clinicians and nurses with a keen eye may recommend epidemiologic studies based on their observations.

The study of toxicology, also known as the science of poisons, focuses on the existence and consequences of chemical agents on human health, especially those that are present in the workplace and surroundings. What happens to dangerous chemicals after they serve their purpose is a major concern for the United States. Previously, a variety of harmful substances (e.g., pesticides) were carelessly dumped into waste sites that were subsequently classified as dangerous. Toxicologic knowledge is useful in determining whether hazardous waste sites contain harmful chemical agents and whether any health effects seen are consistent with known effects of toxic agent exposure. Geneticists may join the research team through the fields of molecular and genetic epidemiology when individual responses to exogenous agents differ. Toxicologists and epidemiologists often work together on environmental and occupational health studies.

The social and behavioral sciences clarify how cultural group membership, education, race, and behavior all contribute to health-related phenomena. Sociology and psychology are social and behavioral science fields that focus on the investigation of behavior and the creation of social theory, respectively. The study of social conditions and disease processes is the focus of social epidemiologic approaches. Additionally, a large portion of the methodology for group comparisons, questionnaire development, design, and delivery, measurement, and sampling comes from the social sciences. Community interventions are increasingly utilizing the wealth of information found in the social sciences. The study of data pertaining to the composition of human populations is known as demography.

Ultimately, the assessment of epidemiologic data depends heavily on the discipline of biostatistics, particularly when attempting to distinguish meaningful observations from coincidental findings. Because the causation of a given disease in a population may involve the interaction of several factors, epidemiology benefits from the interdisciplinary approach. Numerous disciplines' contributions aid in identifying the contributing factors to a given disease.

1.2.1. Methods and Procedures

Quantification of pertinent factors is necessary due to the empirical dimensions of epidemiologic studies. Quantification is the process of converting qualitative perceptions into numerical values. A doctor's observations about the kinds of people who seem to be affected by a disease, for instance, gleaned from their medical practice, are an example of a qualitative source of information about disease. In order to objectify subjective perceptions, epidemiologists count disease cases. Standard epidemiologic measures frequently involve accounting for the number of disease cases and analyzing their distribution based on exposure category, clinical features, and demographic variables like age, sex, and race.

Sometimes epidemiologists present quantified information as tables, maps, charts, and graphs. Both charts and graphs are pictorial illustrations of the frequency of disease.

Key methods for the graphic presentation of data are the use of pie charts, bar graphs, and line graphs. These include: a pie chart (admission diagnoses of discharged hospice care patients); a bar graph (diabetes prevalence among adults); and a line graph (obesity among children). Epidemiologists use these types of graphs to describe characteristics of data, such as subgroup differences and time trends (Figure 1.2).

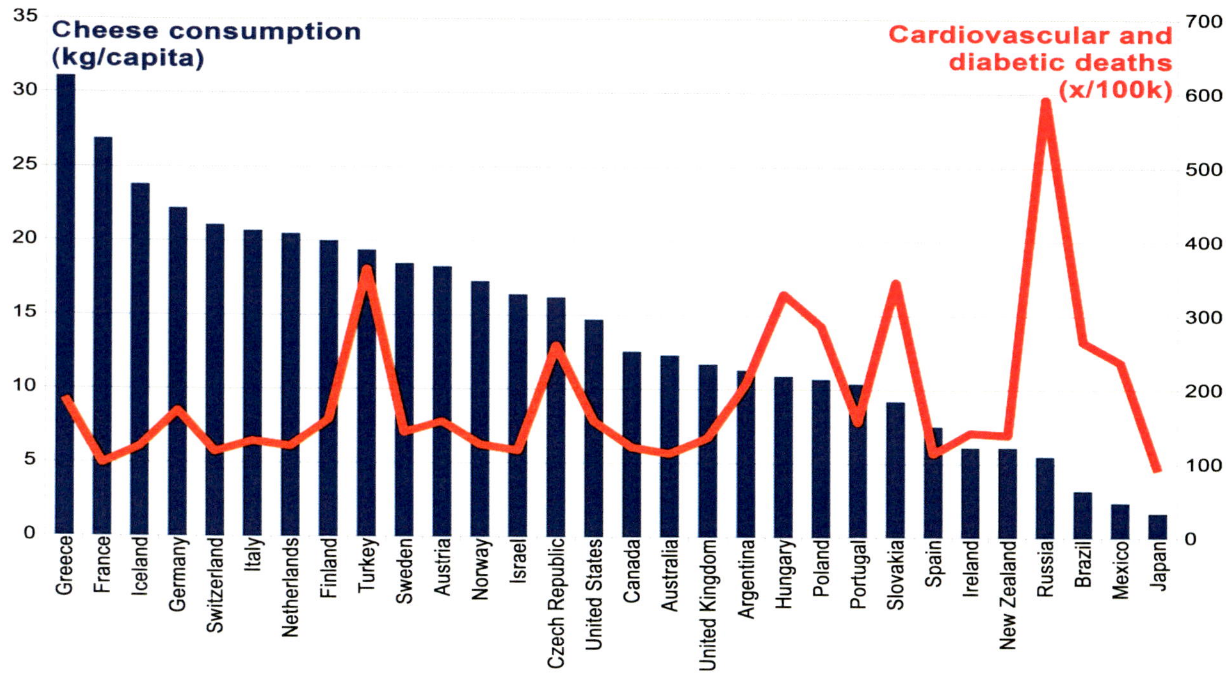

Figure 1.2. *Examples of a presentation of epidemiologic data.*

Source: https://en.wikipedia.org/wiki/File:Epidemiological_data_and_cheese_consumption.png.

1.2.2. Use of Special Vocabulary

A distinct lexicon of terminology is used in epidemiology to characterize the frequency of disease occurrence. Pandemic and epidemic are two terms from this vocabulary.

The definition of an epidemic, according to Dorland's Illustrated Medical Dictionary, is "attacking many people at the same time, widely diffused and rapidly spreading." More specifically, an epidemic is defined as an excessive occurrence of a disease: "The concept of excessive prevalence is stressed in most current definitions of epidemics, both in lay and professional usage." The following passage illustrates this notion by defining an epidemic as:

The occurrence, in a defined community or region, of cases of an illness (or an outbreak) with a frequency clearly in excess of normal expectancy. The number of cases indicating presence of an epidemic varies according to the infectious agent, size and type of population exposed, previous experience or lack of exposure to the disease, and time and place of occurrence; epidemicity is thus relative to usual frequency of the disease.

The term "usual frequency" refers to the disease's normal occurrence in the same location, at the same time, and among the same population. Moreover, an epidemic is indicated when a single case of a contagious disease resurfaces after it has vanished from the population. Additionally, since it implies disease transmission, the occurrence of two cases of a new disease (a "first invasion") that are connected in space and time may be regarded as an epidemic.

According to modern theory, epidemics are not limited to infectious diseases. Consider the Love Canal incident of the late 1970s, which sparked intense public discussion and media attention. In Niagara Falls, New York, there once stood a toxic waste disposal facility called Love Canal. Thousands of chemical-filled drums deposited by Hooker Chemicals and Plastics Corporation were buried there. The landfill was eventually covered over and turned into a residential area. Residents of the area then reported a variety of health effects, such as birth defects, miscarriages, and diminished cognitive abilities. Numerous epidemiological studies and health effects studies were conducted at the Love Canal site. The Superfund was established in 1980 as a result of the threat posed by Love Canal and other hazardous waste sites. Its goal was to encourage hazardous waste cleanup.

The word "pandemic," which describes an epidemic that spreads globally and may affect a large number of people as well as cross international borders, is related to the term "epidemic." Pandemics caused by the flu, like the 1918 pandemic and more recent ones that recur occasionally, are two examples. A disease that is consistently present in a specific geographic area is referred to as endemic. For example, cholera is endemic to less developed nations with poor sanitation, and malaria is endemic to some tropical regions of Asia. In the past, cholera was widespread in Western nations like the United States and England in the 19th century. However, thanks to the implementation of sanitation and other public health initiatives, cholera is no longer an endemic disease in these two nations.

1.2.3. Methods for Ascertainment of Epidemic Frequency of Disease

Continuous surveillance data collection is done by the CDC and state and local vital statistics departments to assess if an epidemic is occurring. The process of gathering data on the prevalence of particular diseases in a systematic manner, analyzing and interpreting that data, and disseminating the combined and processed information to program participants and other interested parties is referred to as surveillance. Tracking influenza, gathering data on infectious and communicable diseases, and keeping an eye on foodborne disease outbreaks are examples of common surveillance activities.

When disease spreads more widely than one would normally expect, it is referred to as an epidemic. To determine epidemic trends, information regarding the typical occurrence of a disease is required. Surveillance serves to provide such information. For instance, let's say a medical professional reports that an epidemic of CHD deaths is occurring, citing 500 reported deaths in an upstate New York community in a given year. The claim that there has been an epidemic of CHD deaths cannot be supported by this data alone. It would be necessary to ascertain the typical frequency of CHD deaths through continuing surveillance programs in the same community at some earlier point in time. Furthermore, it would be necessary to ascertain the population's size, age, and sex distribution. With this data at hand, it would be possible to assess if a CHD death epidemic has broken out.

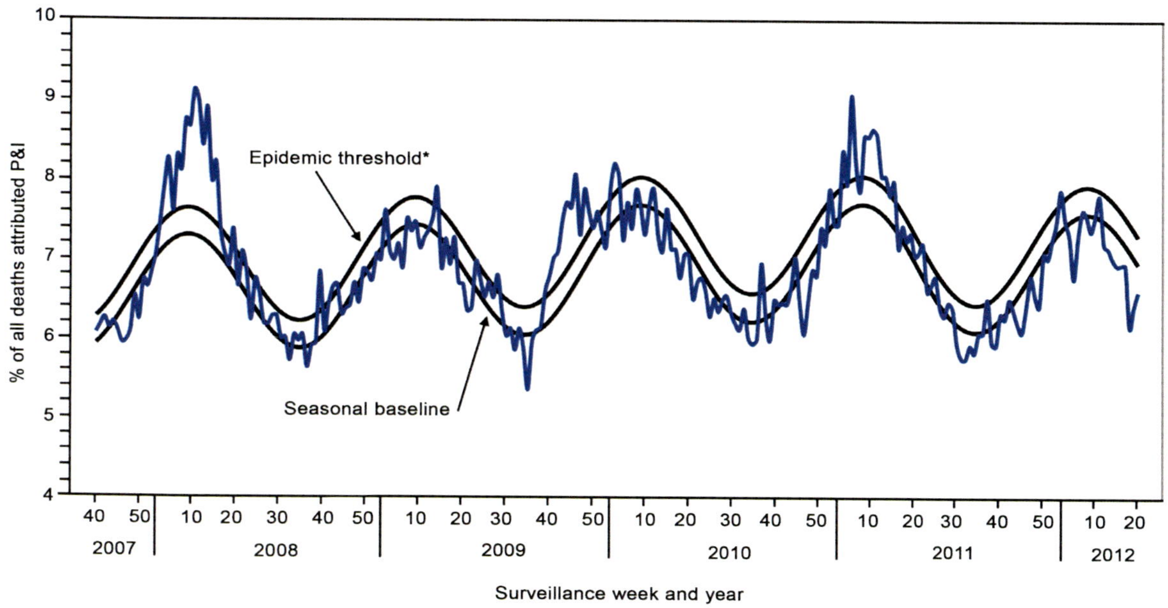

Figure 1.3. *Percentage of all deaths attributable to pneumonia and influenza (P&I), by surveillance week and year—122 Cities Mortality Reporting System, United States, 2007–May 19, 2012.*

Source: Reproduced Centers for Disease Control and Prevention. Update Influenza Activity—United States, 2011–12 Season and Composition of the 2012–13 Influenza Vaccine. MMWR. 2012; 61, 418.

Figure 1.3 provides an additional example of calculating epidemic frequency in relation to deaths from pneumonia and influenza. From winter 2007 to spring 2012, the figure shows the weekly deaths in the United States from influenza and pneumonia. The figure shows that seasonal baselines for influenza (flu) are underlying and reflected in cyclical seasonal increases and decreases in mortality. The winter season is when the flu strikes most people in the Northern Hemisphere, including the United States (i.e., between October and April). As a result, the flu season runs from the end of one calendar year to the beginning of the next (e.g., the flu season of 2011–2012). The lower line in the figure represents the typical annual number of deaths from influenza and pneumonia for each week of the year. The frequency of disease at the epidemic threshold, or the lowest number of fatalities necessary to establish the existence of an epidemic, is shown by an upper parallel line. The threshold for an epidemic is determined by statistical forecasts. Figures 1.3 show that during early 2008, late 2009, and early 2011, the combined number of deaths from influenza and pneumonia reached a significant peak that was above the epidemic threshold.

1.3. Achievements in Epidemiology

1.3.1. Smallpox

Millions of people's health and well-being were significantly improved by the smallpox epidemic, especially in many of the most impoverished communities. The smallpox epidemic highlights both the successes and shortcomings of contemporary public health. It was discovered in the 1790s that cowpox infection offered immunity against the smallpox virus, but it took nearly 200 years for the advantages of this finding to be acknowledged and put to use globally.

An intensive campaign to eliminate smallpox was coordinated over many years by the World Health Organization (WHO). An understanding of the epidemiology of smallpox was central to its eradication, in particular, by:

- providing information about the distribution of cases and the model, mechanisms and levels of transmission;
- mapping outbreaks of the disease;
- evaluating control measures

Along with the low average number of secondary cases infected by a primary case, the absence of an animal host was crucial. In 1967, the WHO proposed a ten-year eradication program, as there were between 10 and 15 million new cases and two million deaths per year in 31 countries. During 1967–1976, the number of countries reporting cases dropped off quickly; by 1976, there were only two countries reporting cases, and the last case of smallpox to occur naturally occurred in 1977 in a woman who had been exposed to the virus in a laboratory. It was declared that smallpox was exterminated on May 8, 1980.

The program's success was attributed to a number of elements, including widespread political support, a clear objective, an exact schedule, skilled personnel, and an adaptable approach. Moreover, the illness possessed numerous characteristics that enabled its eradication, and a potent vaccine that was stable in the heat was accessible. The World Health Organization (WHO) kept 200 million smallpox vaccines in stock in 1979. After that, the stockpile was whittled down to 2.5 million doses; however, the World Health Organization is still making sure that there are enough vaccines on hand because of growing concerns about smallpox being used as a biological weapon.

1.3.2. Methyl Mercury Poisoning

Although mercury was once thought to be dangerous, it has more recently come to represent the risks associated with environmental pollution. Mercury compounds were discharged into a small bay in the 1950s along with water from a factory in Minamata, Japan. As a result, methyl mercury began to build up in fish, which severely poisoned those who consumed them. It took several years of research to determine the precise cause of this first-known outbreak of fish-related methyl mercury poisoning. Currently among the most well-researched environmental diseases is minamata disease. In the 1960s, there was another outbreak in a different region of Japan. Since then, reports from several other nations have indicated less severe mercury poisoning in fish.

1.3.3. Rheumatic Fever and Rheumatic Heart Disease

Poverty, specifically substandard housing and overcrowding, are linked to both rheumatic fever and rheumatic heart disease. These factors facilitate the spread of streptococcal upper respiratory tract infections. The decline in rheumatic fever in many wealthy nations began in the early 1900s, long before the development of useful medications like penicillin and sulfonamides (Figure 1.4). While there are still some areas of comparatively high incidence among socially and economically disadvantaged populations in the majority of high-income countries today, the disease has virtually vanished from these nations.

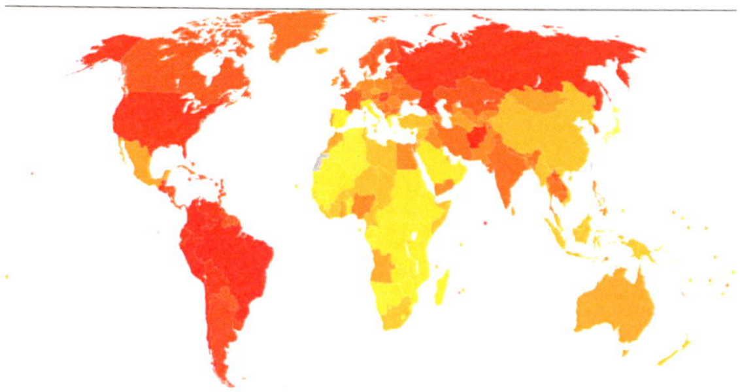

Figure 1.4. *Disability-adjusted life year for RA per 100,000 inhabitants in 2004. no data <40 40–50 50–60 60–70 70–80 80–90 90–100 100–110 110–120 120–130 130–140 >140*

Source: By Lokal_Profil, CC BY-SA 2.5, https://commons.wikimedia.org/w/index.php?curid=8443852.

The contribution of social and economic factors to the spread of streptococcal throat infections and outbreaks of rheumatic fever has been brought to light by epidemiological studies. Compared to methyl mercury poisoning, which has a single specific cause, the causation of these diseases is obviously more complex and multifactorial.

1.3.4. Iodine Deficiency Diseases

A common occurrence in some mountainous areas, iodine deficiency results in insufficient thyroid hormone production, which lowers physical and mental energy. About 400 years ago, the conditions goiter and cretinism were first thoroughly described; however, it wasn't until the 20th century that enough information was gathered to enable efficient prevention and management. The use of iodized salt for goiter control was proposed in Switzerland in 1915, the same year that endemic goiter was named the easiest known disease to prevent. In Ohio, USA, the first extensive iodine trials were conducted shortly afterward on 5,000 girls ages 11 to 18. Impressive preventive and therapeutic benefits led to the widespread introduction of iodized salt in many nations in 1924.

All social classes use salt at about the same rate all year round, which makes the use of iodized salt effective. The efficient production and distribution of salt is essential for success, and quality control, public awareness, and legal enforcement are also necessary.

1.3.5. Tobacco use, Asbestos and Lung Cancer

Formerly uncommon, lung cancer has dramatically increased in incidence since the 1930s, initially striking men. It is now evident that tobacco use is the primary factor contributing to rising lung cancer death rates. In 1950, the first epidemiological studies that connected smoking to lung cancer were published. Five case-control studies found a link between tobacco use and lung cancer in men. The British doctors' study's association should have been strong enough to elicit a strong and quick reaction, especially since other studies have confirmed this association in a wide range of populations. However, the increased burden of lung cancer is also a result of other exposures, including asbestos dust and urban air pollution. Furthermore, smoking and asbestos exposure have a multiplicative effect that raises the risk of lung cancer in workers who smoke and are exposed to asbestos dust.

1.3.6. Hip Fractures

Collaboration between scientists in the domains of epidemiology, social and environmental health, and injury epidemiology is common in injury epidemiological research. Because of the implications for the healthcare needs of an aging population, falls-related injuries, in particular hip fractures (fractures of the neck of the femur) in older adults, have garnered a lot of attention recently. Age-related increases in falls and a reduction in bone mass at the proximal femur cause hip fractures to rise exponentially with age. If efforts are not focused on prevention, it is reasonable to anticipate that the incidence of hip fractures will rise proportionately to the growing number of elderly people in most populations. Hip fractures result in a significant number of hospital days, which translates into high financial expenses. Hip fractures accounted for 20% of all costs associated with injuries in a study on the cost of injuries in the Netherlands, despite ranking only fourteenth in terms of incidence out of 25 listed injuries.

Most hip fractures are the result of a fall, and most deaths associated with falls in elderly people result from the complications of hip fractures. The optimal strategies to prevent hip fractures are unclear. Epidemiologists have a vital role in examining both modifiable and non-modifiable factors in an effort to reduce the burden of hip fractures.

1.3.7. HIV/AIDS

In the United States, the acquired immunodeficiency syndrome (AIDS) was first recognized as a separate medical condition in 1981. It is estimated that 10 million individuals worldwide were infected with the HIV virus by 1990. Since then, the AIDS epidemic has claimed millions of lives and infected 40 million more with HIV, making it one of the most devastating infectious disease epidemics in history (Figures 1.5 & 1.6). Of the 3.1 million deaths from AIDS in 2005, approximately 95% occurred in low- and middle-income countries, with 70% occurring in sub-Saharan Africa and 20% in Asia. Most of the 4.3–6.6 million people newly infected with HIV in 2005 live in these regions.

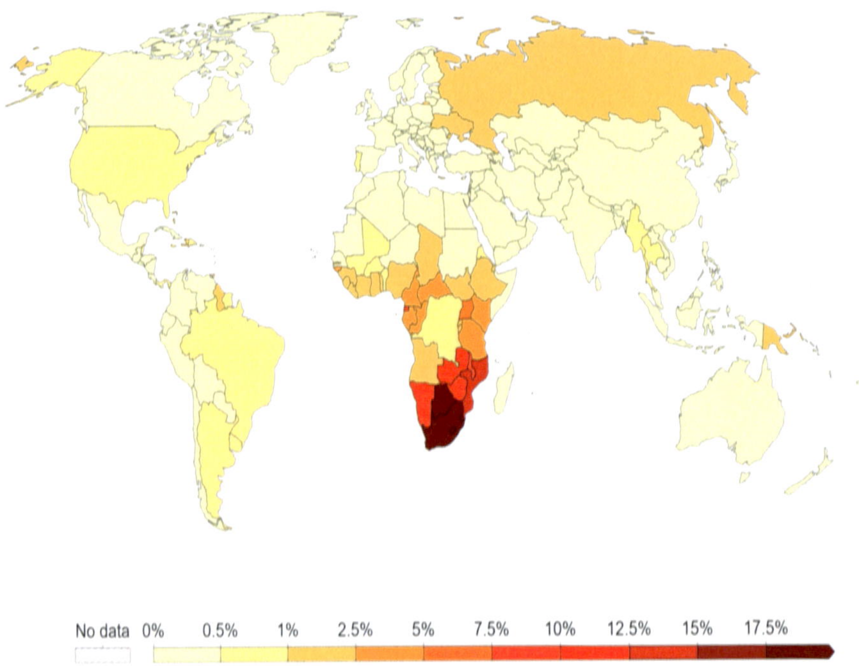

Figure 1.5. *Sourced from our world in data, this map illustrates the prevalence of HIV infection in countries across the world using data collected during 2022.*

Source: By Our world in data – https://ourworldindata.org/hiv-aids, CC BY-SA 4.0, https://commons.wikimedia.org/w/index.php?curid=135466504.

However, within regions or countries themselves, levels of infection and routes of transmission vary considerably. AIDS has a long incubation period and, without treatment, about half of those infected with the causative human immunodeficiency virus (HIV) develop AIDS within nine years of infection. The virus is found in blood, semen and cervical or vaginal secretions. Transmission occurs mainly through sexual intercourse or sharing of contaminated needles, but the virus can also be transmitted through transfusion of contaminated blood or blood products, and from an infected woman to her baby during pregnancy, at birth or through breastfeeding.

1.3.8. SARS

The severe acute respiratory syndrome (SARS) outbreak served as a reminder of the global community's shared susceptibility to new infections, even though it had little bearing on mortality or disease burden. It also emphasized how inadequate public health services are, not just in Asia but even in developed nations like Canada. In November 2002, two patients with atypical pneumonia of unknown cause in southern China were the first cases of SARS. Over the next few months, the virus rapidly spread, leading to over 8,000 cases and roughly 900 deaths in 12 countries. This was made possible by the travel of highly contagious individuals by air. Hospitals, where medical personnel had frequent or close contact with infected patients, had higher death rates than communities where SARS was first discovered.

For instance, SARS has shown that these epidemics can have profound social and economic repercussions that extend well beyond their effects on health. The significance of a serious new illness in a highly mobile and interdependent world is demonstrated by these consequences.

1.4. Epidemiology and Prevention

A major use of epidemiologic evidence is to identify subgroups in the population who are at high risk for disease. Why should we identify such high-risk groups? First, if we can identify these high-risk groups, we can direct preventive efforts, such as screening programs for early disease detection, to populations who are most likely to benefit from any interventions that are developed for the disease. Second, if we can identify such groups, we may be able to identify the specific factors or characteristics that put them at high risk and then try to modify those factors.

It is important to keep in mind that such risk factors may be of two types. Characteristics such as age, sex, and race, for example, are not modifiable, although they may permit us to identify high-risk groups. On the other hand, characteristics such as obesity, diet, and other lifestyle factors may be potentially modifiable and may thus provide an opportunity to develop and introduce new prevention programs aimed at reducing or changing specific exposures or risk factors. In discussing prevention, it is helpful to distinguish among primary, secondary, and tertiary prevention (Table 1.2).

Table 1.2. Effectiveness of Secondary and tertiary Prevention for Violence Against women in Low and Low-Middle Income Countries: A Systematic Review

Study	Country and Setting	Methods	Intervention	Findings
Bernath and Gahongayire 2013	Kigali, Rwanda One stop center in Kacyiru Police Hospital	Mixed-methods evaluation included: • desk review of existing policies, laws, etc. • collection of existing statistical data • interviews with staff and stakeholders • interviews with clients	ISANGE One Stop Centre (IOSC) is a program designed to provide psychosocial, medical, police and legal services to survivors of abuse. It is housed inside a public hospital and offers free 24/7 service.	The quality and availability of medical and forensic services are very high and strong links are present with police. However, weaknesses include: • Difficulty following-up with survivors • Inconsistent legal aid for survivors • Requirement for survivors to report abuse to police to obtain services • Limited data collection and monitoring • Staff training is not systematically planned or monitored
Bhate-Deosthali, Sundari Ravindran, and Vindhya 2012	Mumbai, India Crisis centers at two public hospitals	Mixed-methods evaluation included: • Review of project documents • Interviews with program and hospital staff • Analysis of case records	The Dilaasa Crisis Centers offer counseling (informed by a feminist perspective) to women who have experienced violence and are referred from the hospital or other health facility. They also provide referrals to partner organizations that provide legal assistance and temporary or permanent shelter.	The centers' locations in public hospitals make it possible to reach women from low-income or marginalized groups. Many survivors cited obtaining emotional support from the counseling and some reported improved psychological health. Survivors also stated that the centers helped them to register their complaints with the police. However, the centers faced an ongoing challenge while trying to change the attitudes of health professionals to recognize that domestic violence is an issue they should be concerned about, through ongoing training.

Doucet and Denov 2012	Sierra Leone Rural area in south	6 war-affected women and 4 social workers were purposively selected for open-ended interviews.	Social workers provided psychosocial support to women following the war. The social workers focused on giving advice, as well as principles of solidarity and spirituality in their psychosocial support, rather than clinical diagnostics and psychology.	War-affected women cited the social workers' advice and support as playing an important role in their recovery. No women mentioned foreign professionals as making an impact on recovery, suggesting that local social work practices are valuable, despite being very different from those used in the Global North.
Human Rights Watch 2015	Papua New Guinea	46 interviews were conducted: 27 with survivors of family violence and the remainder with local officials, activists, NGO workers, and other stakeholders.	Interventions include: • Family and Sexual Violence Units (FSVU) in 17 police stations to make police more accessible to victims of gender-based violence • Family Support Centres in 15 hospitals to assist patients seeking care as a result of family violence • Hotline that provides counseling, information, guidance, and referrals for care at local services • Referral Pathway established by government officials in urban areas, designed to ensure that if a survivor accesses one service, they are linked to all other relevant ones	Many of these interventions are relatively new and are said to be effective at increasing support for survivors and access to services. However, barriers remain including: • Lack of awareness about available services • Limited access to services in rural areas • Shortage of safe houses • Service providers not putting the survivor's best interests first (e.g., encouraging reconciliation) • Lack of psychosocial counseling and case management services • Weak law enforcement response. One expert stated that only 7 of the FSVU are functional. • Limited court capacity and legal assistance for survivors • Limited economic opportunities for survivors who leave their partners

Keesbury et al. 2012	Kenya and Zambia One-stop centers (OSC)	A comparative case study was conducted with purposively selected OSCs: 2 in Kenya and 3 in Zambia, representing a range of approaches to the OSC model. Mixed-methods were used, including: • Facility inventory • Record reviews • Key informant interviews	One-stop centers (OSCs) provide integrated, multidisciplinary services for survivors of sexual and gender-based violence in a single physical location. Three major types of OSCs exist: • Health facility-based and hospital-owned OSC, where OSC functions are integrated into routine health center activities • Health facility-based and NGO-owned OSC, where the NGO provides "wrap around" services at the health facility • Stand alone NGO-owned OSC, which provides legal and psychosocial support onsite but refers elsewhere for medical care	The health facility-based and hospital-owned OSC model was found to be better set up to achieve a broader range of legal and health outcomes for survivors, and survivors felt that they were meeting their health needs. Challenges still remain with the OSC model: • Poor integration of OSCs with the legal system • Strengthening of the range of services provided by OSCs and/or linkages to outside services is needed
Kohli et al. 2013	Democratic Republic of Congo Two villages in Walungu Territory	In-depth interviews were conducted with 27 participants, including 13 survivors of sexual violence who were rejected by their families, 3 spouses of survivors, 1 community member, 5 mediators and 5 service providers	Family mediation is a process of resolving family conflict between family members who have rejected a survivor of sexual violence and the survivor.	Reintegrated survivors reported better relationships, improved opportunities for their children, and fewer mental health problems. However, challenges still exist, especially in cases where the survivor has a child from her rapist, or the survivor's partner has remarried. Additional services such as economic support (e.g., children's tuition, livelihood training, etc.) were cited as potential ways to improve reintegration.

GHD Pty Ltd. 2015	Papua New Guinea	In-depth interviews and/or focus group were conducted with staff, survivors, police officers, referral partners and other stakeholders. Limited quantitative data was also aggregated and analyzed.	The Family and Sexual Violence Units (FSVU) are police units that are tasked with responding to the needs of family and sexual violence survivors. They are present in 15 police stations and also provide referrals to other services for these survivors.	The FSVUs have begun to change police response to FSV in PNG, however limitations still remain, including: • Persistent culture of male dominance in police force • Further training needed on how to provide supportive, non-judgmental services for survivors • Improvements to procedures are needed, including timeliness of response, communicating their roles and processes to survivors and making arrest and prosecution protocols consistent across police stations
Manneschmidt and Griese 2009	Afghanistan	109 women who were survivors of war-related violence participated in group evaluations (maximum of 13 participants per group), giving feedback on the intervention	Basic Counselling Training (BCT) uses a group counseling process to provide women with psycho-education, relief from distressing symptoms, new social skills (e.g., problem-solving skills) and new support networks.	Over half of participants mentioned that their social life had improved after the intervention, including their interactions with family members and their stress levels. Many participants also cited being happier or an improvement to their health.
Morel-Seytoux et al. 2010	Zambia	Mixed-methods evaluation included: • Desk review of 36 USAID and CDC monitoring and reporting documents • Key informant interviews with 240 beneficiaries, stakeholders, and ministry officials • 24 site visits/ observations	Coordinated Response Centers (CRCs) in 7 districts provide care and support for survivors to meet their medical, psychological and legal needs.	The coordinated approach is an effective model and provides survivors with more comprehensive services. Coupling of these direct services with public awareness campaigns has improved the public's knowledge of GBV and "broken the silence"

The Population Health and Development (PHD) Group Pvt. Ltd. 2012	Nepal Mobile camps in conflict-affected areas	Mixed-methods evaluation included: • In-depth interviews and focus groups • Analysis of secondary data and reviews • Field visits	Mobile reproductive health camps were conducted for six days (plus four days follow-up) in 14 of the most conflict-affected areas of the country. Survivors of SGBV presenting to the camps were offered psychosocial counseling, legal and medical services, as well as shelter.	The use of reproductive health camps to identify survivors was successful at minimizing stigma for survivors of sexual violence. 86% of survey respondents said the camp services were good and reasons cited included free drugs and services, no wait time, good provider behavior and good counseling. The camps successfully reached marginalized populations with over 66% of clients coming from disadvantaged communities. However, challenges arose, including: • Difficulty filing complaints with police because of politics, fear of family discord, etc. • Challenges tracking survivors because the camps were conducted 5 years after the end of conflict
Wessel and Campbell 1997	Managua, Nicaragua Women's centers in 3 poor neighbo-rhoods	Interviews with 21 survivors of domestic violence and 15 key informants involved in women's centers or related projects.	The Inter-Collective is a group of three women's centers, or *casas de la mujer,* running programs for survivors of domestic violence, including self defense classes, self-help groups, legal information workshops, healthcare for survivors,	As a result of the intervention, survivors cited having new perceptions of women's roles, increased emotional support and knowledge about their health and legal rights, decreased violence by their partners, and increased involvement in programs to help other survivors.
			as well as professional services from lawyers, psychologists and nurses.	

Source: Kirk, L., Terry, S., Lokuge, K. et al. Effectiveness of secondary and tertiary prevention for violence against women in low and low-middle income countries: a systematic review. BMC Public Health 17, 622 (2017). https://doi.org/10.1186/s12889-017-4502-6.

1.4.1. Primary Prevention

Primary prevention is a cornerstone of public health that focuses on preventing the onset of diseases and promoting overall well-being at the population level. Unlike secondary and tertiary prevention, which address diseases in their early or advanced stages, primary prevention aims to avert the occurrence of health issues by eliminating or reducing risk factors and promoting protective factors. In this exploration of primary prevention, we delve into its key principles, strategies, and examples.

1 Key Concepts of Primary Prevention

i. **Health Promotion:** Central to primary prevention is the promotion of health and well-being. This involves fostering environments that support healthy behaviors, encouraging positive lifestyle choices, and addressing social determinants of health to create conditions conducive to overall health.

ii. **Risk Factor Reduction:** Primary prevention seeks to identify and reduce modifiable risk factors that contribute to the development of diseases. This may include interventions targeting lifestyle factors such as diet, physical activity, smoking, and alcohol consumption.

iii. **Immunization:** Vaccination programs represent a classic example of primary prevention. By administering vaccines to individuals, particularly during childhood, the immune system is primed to recognize and fight off specific infections, preventing the occurrence of diseases such as measles, polio, and influenza.

iv. **Education and Awareness:** Providing education and raising awareness about health-related issues are key components of primary prevention. This includes disseminating information about the benefits of healthy behaviors, the risks associated with certain activities, and the importance of regular screenings and check-ups.

v. **Environmental and Policy Interventions:** Primary prevention extends to environmental and policy changes aimed at promoting health. This may involve implementing regulations to reduce exposure to harmful substances, creating safe public spaces, and advocating for policies that support healthy living.

2. Examples of Primary Prevention Strategies

i. **Health Education Programs:** Educational initiatives, ranging from school-based programs to community workshops, aim to inform individuals about healthy lifestyles, the benefits of physical activity, proper nutrition, and the dangers of risky behaviors like smoking and substance abuse.

ii. **Immunization Campaigns:** Immunization is a classic primary prevention strategy. Vaccination programs target infectious diseases such as measles, mumps, rubella, hepatitis, and influenza, preventing their occurrence and reducing the risk of outbreaks within communities.

iii. **Tobacco Control Programs:** Primary prevention efforts in tobacco control focus on reducing smoking initiation, promoting smoking cessation, and implementing policies such as higher taxes on tobacco products and restrictions on tobacco advertising to discourage tobacco use.

iv. **Healthy Eating Initiatives:** Programs promoting healthy eating habits, such as increasing fruit and vegetable consumption and reducing the intake of processed foods, contribute to primary prevention. These initiatives address dietary risk factors associated with chronic conditions like obesity, diabetes, and cardiovascular diseases.

v. **Community Safety Measures:** Primary prevention extends to community safety measures, including the design of pedestrian-friendly neighborhoods, traffic safety regulations, and initiatives to reduce violence and injuries. These measures create safer environments and prevent accidents and injuries.

3. **Challenges and Considerations**

i. **Behavior Change:** Encouraging behavior change is a fundamental challenge in primary prevention. Despite awareness and education, individuals may face barriers to adopting healthier lifestyles due to cultural, economic, or environmental factors. Strategies should consider these factors to be effective.

ii. **Equity and Access:** Ensuring equitable access to primary prevention measures is crucial. Disparities in access to healthcare services, education, and resources may result in certain populations being disproportionately affected by preventable health issues.

iii. **Long-Term Impact:** The impact of primary prevention may not be immediately apparent, and the benefits often manifest in the long term. This can make it challenging to garner sustained public and political support for primary prevention initiatives.

iv. **Environmental Determinants:** Addressing social and environmental determinants of health requires systemic changes, making it complex to implement primary prevention strategies. Advocacy for policies that promote health at the community and societal levels is essential.

1.4.2. Secondary Prevention

Secondary prevention is a critical component of public health that focuses on early detection and timely intervention to mitigate the progression of diseases and reduce their impact on individuals and communities. Unlike primary prevention, which aims to prevent the onset of diseases, secondary prevention targets conditions in their early stages, identifying them before the manifestation of symptoms or complications. This proactive approach allows for prompt intervention, leading to better health outcomes and a decreased burden on healthcare systems. In this exploration of secondary prevention, we delve into its key principles, strategies, and examples.

1. **Key Concepts of Secondary Prevention**

i. **Early Detection:** Central to secondary prevention is the early identification of diseases or risk factors. This often involves screening and diagnostic tests that can detect conditions before symptoms become apparent. Early detection allows for timely intervention and the implementation of appropriate treatment or preventive measures.

ii. **Risk Factor Modification:** Secondary prevention emphasizes the modification of risk factors associated with certain diseases. By addressing lifestyle factors, genetic predispositions, and environmental influences, individuals can reduce their risk of developing specific conditions and improve overall health.

iii. **Screening Programs:** Screening is a key strategy in secondary prevention, involving the systematic application of tests, examinations, or other procedures to detect diseases or conditions in asymptomatic individuals. Common screening programs include those for cancer, cardiovascular diseases, and infectious diseases.

iv. **Early Intervention:** Early detection leads to early intervention, which can significantly alter the course of a disease. This may involve medical treatments, lifestyle modifications, or other interventions aimed at preventing the progression of the condition and reducing the likelihood of complications.

v. **Population-Based Approaches:** Secondary prevention often employs population-based approaches to reach a broader audience. Mass screenings, public health campaigns, and community-based initiatives contribute to the identification of individuals at risk and the implementation of preventive measures.

2. **Examples of Secondary Prevention Strategies**

i. **Cancer Screening:** Cancer screening programs, such as mammography for breast cancer, colonoscopy for colorectal cancer, and Pap smears for cervical cancer, exemplify secondary prevention. These screenings aim to detect cancer at an early, more treatable stage, improving the chances of successful treatment.

ii. **Cardiovascular Risk Assessment:** Assessing cardiovascular risk factors, including blood pressure, cholesterol levels, and diabetes, allows for the early identification of individuals at risk of heart disease. Lifestyle modifications, medications, and other interventions can be initiated to prevent the progression of cardiovascular conditions.

iii. **Infectious Disease Screening:** Screening for infectious diseases, such as HIV, hepatitis, and sexually transmitted infections (STIs), is a crucial aspect of secondary prevention. Early detection enables the prompt initiation of antiretroviral therapy or other treatments, reducing the spread of the infection and improving individual outcomes.

iv. **Genetic Testing:** Genetic testing plays a role in secondary prevention by identifying individuals at risk of hereditary conditions. This information allows for proactive measures, including surveillance, preventive surgeries, or lifestyle modifications, to minimize the impact of genetic disorders.

v. **Osteoporosis Screening:** Bone density screenings for osteoporosis in postmenopausal women represent a secondary prevention strategy. Early detection allows for interventions, such as calcium supplementation, vitamin D, and lifestyle changes, to prevent fractures and complications associated with osteoporosis.

3. **Challenges and Considerations**

i. **Ethical and Social Implications:** Secondary prevention, particularly through genetic testing, raises ethical considerations related to privacy, informed consent, and potential stigmatization. Ensuring that individuals understand the implications of screening and providing appropriate counseling is essential.

ii. **False Positives and Negatives:** Screening tests may yield false positives (indicating a condition that is not present) or false negatives (missing the presence of a condition). Balancing the benefits and harms of screening is crucial to avoid unnecessary interventions or delayed diagnoses.

iii. **Access and Equity:** Disparities in

access to healthcare services and screening programs can undermine the effectiveness of secondary prevention. Efforts must be made to ensure equitable access, especially for vulnerable and underserved populations.

iv. **Overdiagnosis and Overtreatment:** Some screening programs may lead to the identification of conditions that may never progress to cause harm. This can result in overdiagnosis and overtreatment, with potential negative consequences for individuals' physical and psychological well-being.

1.4.3. Tertiary Prevention

Tertiary prevention is the third and final level of the public health model, emphasizing interventions aimed at minimizing the impact of established diseases and preventing further complications or disabilities. Unlike primary and secondary prevention, which focus on disease prevention and early detection, respectively, tertiary prevention is centered around rehabilitation, management, and support for individuals who already have a diagnosed condition.

1. **Key Concepts of Tertiary Prevention**

i. **Rehabilitation:** Tertiary prevention places a significant emphasis on rehabilitation efforts to restore individuals' functioning and quality of life after the onset of a disease or injury. Rehabilitation encompasses a multidisciplinary approach involving healthcare professionals such as physiotherapists, occupational therapists, psychologists, and social workers. The goal is to help individuals regain independence, mobility, and adaptive skills.

ii. **Disease Management:** Managing chronic conditions is a crucial aspect of tertiary prevention. This involves medical treatment, medication adherence, and lifestyle modifications to control the progression of the disease, prevent complications, and improve overall well-being. Chronic diseases like diabetes, cardiovascular conditions, and chronic respiratory diseases often require ongoing management to optimize health outcomes.

iii. **Supportive Care:** Tertiary prevention recognizes the importance of providing ongoing support to individuals dealing with chronic or disabling conditions. This support can come from healthcare professionals, support groups, family, and community resources. Emotional, social, and practical support plays a vital role in helping individuals cope with the challenges posed by their health conditions.

iv. **Preventing Complications:** Another key focus of tertiary prevention is preventing complications and secondary health issues associated with existing diseases. For example, individuals with diabetes may receive education on foot care to prevent complications like ulcers and infections. Regular monitoring and prompt intervention can reduce the impact of complications and enhance overall health.

v. **Quality of Life Improvement:** Enhancing the quality of life is a primary objective of tertiary prevention. This involves addressing not only the physical aspects of health but also the psychosocial and emotional well-being of individuals. Holistic care considers factors such as mental health, social relationships, and the ability to engage in meaningful activities.

2. Examples of Tertiary Prevention Strategies

i. **Cardiac Rehabilitation:** Individuals who have experienced a heart attack or undergone cardiac procedures may participate in cardiac rehabilitation programs. These programs include exercise training, nutritional counseling, and emotional support to improve cardiovascular health and reduce the risk of future cardiac events.

ii. **Stroke Rehabilitation:** Tertiary prevention in stroke care involves rehabilitation programs to help individuals regain motor skills, speech, and cognitive function. Therapists work with stroke survivors to maximize their independence and minimize the long-term impact of the stroke.

iii. **Pulmonary Rehabilitation:** Individuals with chronic respiratory conditions, such as chronic obstructive pulmonary disease (COPD), benefit from pulmonary rehabilitation. This includes exercises to improve lung function, breathing techniques, and education on managing symptoms, contributing to better respiratory health and overall well-being.

iv. **Diabetes Management Programs:** Tertiary prevention for diabetes involves structured management programs that focus on blood sugar control, lifestyle modifications, and education to prevent complications such as diabetic neuropathy, retinopathy, and cardiovascular issues.

v. **Cancer Survivorship Programs:** Cancer survivors often face physical and emotional challenges post-treatment. Tertiary prevention in oncology includes survivorship programs that address ongoing healthcare needs, monitor for potential cancer-related complications, and provide support for coping with the psychological impact of cancer.

3. Challenges and Considerations

i. **Access to Rehabilitation Services:** Disparities in access to rehabilitation services can hinder the effectiveness of tertiary prevention. Ensuring equitable access to rehabilitation programs and healthcare resources is essential for optimizing outcomes.

ii. **Patient Engagement:** Successful tertiary prevention relies on active patient engagement and adherence to prescribed interventions. Educating individuals about the importance of rehabilitation and disease management is crucial for fostering a collaborative approach to healthcare.

iii. **Multidisciplinary Collaboration:** Tertiary prevention often requires collaboration among various healthcare professionals. Effective communication and coordination among physicians, therapists, nurses, and other providers are essential for delivering comprehensive care.

iv. **Healthcare System Integration:** Integrating tertiary prevention into the broader healthcare system is essential. This includes incorporating rehabilitation services into primary care settings and ensuring a seamless transition from acute care to ongoing management and support.

A Closer Look

Achievements in Epidemiology

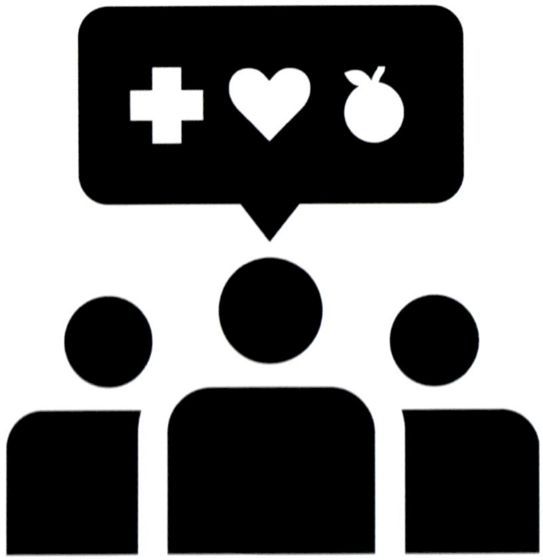

By Edward Boatman – Noun Project – https://thenounproject.com/icon/3746, CC0, https://commons.wikimedia.org/w/index.php?curid=64906637.

Epidemiology has achieved significant milestones in understanding, preventing, and controlling diseases, contributing immensely to public health advancements. One of its notable achievements lies in the eradication and control of infectious diseases. Through epidemiological research, diseases such as smallpox have been eradicated globally, while others like polio have been greatly reduced through vaccination campaigns and surveillance systems. These triumphs demonstrate the effectiveness of epidemiological methods in identifying disease patterns, implementing targeted interventions, and monitoring progress over time.

Furthermore, epidemiology has played a critical role in uncovering the risk factors associated with chronic diseases, such as heart disease, cancer, and diabetes. By conducting large-scale studies and longitudinal research, epidemiologists have identified modifiable risk factors like smoking, poor diet, sedentary lifestyle, and environmental exposures. This knowledge has informed public health campaigns and policies aimed at promoting healthier behaviors and reducing the burden of chronic conditions on society.

In addition, epidemiology has contributed significantly to understanding the complex interplay between genetics, environment, and lifestyle factors in disease development. Through genetic epidemiology studies, researchers have identified genetic markers associated with increased susceptibility to certain diseases, paving the way for personalized medicine approaches and targeted interventions. Similarly, environmental epidemiology has elucidated the impact of pollutants, toxins, and other environmental exposures on health outcomes, informing regulatory policies and public health interventions to mitigate risks.

Moreover, epidemiology has been instrumental in responding to emerging infectious diseases and global health threats. From the HIV/AIDS pandemic to outbreaks of Ebola, Zika, and COVID-19, epidemiologists have played a central role in surveillance, outbreak investigation, and response efforts. By quickly identifying the source of outbreaks, tracking transmission dynamics, and implementing control measures, epidemiologists have helped to contain epidemics and prevent their further spread.

Overall, the achievements of epidemiology underscore its pivotal role in advancing public health and improving population outcomes. By generating evidence-based insights, informing policy decisions, and guiding public health interventions, epidemiologists continue to make significant contributions to disease prevention, control, and health promotion efforts worldwide.

SUMMARY

- Epidemiology is the branch of medical science that deals with the study of the distribution, patterns, and determinants of health and disease conditions in specific populations. It aims to understand how diseases spread, who is affected, and why certain groups of people are more susceptible to particular health conditions than others.
- Epidemiologists study the frequency and distribution of diseases or health-related events within populations over time. This involves calculating rates of diseases (such as incidence and prevalence) and identifying trends.
- The empirical dimensions of epidemiologic studies require quantification of relevant factors. Quantification refers to the translation of qualitative impressions into numbers. Qualitative sources of information about disease may be, for example, a physician's observations derived through medical practice about the types of people among whom a disease seems to be common.
- An epidemic refers to the occurrence of disease in excess of normal expectancy. In order to ascertain epidemic trends, one must have data about the usual occurrence of a disease. Providing such information is the function of surveillance.
- The elimination of smallpox contributed greatly to the health and well-being of millions of people, particularly in many of the poorest populations. Smallpox illustrates both the achievements and frustrations of modern public health. In the 1790s it was shown that cowpox infection conferred protection against the smallpox virus, yet it took almost 200 years for the benefits of this discovery to be accepted and applied throughout the world.
- Mercury was known to be a hazardous substance in the Middle Ages, but has recently become a symbol of the dangers of environmental pollution. In the 1950s, mercury compounds were released with the water discharged from a factory in Minamata, Japan, into a small bay. This led to the accumulation of methyl mercury in fish, causing severe poisoning in people who ate them.
- Epidemiological research on injuries often involves collaboration between scientists in epidemiology and in the social and environmental health fields. Injuries related to falls – particularly fractures of the neck of the femur (hip fractures) in older people – have attracted a great deal of attention in recent years because of the implications for the health service needs of an ageing population.
- Epidemiology and prevention are integral components of public health, working synergistically to understand disease patterns and implement strategies aimed at reducing their impact on populations. Epidemiology, as the cornerstone of these efforts, involves the systematic study of disease distribution, determinants, and risk factors across communities.

References

1. Berggren, U., Fahlke, C., Berglund, K. J., et al. (2010). Dopamine D2 receptor genotype is associated with increased mortality at a 10-year follow-up of alcohol-dependent individuals. *Alcohol Alcoholism*, *45*(1), 1–5.

2. Centers for Disease Control and Prevention. (1980). Red spots on airline flight attendants. *MMWR, 29*, 141.

3. Centers for Disease Control and Prevention. (2001). Ongoing investigation of anthrax—Florida, October 2001. *MMWR, 50*, 877.

4. Centers for Disease Control and Prevention. (2001). Update: Investigation of bioterrorism-related anthrax and interim guidelines for clinical evaluation of persons with possible anthrax. *MMWR, 50*, 941–948.

5. Centers for Disease Control and Prevention. (2001). Update: Investigation of bioterrorism-related anthrax—Connecticut, 2001. *MMWR, 50*, 1077–1079.

6. Centers for Disease Control and Prevention. (2003). Update: Outbreak of severe acute respiratory syndrome—worldwide, 2003. *MMWR, 52*, 244.

7. Centers for Disease Control and Prevention. (2006). Ongoing multistate outbreak of Escherichia coli serotype O157:H7 infections associated with consumption of fresh spinach—United States, September 2006. *MMWR, 55*, 1045–1046.

8. Friis, R. H., Nanjundappa, G., Prendergast, T., et al. (1981). Hispanic coronary heart disease mortality and risk in Orange County, California. *Public Health Reports, 96*, 418–422.

9. Gordis, L. (1985). The virtual disappearance of rheumatic fever in the United States: Lessons in the rise and fall of disease. *Circulation, 72*, 1155–1162.

10. Gottlieb, M. S., Schroff, R., Schanker, H. M., et al. (1981). Pneumocystis carinii pneumonia and mucosal candidiasis in previously healthy homosexual men: evidence of a new acquired cellular immunodeficiency. *New England Journal of Medicine, 305*, 1425–1431.

11. Hansen, B. (1997). The image and advocacy of public health in American caricature and cartoons from 1860 to 1900. *American Journal of Public Health, 87*, 1798–1807.

12. Hughes, J. M., & Gerberding, J. L. (2002). Anthrax bioterrorism: Lessons learned and future directions. *Emerging Infectious Diseases, 8*, 1013–1014.

13. Iffy, L., Kaminetzky, H. A., Maidman, J. E., et al. (1979). Control of perinatal infection by traditional preventive measures. *Obstetrics & Gynecology, 54*, 403–411.

14. Kannell, W. B., & Abbott, R. D. (1984). Incidence and prognosis of unrecognized myocardial infarction: An update on the Framingham study. *New England Journal of Medicine, 311*, 1144–1147.

15. Kass, E. H. (1971). Infectious diseases and social change. *Journal of Infectious Diseases, 123*, 110–114.

16. Keenan, N. L., & Shaw, K. M. (2006). Coronary heart disease and stroke deaths— United States, 2006. *MMWR, 60*, 62–66.

17. Khoury, M. J., Millikan, R., Little, J., & Gwinn, M. (2004). An emergence of epidemiology in the genomics age. *International Journal of Epidemiology, 33*, 936–944.

18. Maillard, J.-M., Fischer, M., McKee, K. T., Jr., et al. (2002). First case of bioterrorism related inhalational anthrax, Florida, 2001: North Carolina investigation. *Emerging Infectious Diseases, 8*(10), 1035–1038.

19. Palmer, L. J. (2004). The new epidemiology: Putting the pieces together in complex disease etiology. *International Journal of Epidemiology, 33*, 925–928.

20. Rose, G. (1985). Sick individuals and sick populations. *International Journal of Epidemiology, 14*, 32–38.
21. Semmelweis, I. P., & Murphy, F. B. (1941). The etiology, the concept and prophylaxis of childbed fever (1861). In *Medical Classics, 5*, 350–773.
22. Syme, S. L. (1974). Behavioral factors associated with the etiology of physical disease: A social epidemiological approach. *American Journal of Public Health, 64*, 1043–1045.
23. Taubenberger, J. K., & Morens, D. M. (2006). 1918 influenza: The mother of all pandemics. *Emerging Infectious Diseases, 12*, 15–22.
24. Wang, M. D., & Jolly, A. M. (2004). Changing virulence of the SARS virus: the epidemiological evidence. *Bulletin of the World Health Organization, 82*, 547, 548.
25. Whitehead, M. (2000). William Farr's legacy to the study of inequalities in health. *Bulletin of the World Health Organization, 78*, 86–96.
26. World Health Organization. (2006). Epidemiology of WHO-confirmed human cases of avian influenza A (H5N1) infection. *Weekly Epidemiological Record, 81*, 249–260.

Chapter

2

MEASURING HEALTH AND DISEASE

Contents

Introduction

Measuring health and disease is at the core of epidemiology, the field dedicated to understanding patterns of health and illness within populations. This discipline relies heavily on quantitative data to assess the prevalence, incidence, distribution, and determinants of diseases.

One fundamental aspect of measuring health and disease is defining and quantifying health outcomes and their associated conditions. Epidemiologists employ various metrics to gauge the presence and severity of diseases, such as morbidity rates, mortality rates, and disability-adjusted life years (DALYs). These measures help in assessing the burden of diseases on populations and prioritizing public health interventions accordingly.

Furthermore, accurate measurement of disease occurrence requires robust surveillance systems capable of capturing data on both diagnosed and undiagnosed cases. Epidemiologists utilize tools like disease registries, health surveys, and electronic health records to gather information on disease prevalence and incidence rates over time.

In addition to measuring the occurrence of diseases, epidemiologists also examine the distribution of health outcomes across different demographic groups, geographic regions, and time periods. Disparities in health outcomes shed light on underlying social, economic, and environmental determinants of health, guiding efforts to address health inequities and improve overall population health.

Overall, measuring health and disease in epidemiology serves as the foundation for understanding the health status of populations, identifying risk factors and protective factors, and informing evidence-based interventions aimed at promoting health and preventing disease. Through rigorous data collection, analysis, and interpretation, epidemiologists play a crucial role in advancing our understanding of health-related phenomena and guiding public health policy and practice.

Orientation and Directional Terms

Term	Definition	Illustration
Preventive Measures	Preventive measures are actions taken to reduce the risk of harm, injury, or undesirable events from occurring. They are proactive strategies implemented to avoid potential problems or mitigate their impact	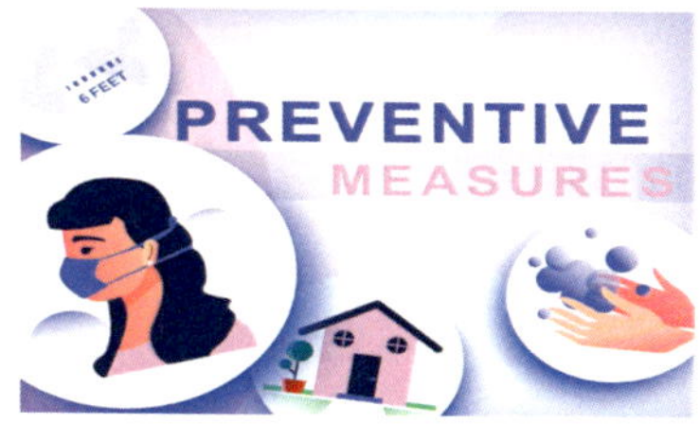
Asbestosis	Asbestosis (as-bes-TOE-sis) is a chronic lung disease caused by inhaling asbestos fibers. Prolonged exposure to these fibers can cause lung tissue scarring and shortness of breath.	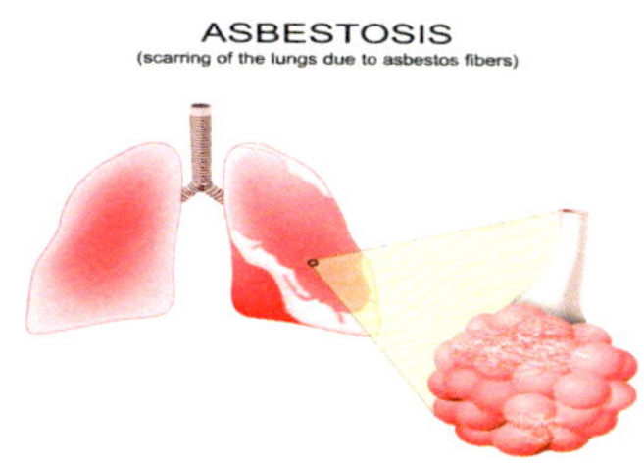
Chest Radiograph	Chest radiograph, chest X-ray, or chest film is a projection radiograph of the chest used to diagnose conditions affecting the chest, its contents, and nearby structures.	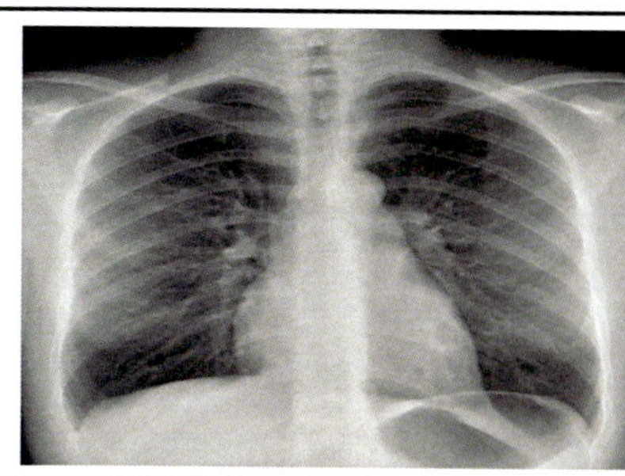
Cervical Cancer	Cervical cancer is a growth of cells that starts in the cervix. The cervix is the lower part of the uterus that connects to the vagina.	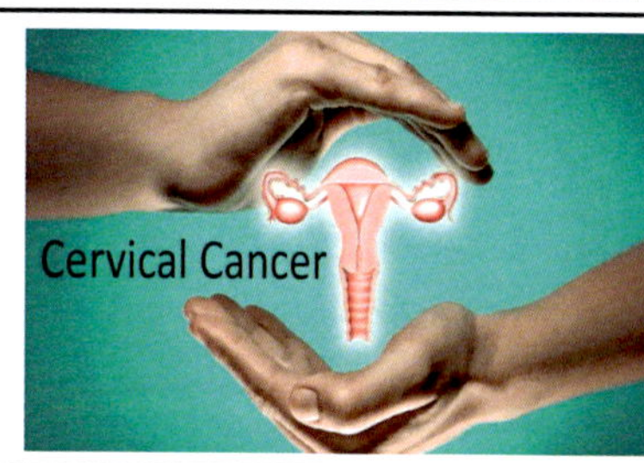
Attack rate	The attack rate is the proportion of an at-risk population that contracts the disease during a specified time interval. It is used in hypothetical predictions and during actual outbreaks of disease.	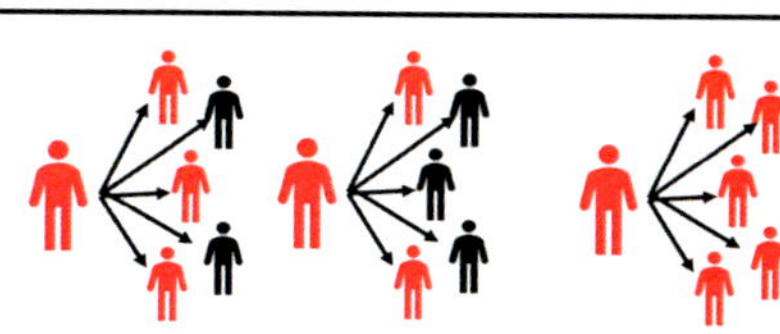

2.1. Defining Health and Disease

The World Health Organization (WHO) defined health as "a state of complete physical, mental, and social well-being and not merely the absence of disease or infirmity" in 1948. This definition is the most ambitious. This definition, which has drawn criticism due to the challenges associated with identifying and quantifying well-being, is still ideal. By the year 2000, everyone should reach a state of health that enables them to lead lives that are both socially and economically productive, according to a resolution made by the World Health Assembly in 1977. This dedication to the "health-for-all" approach was reaffirmed in 1998 and 2003. Practical definitions of health and disease are needed in epidemiology, which concentrates on aspects of health that are easily measurable and amenable to improvement.

2.1.1. Diagnostic Criteria

Typically, test results, history, symptoms, and signs are used to determine the diagnostic criteria.

Table 2.1. Guidelines for the Diagnosis of an Initial Episode of Rheumatic Fever

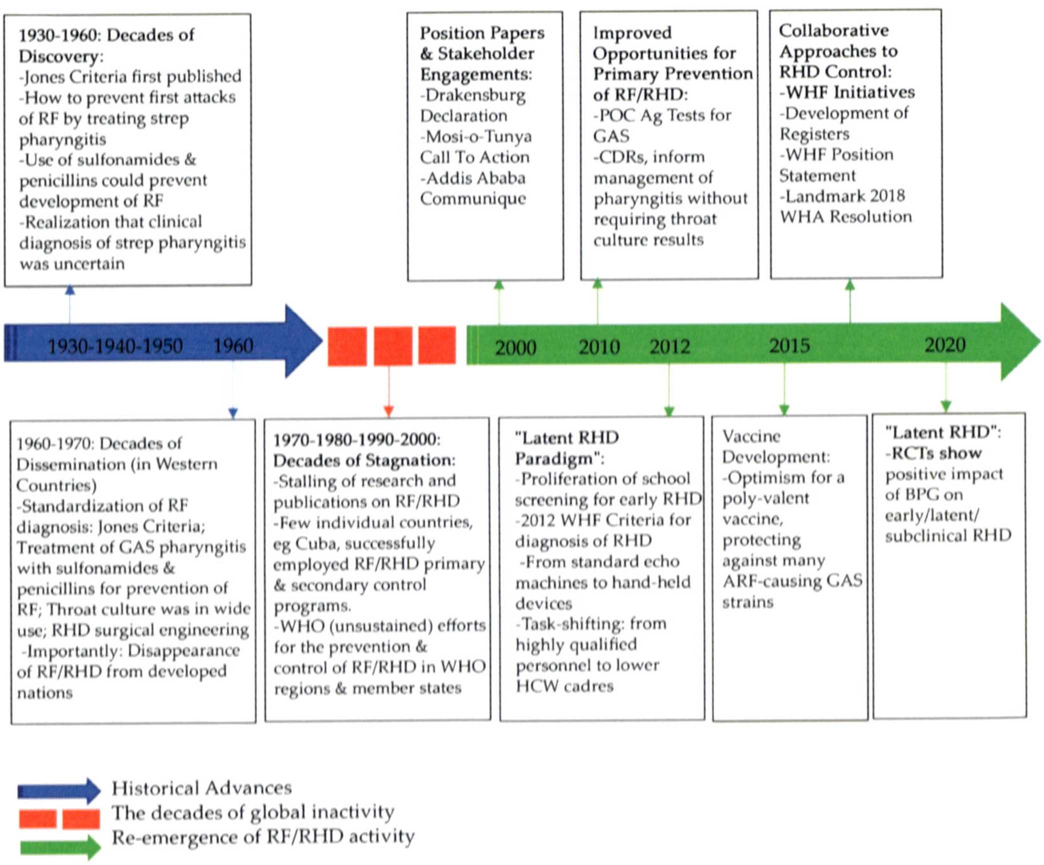

Source: Rwebembera J, Nascimento BR, Minja NW, de Loizaga S, Aliku T, dos Santos LPA, Galdino BF, Corte LS, Silva VR, Chang AY, et al. Recent advances in the rheumatic fever and rheumatic heart disease continuum. Pathogens. 2022; 11(2):179. https://doi.org/10.3390/pathogens11020179.

Hepatitis, for instance, can be recognized by the presence of antibodies in the blood; asbestosis, on the other hand, can be recognized by symptoms and indicators of particular alterations in lung function, radiographic evidence of lung tissue fibrosis or pleural thickening, and a history of asbestos fiber exposure. Table 2.1 illustrates that a number of disease manifestations can be used to diagnose rheumatic fever, with some indications being more significant than others. Certain circumstances justify the use of extremely basic standards. For instance, prompt diagnosis and treatment are essential to lowering the death rate from bacterial pneumonia in children in developing nations. According to WHO case management guidelines, auscultation, chest radiographs, and laboratory testing should not be used in the detection of pneumonia cases; instead, clinical signs alone should be used. A watch is the only piece of equipment needed to time respiratory rate. In situations where bacterial pneumonia is common and it is difficult to rule out other causes due to a lack of resources, the use of antibiotics for children suspected of having pneumonia based solely on a physical examination is advised.

Likewise, a clinical case definition for AIDS in adults was developed in 1985, for use in settings with limited diagnostic resources. The WHO case definition for AIDS surveillance required only two major signs (weight loss ≥ 10% of body weight, chronic diarrhea, or prolonged fever) and one minor sign (persistent cough, herpes zoster, generalized lymphadenopathy, etc.). In 1993, the Centers for Disease Control defined AIDS to include all HIV-infected individuals with a CD4+ T-lymphocyte count of less than 200 per microliter. When knowledge grows or diagnostic methods advance, diagnostic criteria can change quickly. They can also frequently alter depending on the situation in which they are applied. For instance, when an objective technique for evaluating electrocardiograms (the Minnesota Code) was introduced in the 1980s, the original WHO diagnostic criteria for myocardial infarction were changed for use in epidemiological studies. When measuring cardiac enzymes became possible in the 1990s, the criteria underwent further modification.

2.2. Measuring Disease Frequency

The ideas of prevalence and incidence serve as the foundation for many disease frequency metrics. Regretfully, there is still disagreement among epidemiologists regarding the exact meanings of words used in this field.

2.2.1. Population at Risk

Accurately estimating the population under study is crucial for computing disease frequency measures. These figures should ideally only include those who may be at risk for the illnesses under investigation. For example, when determining the frequency of radiation hazard sign (Figure 2.1). The population at risk is made up of individuals who are susceptible to a particular disease and can be identified by environmental, geographic, or demographic factors. For example, occupational injuries happen only to working people, so the workforce is the population at risk; brucellosis only affects people who handle infected animals in some countries, so people who work on farms and in slaughterhouses are the population at risk.

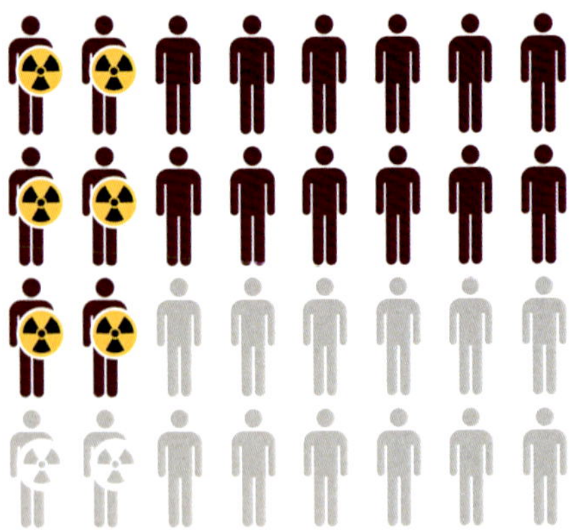

Figure 2.1. *The population at risk radiation hazard sign.*

Source: By Psarka, CC BY-SA 4.0, https://commons.wikimedia.org/w/index.php?curid=72874129.

2.2.2. Incidence and Prevalence

Prevalence is the frequency of existing cases in a defined population at a given point in time, whereas incidence is the rate of new cases arising in a given period in a specified population. Like with diabetes, there could be a low incidence and a high prevalence, or a high incidence and a low prevalence like with the common cold. While diabetes lasts essentially a lifetime, colds occur more frequently but only last temporarily.

Counting cases within specific at-risk populations is a necessary step in measuring prevalence and incidence. To provide an idea of the overall scope of a health issue or of short-term trends in a population, such as during an epidemic, the number of cases reported without reference to the population at risk may be used. Despite their imprecise nature, incidence data in the form of case numbers found in WHO's Weekly Epidemiological Record can provide valuable insights into the evolution of infectious disease epidemics.

During a brief period of time during a disease outbreak in a specifically defined population, the term "attack rate" is frequently used in place of incidence. The number of individuals impacted divided by the total number of exposed is how one can compute the attack rate. For instance, the attack rate for every food consumed can be determined in the event of a foodborne disease outbreak, and the infection source can be found by comparing these rates.

Converting prevalence and incidence data into rates makes them much more useful. A rate is expressed as cases per 10^n people and is computed by dividing the number of cases by the corresponding number of individuals in the population at risk. Some epidemiologists only refer to measurements of disease occurrence per time unit (week, year, etc.) when using the term "rate." We use the term "disease" in a broad sense that encompasses injuries, mental illness, negative biochemical and physiological changes, and clinical disease.

2.2.2.1. Prevalence

Prevalence (P) of a disease is calculated as follows:

Prevalence=incidence x duration

The entire population of the study area is frequently used as an approximation in studies where data on the population at risk are not always available.

Cases per 100 (percentage) or per 1000 population is a common way to express prevalence. P needs to be multiplied by 10^n, the appropriate factor, in this instance. Point prevalence rate, or P, is the number of data collected at a single point in time. Occasionally, it is more practical to employ the "period prevalence rate," which is computed by dividing the total number of cases at any given point in time by the population that is at risk halfway through the period. Likewise, the entire count of individuals known to have had the illness for a portion of their lives is known as their "lifetime prevalence."

Apart from age, several factors determine prevalence (Figure 2.2). In particular:

- The severity of illness (if many people who develop a disease die within a short time, its prevalence is decreased);
- The duration of illness (if a disease lasts a short time its prevalence is lower than if it lasts a long time);
- The number of new cases (if many people develop a disease, its prevalence is higher than if few people do so).

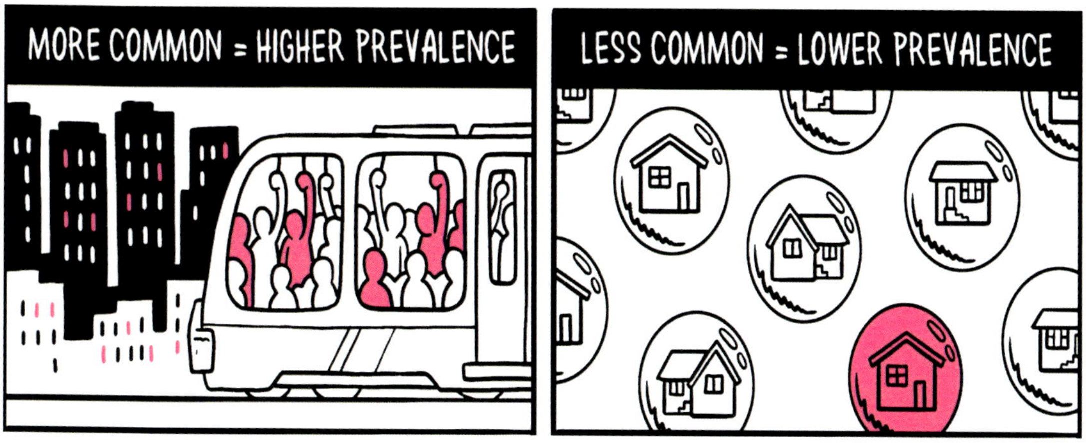

Figure 2.2. *Factors influencing prevalence.*

Source: By Siouxsie Wiles & Toby Morris – https://thespinoff.co.nz/science/29-04-2020/siouxsie-wiles-magic-numbers-and-the-mystery-of-covid-19-silent-spread/, CC BY-SA 4.0, https://commons.wikimedia.org/w/index.php?curid=89917530.

Prevalence studies typically do not offer compelling evidence of causality because a wide range of factors unrelated to the disease's cause can affect prevalence.

Table 2.2. Pooled Prevalence of T2DM, IGT, IFG, and Newly Detected T2DM in South Africa

Condition	Pooled Estimate (95% CI)	I^2, *p* Value
T2DM (%)	15.25 (11.07–19.95)	98.10%, $p < 0.001$
IGT (%)	9.59 (5.82–14.17)	94.18%, $p < 0.001$
IFG (%)	3.55 (0.38–9.61)	98.68%, $p < 0.001$
Newly detected T2DM (%)	8.29 (4.97–12.34)	94.20%, $p < 0.001$

Source: *Pheiffer C, Pillay-van Wyk V, Turawa E, Levitt N, Kengne AP, Bradshaw D. Prevalence of type 2 diabetes in south Africa: a systematic review and meta-analysis. International Journal of Environmental Research and Public Health. 2021; 18(11):5868. https://doi.org/10.3390/ijerph18115868.*

I^2 represents the variation in pooled estimate attributable to heterogeneity. p represents the level of significance. IFG, impaired glucose tolerance; IGT, impaired glucose tolerance; T2DM, type 2 diabetes mellitus.

However, prevalence measures are useful in determining the need for healthcare, preventive measures, and health service planning. When it comes to diseases like maturity-onset diabetes or rheumatoid arthritis, prevalence is a useful indicator of their prevalence. Using the WHO's proposed criteria, the prevalence of type 2 diabetes has been assessed in a variety of populations (Table 2.2). The wide range of results highlights the role that social and environmental factors play in the development of this disease and highlights the differing needs that different populations have for diabetic health services.

2.2.2.2. Incidence

The rate at which new events happen in a population is referred to as its incidence. The variable timespan during which people are disease-free and hence "at risk" of contracting the illness is taken into consideration when calculating incidence. The population at risk of experiencing the event during this period is the denominator in the incidence calculation, which uses the number of new events that occur in a given time period as the numerator. Finding what Last refers to as the "person-time incidence rate" is the most precise method of determining incidence. For each year (or day, week, or month) of observation before the onset of the disease or the participant's loss to follow-up, each individual in the study population adds one person-year to the denominator.

The numerator solely includes the initial occurrences of a disease. Incidence rate units must always include a time component (cases per 10^n as well as cases per day, week, month, year, etc.).

The time of observation for each member of the population is the amount of time that person is free from disease. The total of all the disease-free person-time periods during the population at risk's observation period serves as the denominator for calculating incidence.

The average size of the study population is multiplied by the duration of the study period to approximate the denominator, as it may not be feasible to measure disease-free periods precisely. If the population is large and stable and the incidence is low, as in the case of stroke, this is fairly accurate.

A study conducted in the United States of America analyzed the occurrence of strokes in 118,539 women aged 30–55 who were free of coronary heart disease, stroke, and cancer in 1976. Over the course of eight years of follow-up (totaling 908,447 person-years), 274 cases of stroke were identified. The overall incidence rate of stroke was 30.2 per 100,000 person-years, with smokers having a higher rate compared to non-smokers, and ex-smokers falling in between the two groups (Table 2.3).

Table 2.3. Characteristics of 25 Prospective Cohort Studies of Smoking and Stroke Events

First Author Year (Ref.#)	Cohort	Location/Period	Duration (yrs)	Sample size Male/Female	Outcomes	Events	Adjustment for Covariates	NOS
Coldtiz et al. 1988(18)	Nurse's Health Study	United States 1976-1984	8	F118539	morbidity and mortality of stroke, IS, SAH	274	age,follow-up period,diabetes,hypertension,high cholesterol levels and relative weight.	7
Kawachi et al. 1993(19)	Nurse's Health Study	United States 1976-1988	12	F117006	morbidity of stroke, IS, ICH, SAH	448	age,follow-up period,hypertension,diabetes,high cholesterol levels,BMI,past use of oral contraceptives,postmenopausal estrogen therapy and daily number ofcigarettes consumed.	7
Robbins et al. 1994(20)	Physicians' Health Study	United States 1982-1992	9.7	M22071	morbidity and mortality of stroke, IS, HS	340	age,treatment assignment,angina or revascularization,frequency of vigorous exercise,obesity status,diabetes mellitus,high cholesterol level,high blood pressure and frequency of alcohol consumption.	7
Jacobs et al. 1999(21)	16 cohorts situated in 7 countries	7 countries in Europe, United States, Japan 1957-N/A	25	M12763	mortality of stroke	797	baseline cohort of residence,age,BMI,serum cholesterol level,SBP, and the presence or absense of clinical cardiovascular disease.	8
Shaper et al. 2003(22)	British Regional Heart Study	Great Britain 1978-2000	21.8	M7121	morbidity of stroke	440	age,social class,BMI,physical activity,SBP,serum total cholesterol,alcohol intake and anti-hypertensive treatment.	8
Kurth et al. a 2003(23)	Women's Health Study	United States 1993-2003	9	F39783	HS, ICH, SAH	70	age,exercise and alcohol consumption.	7
Kurth et al. b 2003(24)	Physicians' Health Study	United States 1982-2002	17.8	M22022	HS, ICH, SAH	1069	age, exercise, parental history of MI before 60 years of age, alcohol consumption and randomized treatment assignment.	7
Hsu et al. 2004(25)	Study of Health and Living Status of the Elderly	China 1989-1996	7	M2311/F1738	morbidity of stroke	N/A	demographic and related health factors.	7
Mamun et al. 2004(26)	original Framingham Heart Study cohort	United States 1948-1991	40	M2073/F2650	morbidity and mortality of stroke	N/A	age at baseline or event.	7
Dagenais et al. 2005(27)	Heart Outcomes Prevention Evaluation	Canada, USA, Mexico, Brazil,Argentina and 14 Western European 1993-2000	4.5	total:8905; M:never 54.7%; former83%; current73%	morbidity of stroke	358	age,sex,historyof hypertension,diabetes,total cholestero,HDL-cholesterol,BMI,blood pressure,previous MI,previous stroke,presence of peripheral artery disease,microalbuminuria,left ventricular hypertrophy by electrocardiographic criteria,intervention drugs.	5
Lam et al. 2007(28)	clients in Elderly Health Centres in Hong Kong	China 1998-2005	4.1	M18162/F36052	mortality of stroke	381	age,education,alcohol consumption,physical exercise and active chronic diseases,regular medication,admission to hospital,monthly expenditure,regular contact with relatives,unintentional weight loss,body mass index,self-rated	6
Lawlor et al. 2008(29)	Korean male public servants	Korean 1992-2001	10	M648346	mortality of stroke, IS, ICH, SAH	9475	age,height,blood pressure,BMI,total cholesterol,hyperglycemia,alcohol consumption,regular exercise,income and area of residence.	8
Katanoda et al. 2008(30)	JPHC study,3-pref study,JACC study	Japan 1988-2003	9.6	M140026 F156810	morbidity of stroke, IS, ICH, SAH	N/A	age	7
Lu et al. 2008(31)	Swedish Women's Lifestyle and Health Cohort Study	Sweden 1991-2002	11.4	F45449	morbidity of stroke, IS, ICH	170	age,BMI,education,alcohol intake,age at first birth,ever used OC.	8
Chiuve et al. 2008(32)	Health Professionals Follow-up Study and Nurses'Health Study	United States 1984-2004	20	M43685/F71243	morbidity of stroke, IS, HS	2503	age,calendar year,parental history of MI,regular aspirin use and vitamin E supplementation,plus use of hormone therapy in women.	8
Sandvei et al. 2009(33)	Nord-Trøndelag Health Study	Norway 1984-2005	22	74845 F51.0%	morbidity of SAH	132	sex and age	8
Kondo et al. 2011(34)	Healthy Male Japanese Workers	Japan 2001-2008	7.5	M25464	morbidity of stroke	73	age,SBP,total cholesterol and fasting plasma glucose level.	8
Lindekleiv et al. 2011(35)	Nord-Trøndelag and the Tromsø Health Studies	Norway 1994-2007	N/A	M43437/F49025	morbidity of SAH	120	age, family history of stroke and alcohol consumption.	7
He et al. 2013(36)	workers at a machinery factory in Xi'an	China 1976-2011	14.8	M1124/F572	mortality of stroke, IS, HS	101	age,gender,marital status,occupation,education,alcohol drinking,DBP,triglyceride and total cholesterol levels and BMI.	7
Zhang et al. 2008(37)	Strong Heart Study	United States 1989-2004	13.4	M1846/F2703	morbidity of stroke	258	age,gender,SBP,DBP,BMI,waist circumference,LDL and HDL cholesterol,triglycerides,physical activity,alcohol use,microalbuminuria and macroalbuminuria	7
Pujades-Rodriguez et al. 2014(38)	CALIBER programme	England 1997-2010	5.5	M647400 F766349	morbidity of stroke	9719	age	7
Lindbohm et al. 2016(39)	FINRISK study	Finland 1972-2011	21.1	M31716/F33805	morbidity of SAH	492	age,sex,SBP,BMI,cholesterol,study year and area.	7
Khan et al. 2017(40)	BARI 2D trial	United States,Brazil,Canada,Mexico,Austria and Czech Republic 2001-N/A	5.3	total:2360 M70%/F30%	morbidity of stroke	67	regular exercise,prior MI,ABI,LVEF,CHF,hypertension,hypercholesterolemia,sex,age and prior revascularization.	6
Price et al. 2018(41)	UK Million Women Study	United Kingdom 1999-2015	12.9	F712433	morbidity of stroke, IS, HS, ICH, SAH	11696	age,region of residence,educational attainment,socioeconomic status,use of menopausal hormones,smoking,alcohol consumption,BMI and physical activity.	7
Dinh et al. 2019(42)	Women's Health Initiative	United States 1993-2015	14.01	F109498	morbidity of IS	3534	age,weight change,pack-years,diabetes,education,ethnicity,alcohol,hypertension,high cholesterol,AF,BMI,waist to hip ratio and physical activity.	7

NOTE: NOS, Newcastle–Ottawa Scale; BMI, Body Mass Index; OC, oral contraceptive; LDL, low-density lipoprotein; HDL, High-density lipoprotein; SBP, systolic blood pressure; DBP, diastolic blood pressure; MI, myocardial infarction; ABI, ankle brachial index; LVEF, left ventricular ejection fraction; CHF, congestive heart failure; AF, atrial fibrillation.

Source: Luo J, Tang X, Li F, Wen H, Wang L, Ge S, Tang C, Xu N and Lu L (2022). Cigarette smoking and risk of different pathologic types of stroke: a systematic review and dose-response meta-analysis. Front. Neurol. 12, 772373. doi: 10.3389/fneur.2021.772373.

2.2.2.3. Cumulative Incidence

Cumulative incidence is a simpler measure of the occurrence of a disease or health status. Unlike incidence, it measures the denominator only at the beginning of a study.

The cumulative incidence can be calculated as follows: The distribution of T may be characterized by the cumulative incidence function, $CI(t)=P(T\leq t)$, which is the probability of seeing an event before or at time t.

(Hansen, S.N., Overgaard, M., Andersen, P.K. *et al.* Estimating a population cumulative incidence under calendar time trends. *BMC Med Res Methodol., 17*, 7 (2017). https://doi.org/10.1186/s12874-016-0280-6).

A common way to present cumulative incidence is as cases per 1000 people. Table 2.4 demonstrates that, during the eight-year follow-up, the cumulative incidence of stroke was 2.3 per 1000 (274 stroke cases divided by the 118 539 women who were enrolled in the study). From a statistical perspective, the cumulative incidence represents the likelihood that members of the population will contract the illness within the given time frame.

The duration of the period can vary but typically spans several years or even a person's entire lifetime. The cumulative incidence rate is akin to the concept of "risk of death" commonly utilized in actuarial and life-table calculations. Due to their straightforward nature, cumulative incidence rates are valuable for conveying health information to the public.

2.2.3. Case Fatality

Case fatality is a measure of disease severity and is defined as the proportion of cases with a specified disease or condition who die within a specified time. It is usually expressed as a percentage.

2.2.4. Interrelationships of the Different Measures

Prevalence is dependent on both incidence and disease duration. Provided that the prevalence (P) is low and does not vary significantly with time, it can be calculated approximately as:

P = incidence × average duration of disease

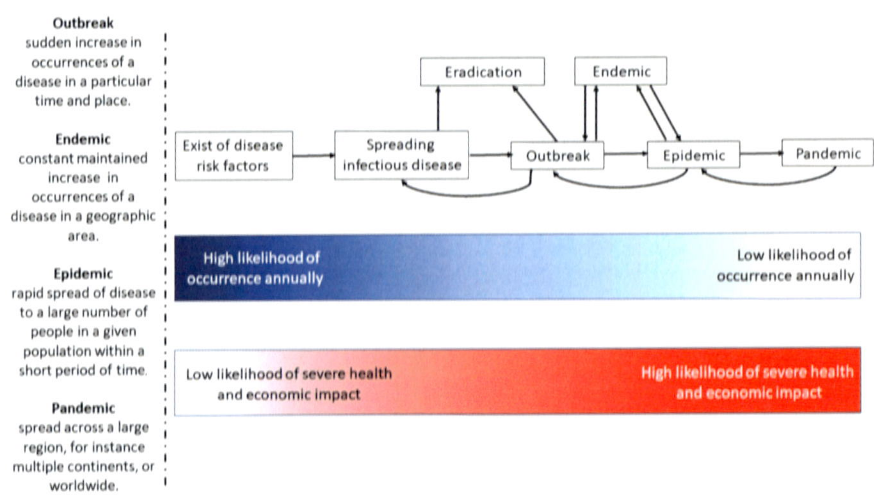

Figure 2.3. *Disease occurrence.*

Source: By Alaa Najjar – Own work, CC BY-SA 3.0, https://commons.wikimedia.org/w/index.php?curid=88074490.

A disease's cumulative incidence rate is determined by the length of the measurement period as well as the incidence. Age-specific incidence rates must be determined because incidence typically varies with age. When the rate is low or the study period is brief, the cumulative incidence rate serves as a helpful approximation of incidence. Figure 2.3 illustrates the various measures of disease. This hypothetical example is based on a study of seven people over seven years.

2.2.5. Using Available Information to Measure Health and Disease

2.2.5.1. Mortality

When examining the health status of a population, epidemiologists frequently begin with data that is regularly gathered. A typical death certificate, which also includes details about the deceased's age, sex, and place of residence, is used in many high-income nations to document the fact and cause of death. Guidelines for categorizing deaths are provided by the International Statistical Classification of Diseases and Related Health Problems (ICD). The methods are used to code causes of death and are updated on a regular basis to consider new illnesses and case definitions.

2.2.5.2. Limitations of Death Certificates

Although data from death statistics are subject to several sources of error, they can frequently offer vital insights into patterns in the health status of a population from an epidemiological standpoint. The accuracy of determining the underlying causes of death and the completeness of the records are two important factors that determine how useful the data is, particularly when it comes to elderly individuals whose autopsy rates are frequently low.

Death statistics are a major source of information for epidemiologists when estimating the burden of disease and monitoring disease trends over time. Unfortunately, basic mortality statistics are unavailable in many nations, typically due to a lack of funding for the establishment of regular vital registration systems. Health services prioritize providing accurate cause-of-death information.

2.2.5.3. Limitations of Vital Registration Systems

The WHO Mortality Database only records one-third of global adult fatalities, most of which occur in wealthy and middle-class nations. Some nations are unable to provide WHO with mortality data, and others have doubts about the data's accuracy. Certain nations only have parts of their countries—urban areas or specific provinces—covered by the vital registration system. Not every death is reported in other nations, even though the vital registration system encompasses the entire nation. In certain nations, such as China and India, the validity of deaths from representative samples of the population is relied upon; in other nations, demographic surveillance sites furnish mortality rates for specific populations.

- **Verbal Autopsy:** Through information gathered from the deceased person's family about symptoms, signs, and circumstances leading up to death, a verbal autopsy is an indirect technique for determining the biological causes of death. For estimating the distribution of causes of death, verbal autopsy is the only method available in many middle-class and low-income countries. Sample registration systems and demographic surveillance are the primary contexts in which verbal autopsies are employed. Comparing cause-of-death statistics across locations and time periods is challenging due to the variety of instruments and techniques employed.

2.2.5.4. Towards Comparable Estimates

Even in countries where underlying causes of death are assigned by qualified staff, miscoding can occur. The main reasons for this are:

- Systematic biases in diagnosis
- Incorrect or incomplete death certificates
- Misinterpretation of ICD rules for selection of the underlying cause
- Variations in the use of coding categories for unknown and ill-defined causes.

Where national vital registration systems do exist and are included in the WHO Mortality Database:

- Death certificates may not be complete
- Poorer segments of populations may not be covered
- Deaths may not be reported for cultural or religious reasons
- The age at death may not be given accurately.

Inaccuracies in reporting or categorizing the cause of death, missing data, and delayed registration are additional elements that lead to untrustworthy registration systems. Since developing high-quality vital registration systems takes time, alternative techniques are frequently employed to estimate mortality and determine the cause of death.

2.2.6. Death Rates

The death rate (or crude mortality rate) for all deaths or a specific cause of death is calculated as follows:

Mortality rates can be seen as calculated using $(d/p)\cdot 10nd/p \times 10^n$, where d represents the deaths from whatever cause of interest is specified that occur within a given time period, p represents the size of the population in which the deaths occur (https://en.wikipedia.org/wiki/Mortality_rate)

The primary drawback of the crude mortality rate is its failure to account for the variation in mortality risk associated with age, sex, race, socioeconomic status, and other variables. In most cases, using it to compare different eras or regions of the world is inappropriate. For instance, mortality trends in recently developed urban areas with a high concentration of young families are probably going to differ significantly from those in seaside resorts, where retired individuals might decide to reside. Age-standardized rates are typically used as the basis for comparisons of mortality rates between groups with different age structures.

- **Age-Specific Death Rates:** Death rates can be expressed for specific groups in a population which are defined by age, race, sex, occupation or geographical location, or for specific causes of death. Fr example, an age- and sex-specific death rate is defined as:
- **Proportionate Mortality:** Proportionate mortality, which is really a ratio representing the number of deaths from a specific cause per 100 or 1000 total deaths in the same period, is sometimes used to describe the mortality in a population. It is not possible to determine the likelihood that a population will become ill or pass away from a disease using proportionate mortality.

Group comparisons of proportionate rates could reveal some intriguing variations. It might not be evident, though, whether a difference between groups is due to differences in the denominators or the numerators unless the crude or age-group-specific mortality rates are known. For instance, even if the lifetime risk of cancer is the same, proportionate death rates from the disease would be significantly higher in high-income nations with a large elderly population than in low- and middle-income nations with a small elderly population.

2.2.6.1. Infant Mortality

The rate of infant mortality is frequently used to gauge the state of health in a community. With the number of live births in the same year serving as the denominator, it calculates the mortality rate for infants in their first year of life.

It is assumed that infant mortality rates are particularly sensitive to changes in socioeconomic conditions and to interventions in healthcare when used as a gauge of a population's general health status. Globally, infant mortality has decreased, but there are still significant differences between and among nations (Figure 2.4).

Infant Mortality Rates are Higher in More Unequal Countries

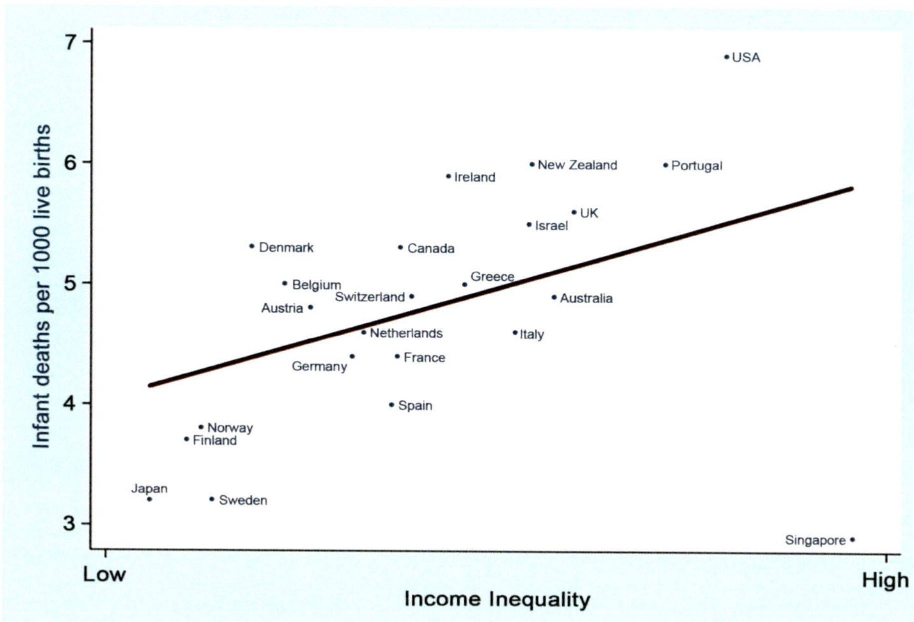

Figure 2.4. *Worldwide trends in infant mortality.*

Source: By The Spirit Level, Wilkinson & Pickett, Penguin 2009., Attribution, https://commons.wikimedia.org/w/index.php?curid=25120853.

2.2.6.2. Child Mortality Rate

Based on deaths of children between the ages of one and four, the child mortality rate, also known as the under-5 mortality rate, is widely used as a fundamental health indicator.

Table 2.4. Country-Wise Estimates

Rank	Country	Infant Mortality Rate (Deaths/1,000 Live Births)
1	Afghanistan	121.63
2	Niger	109.98
3	Mali	109.08
4	Somalia	103.72
5	Central African Republic	97.17
218	Sweden	2.74
219	Singapore	2.65
220	Bermuda	2.47
221	Japan	2.21
222	Monaco	1.80

Source: "Infant mortality rate." CIA – The World Factbook. Archived from the original on November 19, 2012: https://en.wikipedia.org/wiki/Infant_mortality.

In this age range, infectious diseases, malnutrition, and injuries are frequently cited as causes of death. The probability (expressed per 1000 live births) that a child will die before turning five years old is known as the under-5 mortality rate. The death rates for a variety of income brackets are displayed in Table 2.4. The range of uncertainty surrounding the estimates for low- and middle-income nations are displayed in parenthesis.

Table 2.4 contains calculated data that allows for cross-national comparisons of the information. According to exact data, mortality rates for males in Sierra Leone range from 297 (with a wide range of uncertainty: between 250 and 340 per 1000 live births) to as low as 4 for Japan. It is difficult to collect reliable data, so different strategies have been devised.

2.2.6.3. Maternal Mortality Rate

The chance that a mother will pass away from complications related to childbirth or delivery is known as the maternal mortality rate. Due to its difficulty in calculation, this crucial statistic is frequently overlooked.

In high-income nations, the rate of maternal death is approximately 3 per 100,000 live births; in low-income countries, it is over 1500 per 100,000 live births. Even so, this comparison is insufficient to capture the significantly higher lifetime risk of pregnancy-related deaths in developing nations.

2.2.6.4. Adult Mortality Rate

The adult mortality rate is defined as the probability of dying between the ages of 15 and 60 years per 1000 population. The adult mortality rae offers a way to analyze health gaps between countries in the main working age groups. The probability of dying in adulthood is greater for men than for women in almost all countries, but the variation between countries is very large. In Japan, less than 1 in 10 men (and 1 in 20 women) die in these productive age groups, compared with almost 2 in 3 men (and 1 in 2 women) in Angola (Table 2.5).

Table 2.5. World Historical and Predicted Crude Death Rates (1950–2050)

World Historical and Predicted Crude Death Rates (1950–2050) UN, Medium Variant, 2012 rev. (Mathers, Ma Fat, Inoue, Rao & Lopez, 2005)			
Years	**CDR**	**Years**	**CDR**
1950–1955	19.1	2000–2005	8.4
1955–1960	17.3	2005–2010	8.1
1960–1965	16.2	2010–2015	8.1
1965–1970	12.9	2015–2020	8.1
1970–1975	11.6	2020–2025	8.1
1975–1980	10.6	2025–2030	8.3
1980–1985	10.0	2030–2035	8.6
1985–1990	9.4	2035–2040	9.0
1990–1995	9.1	2040–2045	9.4
1995–2000	8.8	2045–2050	9.7

Source: "UNdata – record view – Crude death rate (deaths per 1,000 population)." data.un.org https://en.wikipedia.org/wiki/Mortality_rate.

2.2.6.5. Life Expectancy

Another quick indicator of a population's health is life expectancy. It is defined as the average number of years that, under current mortality rates, a person of a given age should expect to live. Understanding the causes of the variations in life expectancy amongst nations is not always simple; the metrics employed may cause distinct trends to appear.

For the world as a whole, life expectancy at birth has increased from 46.5 years during the period 1950–1955 to 65.0 years during the period 1995–2000 (Figure 2.5). Reversals in life expectancy have occurred in some sub-Saharan countries largely due to AIDS. Similar reversals in life expectancy have also occurred in middle-aged men in the former Soviet Union, where almost 1 in 2 men die between the ages of 15 and 60 years, largely due to changes in the use of alcohol and tobacco.

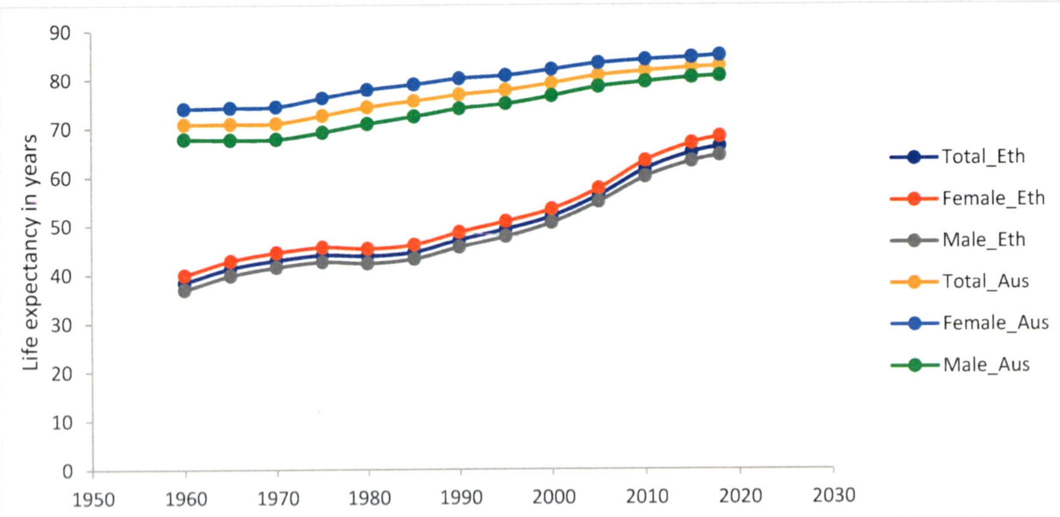

Figure 2.5. *Life expectancy trend by gender in Australia and Ethiopia, 1960–2018.*

Source: Baum F, Musolino C, Gesesew HA, Popay J. New perspective on why women live longer than men: an exploration of power, gender, social determinants, and capitals. International Journal of Environmental Research and Public Health. 2021; 18(2):661. https://doi.org/10.3390/ijerph18020661.

As a general indicator of health status, life expectancy at birth gives more weight to infant deaths than to deaths during later life. Data for specific countries are provided in Table 2.6. Since the data are derived from current age-specific death rates, further computation is required to enable cross-national comparability; the estimates' uncertainty is indicated in parenthesis. Confidence intervals can be fairly wide, as in Zimbabwe, but they can also be very accurate in nations with comprehensive vital registration, like Japan.

Table 2.6. Life Expectancy and Life Expectancy Difference (in Years) by Country Income

Countries Grouped by Income Level	Life Expectancy, Total, at Birth	Life Expectancy, Female, at Birth	Life Expectancy, Male, at Birth	Gender Life Expectancy Difference
Low-income	63.49	65.41	61.59	3.82
Middle-income	71.86	74.11	69.75	4.36
High-income	80.66	83.35	78.13	5.22
World	72.56	74.87	70.39	4.48

Source: World Bank database (2018); Baum F, Musolino C, Gesesew HA, Popay J. New perspective on why women live longer than men: an exploration of power, gender, social determinants, and capitals. International Journal of Environmental Research and Public Health. 2021; 18(2):661. https://doi.org/10.3390/ijerph18020661.

2.2.6.6. Age-Standardized Rates

An age-standardized death rate (also referred to as an age-adjusted rate) is a summary measure of the death rate that a population would have if it had a standard age structure. The standardization of rates can be done either directly or indirectly. Comparisons between populations with varying age structures are made possible by age-standardized rates. Standardization is possible for variables other than age as well. This is required when comparing two or more populations that differ in fundamental ways that independently affect mortality risk (e.g., age, race, socioeconomic status, etc.).

Frequently used standard populations include:

- The Segi world population
- The European standard population is based on the Swedish population
- The WHO World Standard Population, which is based on the world overall average projected population 2000–2025.

The impact of varying age distributions on the morbidity or mortality rates under comparison is removed through the age-standardization of rates. For instance, Table 2.7 illustrates reported crude mortality rates for heart disease in a study. Although Brazil's crude heart disease death rate is about three times lower than Finland's, the country's standardized rate is the same. Likewise, the crude rate in the United States of America is more than twice as high as that in Brazil; however, age-standardized rates are comparable. As a result, despite what the crude rates would seem to indicate, there is less of a difference between these nations.

Compared to low- and middle-income countries, high-income countries have a significantly higher percentage of elderly citizens, and these citizens also have higher rates of cardiovascular disease. The accuracy of the initial cause-of-death data affects all of these death rates.

Table 2.7. Joinpoints and Annual Percentage Changes of IHD Mortality Among Females

Country	Period	APC	Period	APC	Period	APC	Period	APC
Spain	1985–1998	−0.61	1998–2003	−3.40	2003–2019	−4.88 *		
France	1985–1994	−3.86 *	1994–2003	−2.27 *	2003–2011	−6.37 *	2011–2017	−3.61 *
Croatia	1985–1990	−0.27	1990–1993	+46.08 *	1993–2019	−1.91 *		
Italy	1985–2004	−1.58 *	2004–2019	−4.24 *				
Slovenia	1985–1987	−22.48 *	1987–1991	+21.55 *	1991–2019	−5.06 *		

APC = annual percentage changes; * $p < 0.05$.

Source: Biloglav Z, Medaković P, Ćurić J, Padjen I, Vidović D, Migo WAA, Škrlec I. Morbidity and mortality trends of ischemic heart disease and medical interventions in mediterranean countries—pre-COVID analysis: croatia, slovenia, France, Italy, and Spain. Applied Sciences. 2024; 14(6):2581. https://doi.org/10.3390/app14062581.

2.2.7. Morbidity

To research diseases with a high case-fatality, death rates are especially helpful. Many diseases, though, like the majority of mental illnesses, musculoskeletal disorders, rheumatoid arthritis, chickenpox, and mumps, have low case-fatality rates. Morbidity (illness) data are more helpful in this case than death rates.

Statistics on morbidity can be very useful in elucidating the causes of specific patterns in death. Variations in case fatality or morbidity rates may be the cause of shifts in death rates. For instance, the recent decline in the mortality rates from cardiovascular disease in many developed nations may be the result of a decline in case-fatality (which suggests improvements in treatment) or incidence (which suggests improvements in primary prevention). Time-trend analyzes should be based on age-standardized rates of morbidity and mortality because population age structures are dynamic.

Other sources of morbidity data include:

- Hospital admissions and discharges
- Outpatient and primary healthcare consultations
- Specialist services (such as injury treatment)
- Registers of disease events (such as cancer and congenital malformations).

For epidemiological studies, the data must be easily obtainable and pertinent. Hospital data may not be available for epidemiological research in some nations due to the private nature of patient medical records. The epidemiological value of routine health service data may be reduced by a recording system that prioritizes administrative or financial data over individual and diagnostic features. Aside from population morbidity, other factors that affect hospital admission rates include bed availability, hospital admission policies, and social factors. Many epidemiological studies of morbidity rely on the collection of new data using specially designed questionnaires and screening techniques because routinely recorded morbidity data have several limitations. This increases the confidence that investigators have in the data and the rates that are derived from it.

2.2.7.1. Disability

In addition to the incidence of disease, epidemiologists are interested in its aftereffects, such as impairments, disabilities, and handicaps. The WHO's International Classification of Functioning, Disability, and Health (ICF) has defined these.

ICF explains how individuals manage their health condition. An inventory of environmental factors is also included in the ICF because an individual's functioning and disability occur within a framework. ICF is a helpful tool for calculating and comprehending health-related outcomes. It can be applied to individuals or populations in clinical settings, health services, or surveys.

The key parameters of ICF are as follows:

- **Impairment:** any loss or abnormality of psychological, physiological or anatomical structure or function;
- **Disability:** any restriction or lack (resulting from an impairment) of ability to perform an activity in the manner or within the range considered normal for a human being;
- **Handicap:** a disadvantage for a given individual, resulting from an impairment or a disability, that limits or prevents the fulfillment of a role that is normal (depending on age, sex, and social and cultural factors) for that individual.

2.2.8. Health Determinants, Indicators, and Risk Factors

2.2.8.1. Health Determinants

The underlying social, economic, cultural, and environmental factors that cause health and disease are commonly referred to as health determinants, and the majority of these factors are not related to the health sector.

2.2.8.1. Health Indicators

A health indicator is a variable that can be used to measure and represent the overall health of a community. Every year, WHO releases the most recent information on 50 health indicators. Additionally, a more comprehensive social development index can be calculated using health indicators as constituents. The Human Development Index is a prime example; it rates nations annually based on a composite of economic development, life expectancy, literacy, and education.

2.2.8.2. Risk Factors

A risk factor is a characteristic of one's behavior or exposure to the environment that is linked to a higher chance of contracting an illness. Since risk factors are typically modifiable, taking action to change them for the better can lower the likelihood that a disease will manifest. Repeated measurements with the same definitions and methods can be used to assess the effectiveness of these interventions.

2.2.9. Other Summary Measures of Population Health

In addition to having to forecast future priorities, policymakers must respond to the pressing issues of disease prevention and control today. These choices ought to be supported by summary metrics that express the magnitude of illness at the community level. These metrics must employ a common unit of measurement and combine deaths and time spent unwell in an internally consistent manner. These summary metrics provide a standard by which to report the burden of disease within populations. They offer a means of keeping an eye on and assessing population health, enabling prompt intervention and control measures when needed.

Mortality alone does not provide a full picture of how different causes affect population health. Duration of life combined with some notion of its quality are reflected in the following population measures:

- Years of potential life lost (PLL) based on the years of life lost through premature death (before an arbitrarily determined age);
- Healthy life expectancy (HALE);
- Disability-free life expectancy (DFLE);
- Quality-adjusted life years (QALYs);
- Disability-adjusted life years (DALYs).

2.2.9.1. Disability-Adjusted Life Years

The Global Burden of Disease project combines the impact of premature mortality with that of disability. It captures the population impact of important fatal and non-fatal disabling conditions through a single measure. The major measure used is disability-adjusted life years (DALYs) which combines:

- **Years of Lost Life (YLL):** calculated from the number of deaths at each age multiplied by the expected remaining years of life according to a global standard life expectancy
- **Years Lost to Disability (YLD),** where the number of incident cases due to injury and illness is multiplied by the average duration of the disease and a weighting factor reflecting the

severity of the disease on a scale from 0 (perfect health) to 1 (dead).

A disease-adjusted life year (DALY) represents one year of lost "healthy" life, and the measured disease burden is the difference between the current health status of a population and the ideal situation, in which all individuals live to an old age without disability. For females and males, respectively, the normative reference population has a life expectancy at birth of 82.05 and 80.0 years. Standard DALYs are calculated using time-discounting and non-uniform age weights, which assign less weight to years lived at younger and older ages, as stated in recent WHO World Health Reports. A death in infancy corresponds to 33 DALYs with age weights and time discounting, and a death between the ages of 5 and 20 to approximately 36 DALYs. A population with a disease burden of 3300 DALYs would therefore experience 100 infant deaths or roughly 5500 blind individuals living for a year (disability weighting = 0.6).

DALYs were created to inform global priority settings for health research and international health programs, as well as to direct World Bank investment policies for health. New insights into the relative significance of various disease prevention strategies have been provided by analysis of DALYs resulting from a range of causes and risk factors.

2.3. Comparing Disease Occurrence

The first stage in the epidemiological process is to measure the prevalence of disease or other health states. Comparing the occurrence in two or more groups of people with different exposures is the next step. A factor under investigation can either expose or unexpose a person. A reference group that has not been exposed is frequently utilized. Different exposure levels and times can affect those who have been exposed. The term "dose" refers to the total quantity of a factor that reaches a specific person." The risk that an exposure will have a negative impact on one's health can then be determined by comparing occurrences. The measures indicate the degree of an association between exposure and outcome, so we can compare in both absolute and relative terms.

2.3.1. Absolute Comparisons

2.3.1.1. Risk Difference

The difference in the rates of occurrence between exposed and unexposed groups in the population is known as the risk difference, or excess risk. It is a helpful indicator of the scope of the exposure-related public health issue. For instance, Table 2.4's data indicates that there is a risk difference of 31.9 per 100,000 person-years between the incidence rate of stroke in women who smoke and the rate of stroke in women who have never smoked.

With the exception of the factor under study, two or more groups must be as similar as possible when compared. If the groups are different in terms of gender, age, etc. It is not possible to compare without first standardizing the rates.

2.3.1.2. Attributable Fraction (Exposed)

The percentage of all cases that can be linked to a specific exposure is called the attributable fraction (exposed), also referred to as the etiological fraction (exposed). By dividing the risk (or attributable) difference by the incidence within the exposed population, we can calculate the attributable fraction (AF). The attributable fraction of smoking for stroke in smokers according to Table 2.4 data is ((49.6 – 17.7)/49.6) ×100 = 64%

The attributable fraction is the percentage of a disease in a given population that would disappear if a particular exposure were to be eliminated when that exposure is thought to be the cause of the disease. Assuming that smoking is both causative and preventable, quitting smoking would result in a 64% reduction in the risk of stroke among the female smokers in the aforementioned example. It is helpful to evaluate priorities for public health action using attributable fractions. For instance, smoking and air pollution are both known to cause lung cancer, but smoking's contribution to the disease is typically far higher than air pollution's. Lung cancer is most likely to be caused by severe air pollution, which is only likely to occur in areas with very low smoking prevalence. For the majority of nations, programs aimed at preventing lung cancer should prioritize smoking cessation.

2.3.1.3. Population Attributable Risk

The incidence of a disease in a population linked to (or attributed to) exposure to a risk factor is known as the population attributable risk, or PAR. The relative significance of exposures for the whole population can be ascertained with the help of this measure. It is the amount that, in the event that exposure were stopped, would lower the incidence rate of the outcome across the board.

It is calculated as $AFp=(Ip-Iu)/Ip$Ip-Iu/Ip, where IpIP is the incidence in the population, and IuIu is the incidence in the unexposed group.

2.3.2. Relative Comparisons

2.3.2.1. Relative Risk

The ratio of the risk of an illness occurring among those who have been exposed to it to that among those who have not is known as the relative risk, or risk ratio.

Since the risk ratio is expressed in relation to a baseline level of occurrence, it serves as a more reliable indicator of the strength of an association than the risk difference. It is dependent on the size of the baseline incidence rate, unlike the risk difference, which means that populations with similar risk differences may have very different risk ratios. When determining whether an association indicates a causal relationship, the risk ratio is utilized. For instance, there is roughly a 20% risk of lung cancer among long-term heavy smokers compared to non-smokers. This is extremely high and suggests that there is little chance that this relationship was discovered by accident. Smaller risk ratios can, of course, also point to a causal relationship; however, one must be careful to rule out alternative theories.

2.3.2.2. Attributable Risk

The rate (proportion) of an illness or other consequence in those who have been exposed that can be linked to the exposure is known as the "attributed risk." For the sake of public health, this term is more helpful since it indicates the degree—typically given as a percentage—by which the risk of an illness is decreased through the removal or management of a specific exposure. By deducting the rate of the outcome (often incidence or mortality) among the unexposed from the rate among the exposed individuals, one can use attributable risk to estimate the number of people spared the consequences of exposure. For instance, the attributable risk would be 5 per 100 if there were 6 deaths per 100 smokers and 1 death per 100 non-smokers. This presupposes that the exposed and unexposed groups have been equally impacted by causes other than the one being investigated.

A Closer Look

Measuring Population Health

Measuring population health is essential for understanding the overall well-being of communities and identifying areas for improvement. Several key indicators and measures are used to assess population health comprehensively.

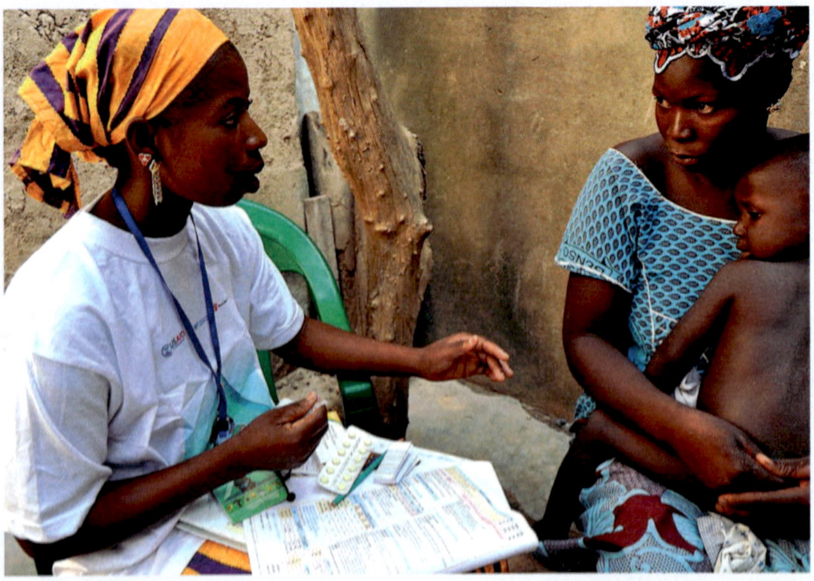

Source: By President's Malaria Initiative – Community Health Worker treats child, Public Domain, https://commons.wikimedia.org/w/index.php?curid=72085321.

One fundamental measure is life expectancy, which provides an overall snapshot of the health status and longevity of a population. Life expectancy at birth reflects the average number of years a person can expect to live, taking into account mortality rates across different age groups. It serves as a widely recognized indicator of overall population health and is influenced by factors such as access to healthcare, socioeconomic conditions, and lifestyle behaviors.

Another important measure is the infant mortality rate, which refers to the number of deaths of infants under one year of age per 1,000 live births. High infant mortality rates often indicate underlying health disparities, inadequate access to prenatal care, and socio-economic challenges within a population. Conversely, decreasing infant mortality rates are often seen as a sign of improvements in healthcare services and public health interventions. Additionally, morbidity indicators, such as the prevalence of chronic diseases, infectious diseases, and injuries, provide insights into the burden of illness within a population. Chronic disease prevalence rates, for example, help identify the prevalence of conditions like diabetes, heart disease, and cancer, which are major contributors to morbidity and mortality globally. Tracking infectious disease incidence rates allows for early detection of outbreaks and informs targeted intervention strategies, such as vaccination campaigns and disease surveillance systems.

Furthermore, measures of disability-adjusted life years (DALYs) and quality-adjusted life years (QALYs) combine information on morbidity and mortality to quantify the overall burden of disease and assess the impact of interventions on population health. DALYs represent the years of healthy life lost due to premature death and disability, while QALYs incorporate measures of health-related quality of life. These measures help policymakers prioritize health interventions and allocate resources effectively to maximize population health outcomes.

Social determinants of health, such as education, income, housing, and access to healthcare, also play a crucial role in shaping population health indicators. Therefore, a comprehensive assessment of population health requires consideration of both health outcomes and the underlying socio-economic determinants that influence them.

SUMMARY

- Measuring health and disease involves a complex interplay of various factors, from physiological markers to societal well-being indicators. At its core, health is often quantified by assessing the functioning of bodily systems, such as cardiovascular health, immune function, and neurological status.
- Accurately estimating the population under study is crucial for computing disease frequency measures. These figures should ideally only include those who may be at risk for the illnesses under investigation.
- Prevalence is the frequency of existing cases in a defined population at a given point in time, whereas incidence is the rate of new cases arising in a given period in a specified population. Like with diabetes, there could be a low incidence and a high prevalence, or a high incidence and a low prevalence like with the common cold. While diabetes lasts essentially a lifetime, colds occur more frequently but only last temporarily.
- The rate of infant mortality is frequently used to gauge the state of health in a community. With the number of live births in the same year serving as the denominator, it calculates the mortality rate for infants in their first year of life.
- The adult mortality rate is defined as the probability of dying between the ages of 15 and 60 years per 1000 population. The adult mortality rae offers a way to analyze health gaps between countries in the main working age groups.
- An age-standardized death rate (also referred to as an age-adjusted rate) is a summary measure of the death rate that a population would have if it had a standard age structure. The standardization of rates can be done either directly or indirectly.
- In addition to the incidence of disease, epidemiologists are interested in its aftereffects, such as impairments, disabilities, and handicaps. The WHO's International Classification of Functioning, Disability, and Health (ICF) has defined these.
- A health indicator is a variable that can be used to measure and represent the overall health of a community. Every year, WHO releases the most recent information on 50 health indicators. Additionally, a more comprehensive social development index can be calculated using health indicators as constituents.
- The rate (proportion) of an illness or other consequence in those who have been exposed that can be linked to the exposure is known as the "attributed risk." For the sake of public health, this term is more helpful since it indicates the degree—typically given as a percentage—by which the risk of an illness is decreased through the removal or management of a specific exposure.

References

1. Alpert, J. S., Thygesen, K., Antman, E., & Bassand, J. P. (2000). Myocardial infarction redefined—a consensus document of The Joint European Society of Cardiology/American College of Cardiology Committee for the redefinition of myocardial infarction. *Journal of the American College of Cardiology, 36*(3), 959–969.

2. Armstrong, T., & Bonita, R. (2003). Capacity building for an integrated noncommunicable disease risk factor surveillance system in developing countries. *Ethnicity & Disease, 13*(2 Suppl 2), S2-13–S2-18.
3. Barford, A., Dorling, D., Davey Smith, G., & Shaw, M. (2006). Life expectancy: women now on top everywhere. *BMJ, 332*(7545), 808.
4. Bonita, R., Winkelmann, R., Douglas, K. A., & de Courten, M. (2003). The WHO STEP wise approach to surveillance (STEPS) of noncommunicable disease risk factors. In McQueen, D. V., & Puska, P. (Eds.), *Global risk factor surveillance* (pp. 9–22). New York: Kluwer Academic/ Plenum Publishers.
5. Brett, A. S. (1989). Treating hypercholesterolemia: How should practicing physicians interpret the published data for patients? *New England Journal of Medicine, 321*(10), 676–680.
6. Centers for Disease Control and Prevention. (1993). Revised classification system for HIV infection and expanded surveillance case definition for AIDS among adolescents and adults. *MMWR Recommendations and Reports, 41*(RR–17), 1–19.
7. Colditz, G. A., Bonita, R., Stampfer, M. J., Willett, W. C., Rosner, B., Speizer, F. E., et al. (1988). Cigarette smoking and risk of stroke in middle-aged women. *New England Journal of Medicine, 318*(15), 937–941.
8. Evans, A. S. (1978). Causation and disease: A chronological journey. *American Journal of Epidemiology, 108*(4), 249–258.
9. Hill, A. B. (1965). The environment and disease: Association or causation? *Proceedings of the Royal Society of Medicine, 58*(5), 295–300.
10. Irwin, A., Valentine, N., Brown, C., Loewenson, R., Solar, O., et al. (2006). The Commission on Social Determinants of Health: Tackling the social roots of health inequities. *PLoS Medicine, 3*(6), e106.
11. King, H., & Rewers, M. (1993). Global estimates for prevalence of diabetes mellitus and impaired glucose tolerance in adults. WHO Ad Hoc Diabetes Reporting Group. *Diabetes Care, 16*(1), 157–177.
12. Lee, J. W. (2005). Public health is a social issue. *Lancet, 365*(9464), 1005–1006.
13. Marmot, M. (2005). Social determinants of health inequalities. *Lancet, 365*(9464), 1099–1104.
14. Mathers, C. D., Ma Fat, D., Inoue, M., Rao, C., & Lopez, A. D. (2005). Counting the dead and what they died from: an assessment of the global status of cause of death. *Bulletin of the World Health Organization, 83*(3), 171–177.
15. McKee, M., & Zatonski, W. (2003). Public health in Eastern Europe and the former Soviet Union. In Beaglehole, R. (Ed.), *Global Public Health: A New Era* (pp. 217–236). Oxford: Oxford University Press.
16. Moser, K., Shkolnikov, V., & Leon, D. A. (2005). World mortality 1950–2000: divergence replaces convergence from the late 1980s. *Bulletin of the World Health Organization, 83*(3), 202–209.
17. Murphy, M., Hultgren, H. N., Detre, K., et al. (1977). Treatment of chronic stable angina: A preliminary report of survival data of the randomized Veterans Administration Cooperative Study. *New England Journal of Medicine, 297*(13), 621–627.

18. Pekkanen, J., Linn, S., Heiss, G., et al. (1990). Ten-year mortality from cardiovascular disease in relation to cholesterol level among men with and without preexisting cardiovascular disease. *New England Journal of Medicine, 322*(24), 1700–1707.

19. Setel, P. W. (2005). Sample registration of vital events with verbal autopsy: a renewed commitment to measuring and monitoring vital statistics. *Bulletin of the World Health Organization, 83*(8), 611–617.

20. Shibuya, K. (2006). Counting the dead is essential for health. *Bulletin of the World Health Organization, 84*(3), 170–171.

21. Shibuya, K., & Boerma, T. (2005). Measuring progress towards reducing health inequalities. *Bulletin of the World Health Organization, 83*(3), 162.

22. Sibai, A. M. (2005). Mortality certification and cause of death reporting in developing countries. *Bulletin of the World Health Organization, 83*(3), 83.

23. Soleman, N., Chandramohan, D., & Shibuya, K. (2006). Verbal autopsy: current practices and challenges. *Bulletin of the World Health Organization, 84*(3), 239–245.

24. Special Writing Group of the Committee on Rheumatic Fever, Endocarditis, and Kawasaki Disease in the Young of the American Heart Association. (1992). Guidelines for the diagnosis of rheumatic fever. Jones criteria, 1992 update. *JAMA, 268*(15), 2069–2073.

25. Susser, M. (1977). Judgment and causal inference: Criteria in epidemiologic studies. *American Journal of Epidemiology, 105*(1), 1–15.

26. Tolonen, H., Dobson, A., Kulathinal, S., for the WHO MONICA Project. (2005). Assessing the quality of risk factor survey data: lessons from the WHO MONICA Project. *European Journal of Cardiovascular Prevention & Rehabilitation, 12*(2), 104–114.

27. Tunstall-Pedoe, H., Vanuzzo, D., Hobbs, M., Mahonen, M., Cepaitis, Z., Kuulasmaa, K., et al. (2000). Estimation of contribution of changes in coronary care to improving survival, event rates, and coronary heart disease mortality across the WHO MONICA Project populations. *Lancet, 355*(9205), 688–700.

28. Winkelstein Jr., W. (1995). Invited commentary on "Judgment and causal inference: Criteria in epidemiologic studies." *American Journal of Epidemiology, 141*(8), 699–700.

Chapter

STUDY DESIGNS IN EPIDEMIOLOGY

3

Contents

Introduction

Epidemiology is a branch of public health that looks at patterns of disease occurrence and the factors that affect them in populations using a variety of study designs. The framework for methodically collecting and evaluating data to comprehend the distribution, causes, and consequences of health-related events is provided by these designs. Cross-sectional, case-control, and cohort studies are examples of observational studies, which are among the basic study designs in epidemiology.

Cross-sectional studies are conducted at a single point in time to assess the prevalence of a disease or health-related condition within a population. By collecting data on both the exposure and outcome simultaneously, cross-sectional studies provide a snapshot of the relationship between variables at a specific moment. However, they cannot establish causality or temporal relationships between exposure and outcome. Case-control studies are retrospective observational studies that compare individuals with a particular health outcome (cases) to those without the outcome (controls). Researchers examine the differences in exposure history between cases and controls to identify potential risk factors for the disease of interest. Case-control studies are efficient for studying rare diseases or outcomes with long latency periods but may be susceptible to recall bias and selection bias.

Cohort studies are prospective observational studies that follow a group of individuals over time to assess the association between exposure and disease incidence. Participants are categorized based on their exposure status at the beginning of the study and followed up to measure the occurrence of the outcome. Cohort studies provide stronger evidence for establishing causality and temporal relationships but can be resource-intensive and subject to loss to follow-up.

In addition to observational designs, epidemiological research also utilizes experimental or interventional study designs, such as randomized controlled trials (RCTs). These RCTs involve randomly assigning participants to intervention and control groups to evaluate the effectiveness of a preventive or therapeutic intervention. While RCTs are considered the gold standard for assessing causality, they may not always be feasible or ethical, especially for studying long-term outcomes or exposures.

Overall, the choice of study design in epidemiology depends on various factors, including the research question, resources, ethical considerations, and the strength of evidence needed to inform public health policies and interventions. By employing a combination of study designs, epidemiologists can systematically investigate the complex interactions between biological, behavioral, environmental, and social factors that influence population health.

Orientation and Directional Terms

<table>
<tr><th>Term</th><th>Definition</th><th>Illustration</th></tr>
<tr><td>Cohort Study</td><td>A cohort study is a particular form of longitudinal study that samples a cohort, performing a cross-section at intervals through time. It is a type of panel study where the individuals in the panel share a common characteristic.</td><td>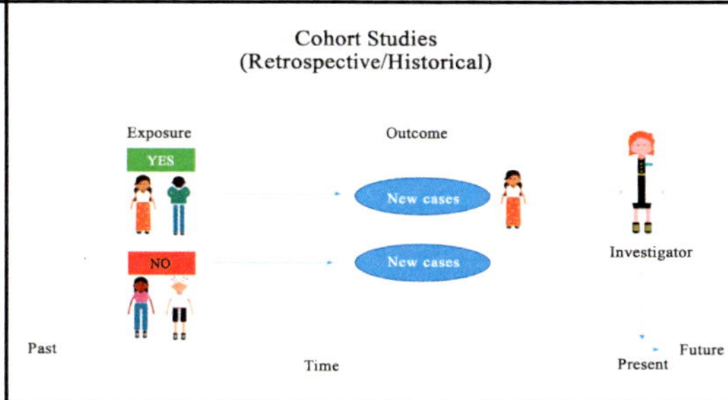
</td></tr>
<tr><td>Case-Control Study</td><td>Case-control study is a type of observational study commonly used to look at factors associated with diseases or outcomes. The case-control study starts with a group of cases, which are the individuals who have the outcome of interest.</td><td>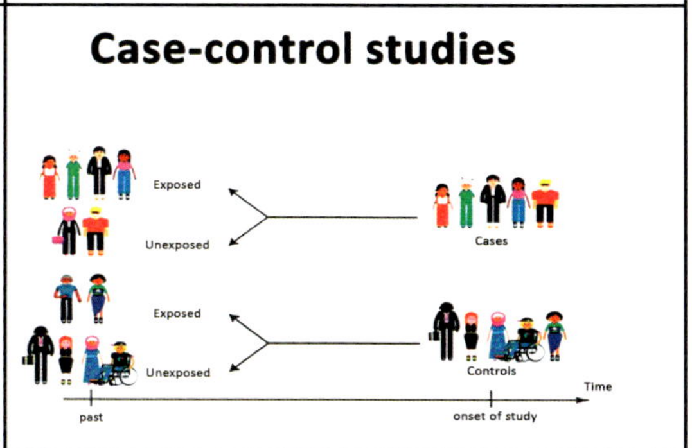
</td></tr>
<tr><td>Cross-Sectional Studies</td><td>Cross-sectional studies are observational studies that analyze data from a population at a single point in time. They are often used to measure the prevalence of health outcomes, understand determinants of health, and describe features of a population.</td><td>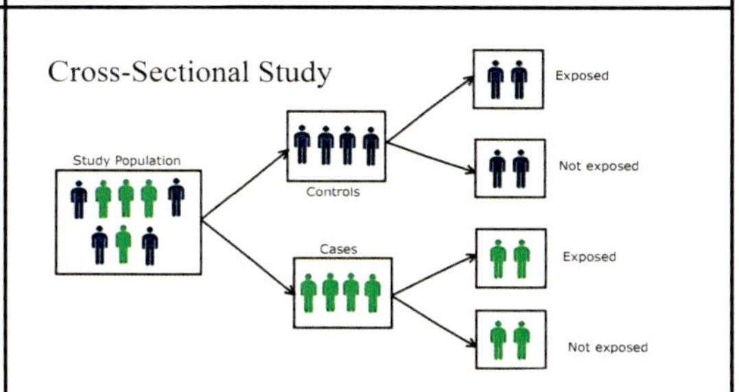
</td></tr>
<tr><td>Randomized Controlled Trials (RCTs)</td><td>Randomized controlled trials (RCTs) are the best way to study the safety and efficacy of new treatments. RCTs are used to answer patient-related questions and are required by governmental regulatory bodies as the basis for approval decisions.</td><td>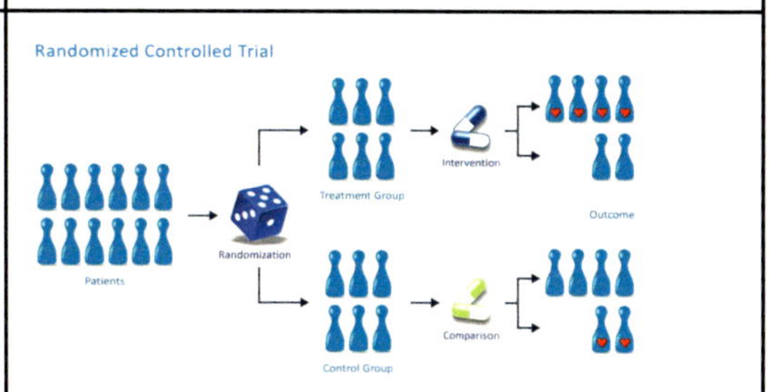
</td></tr>
<tr><td>Respiratory Health</td><td>The respiratory community generally defines respiratory health as the absence of overt lung disease.</td><td>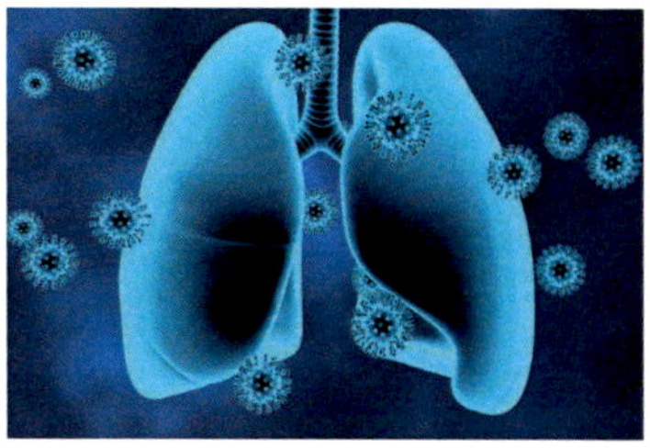</td></tr>
</table>

3.1. Ecologic Studies

Ecologic studies, also known as aggregate studies or population studies, focus on analyzing data at the level of groups or populations rather than individuals. These studies examine the relationship between exposure variables (e.g., environmental factors, socioeconomic indicators, public health policies) and health outcomes (e.g., disease incidence, mortality rates) across different geographical regions or time periods.

In ecologic studies, exposure and outcome data are collected and analyzed at the same level of aggregation, such as communities, counties, states, or countries. Researchers typically use existing databases, registries, surveys, or vital statistics to obtain population-level data on both exposures and outcomes. Statistical methods are then employed to explore associations, often using correlation or regression analyzes to assess the strength and direction of relationships between variables.

3.1.1. Types of Ecologic Study Designs

There are three main types of ecologic study designs: cross-sectional ecologic studies, time-trend ecologic studies, and solely descriptive ecologic studies.

- Cross-sectional ecologic studies compare aggregate exposures and outcomes over the same time period. An example of this study design is an investigation comparing bladder cancer mortality rates in cities with surface drinking water sources that contain chlorine by-products compared to rates in cities with ground drinking water sources that contain little or no chlorine by-products.
- Time-trend ecologic studies compare variations in aggregate exposures and outcomes over time within the same community. A study investigating whether hospital admissions for cardiac disease in Los Angeles increase on days when carbon monoxide levels are higher would be an example of this type of study.
- Solely descriptive ecologic studies investigate disease or risk factor differences between communities at the same time, or within the same community over time.

3.1.2. Limitations of Ecologic Studies

Ecologic studies are subject to numerous biases and limitations. Most notably, these study designs are subject to the ecologic fallacy, which occurs by inferring that associations at the aggregate level are true at the individual level. Ecologic studies are also more often subject to confounding bias than are individual risk studies. Confounding is a mixing of the effects of other risk factors with the exposure of interest. Confounding bias may occur in an ecologic study if the confounding factor is correlated with the background rate of disease (the disease rate among unexposed persons in each study community). Cross-level bias occurs when the confounding factor is associated with the background rate of disease differentially across groups. The ecologic fallacy may occur as a result of cross-level bias.

3.1.3. Advantages of Ecologic Studies

1. **Efficiency:** Ecologic studies are often more efficient than individual-level studies since they utilize existing population-level data sources, reducing the need for extensive data collection efforts and resource-intensive follow-up procedures.
2. **Cost-Effectiveness:** By utilizing readily available aggregate data, ecologic studies are generally less expensive to conduct compared to individual-level studies, making them a cost-effective option for investigating broad population trends and associations.
3. **Hypothesis Generation:** Ecologic studies can generate hypotheses and identify potential associations between population-level exposures and health outcomes, providing valuable insights for further investigation through more rigorous study designs.
4. **Examination of Population Trends:** Ecologic studies allow researchers to examine temporal and geographical trends in health outcomes and exposures, providing a broader perspective on public health patterns and disparities across different regions or time periods.
5. **Policy Implications:** Findings from ecologic studies can inform public health policies and interventions by identifying modifiable risk factors at the population level and guiding resource allocation to address specific health concerns in different communities or regions.
6. **Exploration of Ecologic Fallacy:** Ecologic studies provide an opportunity to explore the ecologic fallacy, which occurs when associations observed at the population level do not necessarily reflect individual-level relationships. By comparing ecologic findings with those from individual-level studies, researchers can gain insights into the potential biases and limitations of both approaches.

3.1.4. Disadvantages of Ecologic Studies

1. **Ecologic Fallacy:** One of the primary limitations of ecologic studies is the risk of ecologic fallacy, wherein associations observed at the population level may not accurately represent relationships at the individual level. This discrepancy can occur due to the ecological nature of the data, which does not account for individual-level variability or confounding factors.
2. **Inability to Establish Causality:** Similar to other observational study designs, ecologic studies cannot establish causality due to the absence of randomization and potential confounding variables. Associations observed in ecologic analyzes may be influenced by unmeasured factors or ecological biases, making it challenging to infer causal relationships.
3. **Ecological Bias:** Ecologic studies are susceptible to ecological bias, wherein associations between exposures and outcomes are distorted by group-level factors or artifacts. This bias can arise from aggregation effects, data inaccuracies, or ecological

confounding, leading to erroneous conclusions about the true relationship between variables.

4. **Data Aggregation Issues:** Aggregating data at the population level can obscure individual-level variability and heterogeneity within groups, potentially masking important associations or disparities that exist at smaller geographical or social scales.
5. **Limited Control for Confounding:** Ecologic studies often lack individual-level data on potential confounders, making it challenging to control for factors that may influence both exposure and outcome relationships. This limitation can lead to residual confounding and undermine the validity of ecologic findings.
6. **Ecological Fallacy in Policy Development:** Policy decisions based solely on ecologic study findings may overlook individual-level factors and fail to address the specific needs of vulnerable populations or subgroups within communities. The ecological fallacy can thus impact the effectiveness and equity of public health interventions.

3.1.5. Applications of Ecologic Studies

1. **Environmental Epidemiology:** Ecologic studies are widely used in environmental epidemiology to investigate the relationship between environmental exposures (e.g., air pollution, water quality, climate) and health outcomes (e.g., respiratory diseases, cancer, cardiovascular mortality) at the population level. These studies help identify environmental risk factors and inform regulatory policies to mitigate public health risks.
2. **Social Epidemiology:** Ecologic studies are employed in social epidemiology to explore the impact of social determinants (e.g., socioeconomic status, education, employment) on health outcomes and health disparities within populations. By analyzing population-level data on social indicators and health metrics, researchers can identify socioeconomic gradients in health and advocate for interventions to address underlying social inequalities.
3. **Policy Evaluation:** Ecologic studies play a role in evaluating the effectiveness of public health policies and interventions by examining changes in population-level exposures and health outcomes before and after policy implementation. These studies assess the impact of interventions such as smoking bans, vaccination campaigns, or health promotion initiatives on population health indicators and guide future policy decisions.
4. **Global Health Research:** Ecologic studies contribute to global health research by analyzing cross-national variations in health outcomes, healthcare systems, and population health determinants. These studies compare health indicators across countries or regions to identify patterns, disparities, and potential drivers of population health differences, informing international health policies and interventions.

3.1.6. Examples of Ecologic Studies

1. **Smoking and Lung Cancer Rates:** Early ecologic studies in the mid-20th century explored the association between smoking prevalence and lung cancer mortality rates across different countries or regions. These studies provided evidence of a strong ecological relationship between smoking rates and lung cancer incidence, contributing to the recognition of smoking as a major risk factor for lung cancer and the implementation of tobacco control policies worldwide.
2. **Air Pollution and Respiratory Health:** Ecologic studies have investigated the impact of air pollution on respiratory health outcomes, such as asthma prevalence, hospital admissions for respiratory conditions, and mortality rates from respiratory diseases. By analyzing population-level exposure data from air quality monitoring stations and health outcome registries, these studies have highlighted the detrimental effects of air pollution on respiratory health and informed regulatory efforts to reduce pollution levels.
3. **Income Inequality and Health Disparities:** Ecologic studies have examined the relationship between income inequality and health outcomes at the population level, demonstrating higher rates of morbidity and mortality in areas with greater income disparities. These studies have underscored the importance of addressing socioeconomic inequalities as a determinant of population health and have informed policies aimed at reducing health disparities within communities.
4. **Public Health Interventions and Disease Control:** Ecologic studies have evaluated the impact of public health interventions on disease control and prevention efforts, such as vaccination programs, sanitation improvements, or access to clean water. By analyzing changes in population-level disease incidence or mortality rates following the implementation of interventions, these studies have demonstrated the effectiveness of targeted public health strategies in reducing the burden of infectious diseases and improving population health outcomes.
5. **Climate Change and Health Effects:** Ecologic studies have investigated the health impacts of climate change, including changes in temperature, precipitation patterns, and extreme weather events. These studies have explored associations between climatic factors and health outcomes such as heat-related illnesses, vector-borne diseases, and food insecurity, informing adaptation strategies and public health interventions to mitigate the adverse effects of climate change on human health.

3.2. Cross-Sectional Studies

The first study design discussed in this chapter is the cross-sectional study, also known as a prevalence study, which collects data on exposure and disease at the individual level. First, a sample of subjects (N) is chosen, and the distribution of exposure and disease is then ascertained. It is not necessary for cross-sectional studies to evaluate exposure and disease, though. Certain studies might only be intended to give an estimate of the disease burden within a population, while other studies might only concentrate on how specific exposures are distributed.

One observation period is one of the characteristics of this kind of study design (Figure 3.1). As illustrated in Figure 3.1, exposure and disease histories are gathered concurrently and may involve an evaluation of exposure or disease history. Individuals are the unit of observation and analysis in cross-sectional studies. While secondary data, such as medical and school records, may be added, the majority of the data are initially gathered, mainly for the study's objectives. Information gathered from nationwide surveys conducted by the U. S. government are regularly employed.

Cross-sectional studies are usually descriptive in nature. They are primarily useful for producing quantitative estimates of the size of an issue, but they are not useful for measuring the temporal ordering of cause and effect. There are two main ways to quantify the scope of a public health issue: Gather information on every individual in the population (i.e., a census, which is widely used in prevalence studies) or draw conclusions about the population as a whole from a sample of the population. The second approach is more popular, though, as it allows for more accurate estimations of the scope of a health issue to be obtained much more quickly and at a lower cost by surveying a subset of the population.

- **Sample Designs:** Sampling schemes for cross-sectional studies comprise two main types: probability samples and nonprobability samples. They are defined as follows:

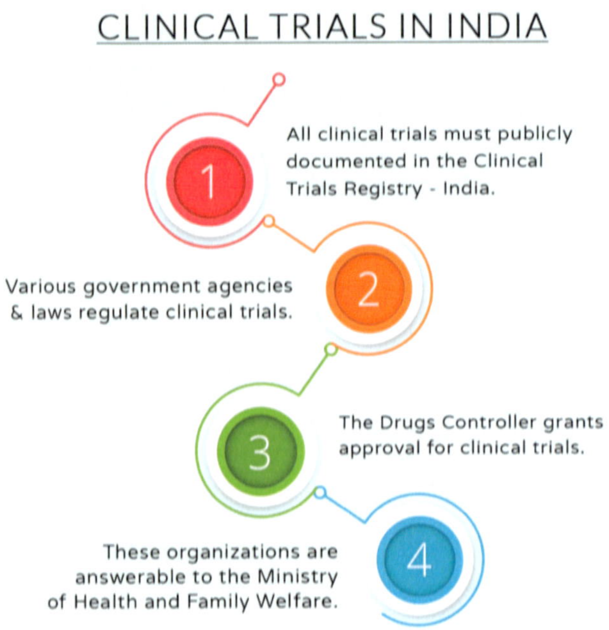

Figure 3.1. *Illustration of subject selection in a cross-sectional study.*

Source: By AbhiSuryawanshi – Own work, CC BY-SA 4.0, https://commons.wikimedia.org/w/index.php?curid=97271820.

A probability sample has the characteristic that every element in the population has a nonzero probability of being included in the sample. A nonprobability sample is one based on a sampling plan that does not have that feature.

Simple random samples, systematic samples, and stratified samples are a few types of probability samples. Simple random samples are those in which there is an equal chance of selection for every member of the population (or other group). Simple random samples necessitate counting every possible subject before sampling, which is a costly procedure that might not be possible to carry out. The process of choosing individuals based on a basic, methodical rule—for example, all those whose names start with a particular alphabetic letter, all those born on specific dates, or all those situated at specific locations on a master list—is known as a systematic sample. The entire number of sampling units need not always be known before creating a systematic sample. "That element or set of elements considered for selection in some stage of sampling" is the definition of a sampling unit. A sampling unit in epidemiologic research is typically a particular subject chosen for the investigation. Of all the sampling procedures, systematic sampling is the most commonly used because it can be done concurrently with the construction of the sampling frame. The actual list of sampling units from which the sample or a portion of the sample is chosen is known as a sampling frame."

Let's say that estimates of the severity of a health issue in a comparatively small portion of the population are sought after. There is no guarantee that this subgroup will be sufficiently represented in simple random samples or systematic samples to allow for the derivation of meaningful estimates. The population must be split into exhaustive and mutually exclusive strata in order to use a stratified sampling approach. Within each stratum, sampling is done (strata are defined as "distinct subgroups according to some important characteristic, such as age or socioeconomic status.").

Samples that are not probability-based comprise judgmental and quota samples. When interviewers are required to gather data from a predetermined number of subjects who possess specific attributes, regardless of their distribution within the population, this is an example of a quota sample design. When choosing subjects for a judgmental sample, the investigator bases their decision on their belief that the individuals included in the sample will accurately reflect the population at large. Cross-sectional studies should not employ nonrandom samples as they do not allow for the evaluation of the reliability of the estimates derived from them.

3.2.1. Examples of Cross-Sectional Studies

The prevalence of neurodevelopmental disorders, the health needs of minority populations, the extent of smokeless tobacco use, and changes in risk factors for disease are a few subjects covered by cross-sectional studies. Murray along with others. Fifteen ninth graders from four Minneapolis–Saint Paul school districts participated in a survey on smokeless tobacco use. Minnesota metropolitan area of St. Paul.

In the fall of 1985, a questionnaire was given out in the classroom to determine the prevalence of usage and to find usage correlates that might indicate which teenagers were more likely than their peers to use smokeless tobacco. According to the study, only 18% of boys and 24% of girls had used smokeless tobacco in the previous week, despite the fact that 24% of girls and nearly 63% of boys had ever used it. Additionally, the prevalence of usage was linked to ethnicity, particularly in boys. The self-reported prevalence varied by ethnicity: low among Asians and African Americans was 21% and 22%, respectively; medium among whites was 45.5%; and high among Native Americans was 60.8%. Boys from two-parent households had a prevalence of 42.1%; boys from single-parent households had a prevalence of 41.3%; and boys from father-only households had a prevalence of 54.5%. When compared to nonsmokers, smokers of cigarettes used smokeless tobacco far more frequently. Compared to 16% of smoking girls, only 6% of nonsmoking girls reported using smokeless tobacco. The boys' differences were similarly significant, with 34.5% and 56.1% of them being smokers and nonsmokers, respectively. Further examinations demonstrated a clustering of harmful conduct among teenagers who smoked, drank alcohol, and used marijuana. Compared to non-consumers, their rate of smokeless tobacco use was over seven times higher, at 50.8% versus 60.9%, respectively.

The example that came before it was based on a survey that was conducted among students in one large city. It is also possible to conduct prevalence studies using a far larger sample frame. For instance, data on the prevalence of sterilization has mostly come from surveys of women, despite the fact that surgical sterilization has many advantages over other methods of contraception.

Therefore, in order to determine the factors linked to sterilization and estimate the prevalence of vasectomy, a nationally representative survey of male U. S. residents between the ages of 15 and 44 in 2002. According to the survey, 13% of married men said they had undergone a vasectomy, and 13% said their partners had undergone tubal sterilization. Vasectomy rates rose with age, number of biological children, non-Hispanic white ethnicity, and family planning clinic visits in the past. Women who had previously given birth naturally were more likely to use tubal sterilization; many of these women's male partners were older and had not gone to college. As a result, one in eight married men said they had had vasectomies; men who relied on vasectomies differed slightly from men whose partners had tubal ligations.

A spectrum of complex neurodevelopmental disorders known as autism spectrum disorder (ASD) is typified by limited repetitive behavior patterns and mild to severe difficulties with social interaction and communication. The symptoms of ASD start before the age of three and persist into adulthood, though they may gradually get better. The American Academy of Pediatrics advises early behavioral intervention once a child is diagnosed with ASD, even though there isn't a single best course of action. The majority of kids (94%) who have ASD need additional health or related services on top of what kids typically need.

A nationally representative survey on children with special healthcare needs (NSCSHCN) aged 6–17 years who have ever been diagnosed with autism spectrum disorder (ASD), intellectual disability, or developmental delay is called the Survey of Pathways to Diagnosis and Services.

Parents or guardians who indicated that their child had ever been diagnosed with at least one of the three chosen developmental conditions and who had previously taken part in the 2009–2010 National Survey–CSHCN (supported by the Maternal and Child Health Bureau) were contacted again by phone or landline to take part in the Pathways survey. The CSHCN had to be between the ages of 6 and 17 at the time of the Pathways interview and still residing in the same home as the parent or guardian who had been contacted again in order to be eligible. 71% of the parents or guardians with qualifying CSHCN were able to get in touch with them again, and 87% of them consented to take part. From February to May 2011, 4,032 interviews were conducted, with an average of 9 months elapsed since the first interview.

According to the survey, school-aged children with autism spectrum disorder (ASD) and special healthcare needs (CSHCN) were first diagnosed at a median age of five years. Children under the age of five were more frequently identified by generalists and psychologists, whereas children five years of age and older were more frequently identified by psychologists and psychiatrists. Nine out of ten school-aged CSHCN with ASD use one or more services to meet their developmental needs; nearly three-fifths of these children use speech or language therapy and social skills training. Lastly, a majority of CSHCN with ASD who are school-age use psychotropic medication (Figure 3.2).

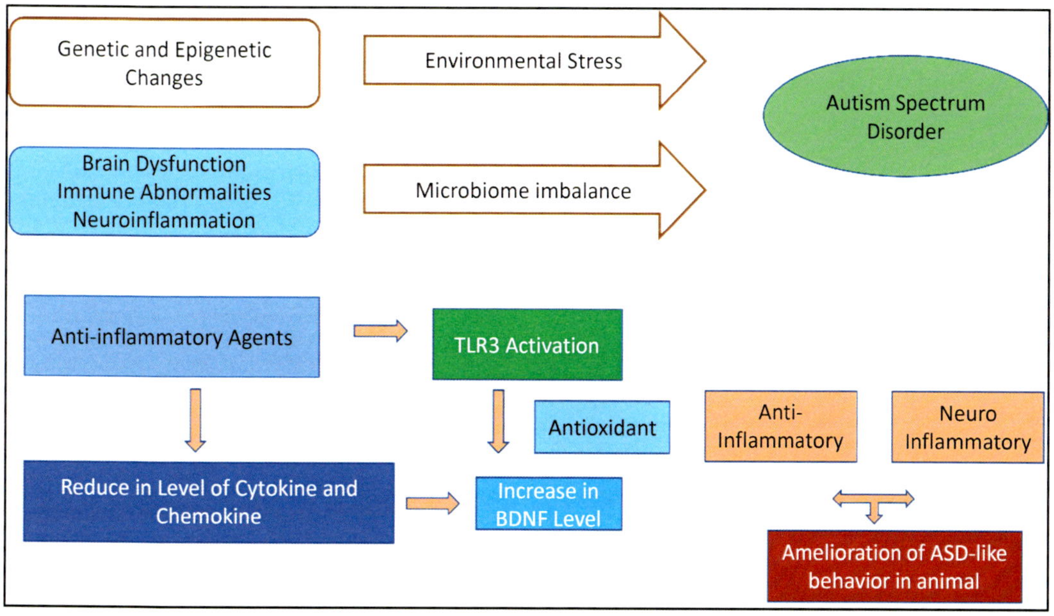

Figure 3.2. *Autism spectrum disorderhealthcare.*

Source: Singh R, Kisku A, Kungumaraj H, Nagaraj V, Pal A, Kumar S, Sulakhiya K. Autism spectrum disorders: A recent update on targeting inflammatory pathways with natural anti-inflammatory agents. Biomedicines. 2023; 11(1):115. https://doi.org/10.3390/biomedicines11010115healthcare.

Finding the resources needed for health interventions can be aided by prevalence surveys. For instance, Friis et al. carried out a cross-sectional prevalence survey in Long Beach, California, to find out how many Cambodian Americans smoke cigarettes. 1,414 adult respondents were chosen at random from a stratified random sample drawn from 15 census tracts with significant populations of Cambodian Americans. There was a sex-specific smoking prevalence of 54% among women and 24.4% among men. The factors of gender, age, education, marital status, and health were significant covariates of current smoking. Compared to other males in California, men of Cambodian American descent smoked more frequently. According to the research, culturally appropriate interventions are required to address the high rate of smoking among Americans of Cambodian descent. There appears to be a correlation between the high prevalence of smoking in Cambodia and a number of cultural aspects, including the high regard for religion, elders, and peers.

3.2.2. Advantages of Cross-Sectional Studies

1. **Efficiency:** Cross-sectional studies are efficient in terms of time and resources since they provide a snapshot of the population's health status at a single time point, eliminating the need for long-term follow-up or data collection procedures.
2. **Cost-Effectiveness:** Compared to longitudinal studies, which require continuous follow-up of participants over time, cross-sectional studies are generally less expensive to conduct, making them a cost-effective option for investigating prevalence and associations in large populations.
3. **Hypothesis Generation:** Cross-sectional studies can generate hypotheses about potential associations between exposure variables and health outcomes by examining prevalence patterns within the population. These hypotheses can guide further research using longitudinal or experimental study designs to establish causal relationships.
4. **Population Surveillance:** Cross-sectional studies serve as valuable tools for population surveillance by monitoring trends in health-related variables over time and identifying emerging public health issues or disparities within communities. Surveillance data from cross-sectional studies inform public health policies and interventions aimed at improving population health outcomes.
5. **Comparative Analysis:** Cross-sectional studies allow for comparative analysis of health-related variables across different population subgroups (e.g., age groups, gender, socioeconomic status), enabling researchers to identify disparities, risk factors, and health inequities within the population.
6. **Prevalence Estimation:** Cross-sectional studies provide estimates of disease prevalence and the prevalence of risk factors or protective factors within the population, which are essential for planning and prioritizing public health interventions and resource allocation.

3.2.3. Disadvantages of Cross-Sectional Studies

1. **Inability to Establish Temporality:** One of the primary limitations of cross-sectional studies is their inability to establish temporal relationships or causality between exposure variables and health outcomes. Since data are collected at a single time point, it is challenging to determine whether the exposure preceded the outcome or vice versa.
2. **Susceptibility to Prevalence-Incidence Bias:** Cross-sectional studies may be susceptible to prevalence-incidence bias, wherein prevalent cases with longer disease duration are overrepresented compared to incident cases, leading to biased estimates of disease prevalence and associations with exposure variables.
3. **Selection Bias:** Selection bias may occur in cross-sectional studies if the sample is not representative of the target population, leading to biased prevalence estimates and

associations. Non-response bias, self-selection bias, and sampling methods can contribute to selection bias and undermine the validity of study findings.

4. **Recall Bias:** Cross-sectional studies rely on self-reported data from participants, which may be subject to recall bias or social desirability bias. Participants may inaccurately recall past exposures or health-related behaviors, leading to misclassification and biased estimates of associations with health outcomes.
5. **Confounding:** Confounding variables, which are factors associated with both the exposure and the outcome of interest, can distort the observed associations in cross-sectional studies. Without controlling for potential confounders, researchers may overestimate or underestimate the true relationship between exposure variables and health outcomes.
6. **Limited Generalizability:** Cross-sectional studies may have limited generalizability to the broader population if the sample is not representative or if certain population subgroups are underrepresented. Generalizability issues can arise from sampling methods, non-response bias, or exclusion criteria, affecting the external validity of study findings.

3.3. Case-Control Studies

To ascertain whether there is a connection between an exposure and a particular health outcome, case-control studies are utilized. These research start with the effect (e.g., health result, state, or illness) to induce (exposure). By evaluating whether exposure is disproportionally distributed between the cases and controls, case-control studies can determine whether an exposure is associated with a higher risk of the health outcome they are studying. Researching uncommon health outcomes or diseases usually involves the use of case control studies.

3.3.1. Design of a Case-Control Study

Figure 3.3 illustrates how a case-control study is designed. In order to investigate the potential relationship between exposure to a particular disease and its outcome, we first identify a group of people who have the disease (referred to as cases) and a control group of people who do not have the disease (referred to as controls). We ascertain the fraction of cases that were exposed and the fraction that wasn't.

Additionally, we ascertain which percentage of the controls were exposed and which percentage was not. In the case of the children with cataracts, the children without cataracts would be the controls, and the children with cataracts would be the cases. Then, it would be required to determine whether or not the mother was exposed to rubella while carrying that child for each child.

If the disease (cataracts) is indeed caused by the exposure (rubella), then we expect that the prevalence of exposure history in the cases—children who have cataracts—will be higher than in the controls—children who do not have cataracts. Therefore, if there is a correlation between an exposure and a disease in a case-control study, the prevalence of exposure history should be higher in individuals with the disease (cases) than in individuals without the disease (controls).

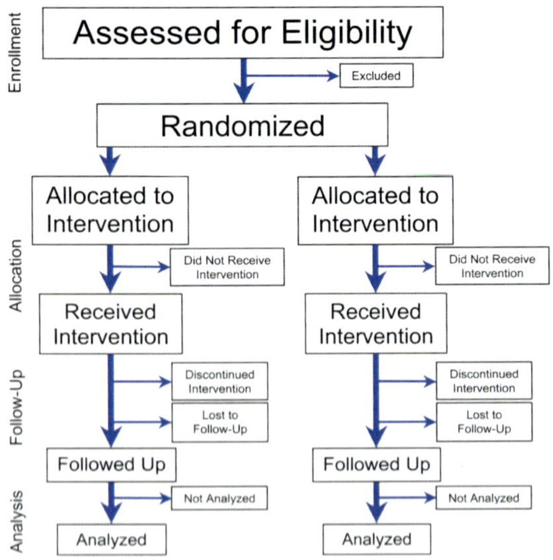

Figure 3.3. *Design of a case-control study.*

Source: By PrevMedFellow – Own work, CC BY-SA 3.0, https://commons.wikimedia.org/w/index.php?curid=9841081.

Let us see how a case-control study is conducted. We begin by selecting cases (with the disease) and controls (without the disease), and then measure past exposure by interview and by review of medical or employee records or of results of chemical or biological assays of blood, urine, or tissues. If exposure is dichotomous, that is, exposure has either occurred (yes) or not occurred (no), breakdown into four groups is possible: There are cases who were exposed and c cases who were not exposed. Similarly, there are b controls who were exposed and d controls who were not exposed. Thus the total number of cases is (a + c) and the total number of controls is (b + d). If exposure is associated with disease, we would expect the proportion of the cases who were exposed, to be greater than the proportion of the controls who were exposed.

Take an example of a case-control study that is hypothetical. We are investigating the potential link between smoking and coronary heart disease (CHD) using a case-control study. We begin by comparing 200 individuals (cases) with congestive heart failure to 400 individuals (controls). In the event that smoking and CHD are related, we would expect that a higher percentage of CHD cases than controls were smokers (exposed). Assume that out of the 200 cases of CHD, 112 smokers and 88 nonsmokers were identified. 176 of the 400 controls smoked, while the remaining 224 did not smoke. Consequently, compared to 44% of the control group, 56% of CHD cases had a smoking history. This computation is merely the initial phase.

Parenthetically, it is of interest to note that if we use only the data from a case-control study, we cannot estimate the prevalence of the disease. In this example, we had 200 cases and 400 controls, but this does not imply that the prevalence is 33%. The decision as to the number of controls to select per case in a case-control study is in the hands of the investigator and does not reflect the prevalence of disease in the population. In this example, the investigator could have selected 200 cases and 200 controls (1 control per case), or 200 cases and 800 controls (4 controls per case). Because the proportion of the entire study population that consists of cases is determined by the ratio of controls per case, and this proportion is determined by the investigator, it clearly does not reflect the true prevalence of the disease in the population in which the study is carried out.

It is important to note that the case-control study's defining characteristic is that it starts with individuals who have the illness (called cases) and contrasts them with individuals who do not (called controls). A cohort study, on the other hand, starts with a group of exposed individuals and compares them to a nonexposed group. There is a misconception among certain individuals that the two types of study designs are different in that case-control studies move backward in time while cohort studies move forward in time. This distinction is untrue; in fact, it is regrettable that case-control studies have been referred to as retrospectives, as the term falsely suggests that calendar time is what sets case-control apart from cohort design. Calendar time, then, is not the feature that sets a case-control study apart from a cohort study. The starting points for the two study designs are either exposed and nonexposed individuals (cohort study) or diseased and nondiseased individuals (case-control study).

The findings of a case-control investigation on the association between bladder cancer and artificial sweeteners can be taken as another example. There were 5,776 controls in this study who did not have bladder cancer and 3,000 cases with bladder cancer. The most likely reason for the unusually high number of controls is that the investigation was designed to include two controls per case, or 6,000 controls in total, and some of the controls were not used. 2,455 out of 5,776 controls and 1,293 out of the 3,000 cases (43.1%) had used artificial sweeteners. (42.5%). These findings, which had generated a great deal of controversy and had significant policy implications for government regulation, were not confirmed by the researchers in this study, although the proportions are extremely close. One of the earliest studies of cigarette smoking and lung cancer was conducted by Sir Richard Doll (1912–2005) and Sir Austin Bradford Hill (1897–1991). Doll was an internationally known epidemiologist, and Hill was a well-known statistician and epidemiologist who developed the "Bradford Hill" guidelines for evaluating whether an observed association is causal. Both men were knighted for their scientific work in epidemiology and biostatistics.

Data from their study of 1,357 males with lung cancer and 1,357 controls based on daily average number of cigarettes smoked in the ten years prior to the current illness can be considered next. A strong correlation between smoking and lung cancer is suggested by the observation that there are fewer heavy smokers among the controls and relatively few nonsmokers among the lung cancer cases.

Table 3.1. Increase in Lung Cancer Incidence Rate Per 100,000 for the Increase of One Cigarette Per Person Per Day

	Men	Women
Canada	3.85	1.96
Norway	3.66	5.40
Sweden	2.42	3.03
	3.31 ± 0.78	3.46 ± 1.76

Source: Chen J. A Comparative analysis of lung cancer incidence and tobacco consumption in Canada, Norway and Sweden: A population-based study. International Journal of Environmental Research and Public Health. 2023; 20(20):6930. https://doi.org/10.3390/ijerph20206930.

Unlike the preceding example, exposure in this study is further stratified according to dose, which is determined by the quantity of cigarettes smoked daily, rather than being simply dichotomized (exposed or not exposed). Given that many of the environmental exposures that we currently worry about are not all-or-nothing situations, it is crucial to explore the possibility of conducting research and analysis that considers exposure dose (Table 3.1).

3.3.2. Potential Biases in Case-Control Studies

3.3.2.1. Selection Bias

- **Sources of Cases:** Patients from a range of sources, such as clinics, hospitals, and doctor's offices, can be chosen as cases for a case-control study. A great source of cases for these types of studies is the patient registries that are kept up to date by many communities for specific diseases, like cancer.

The selection of cases for a case-control study involves taking into account a number of issues. The results may not apply to all patients with the disease if cases are chosen from a single hospital because any risk factors that are found there may be specific to that hospital due to referral patterns or other factors. As such, it is preferable to choose hospitalized cases from multiple local hospitals if they are to be used. Moreover, any risk factors found in the study might only apply to patients with severe forms of the disease if the hospital from which the cases are drawn is a tertiary care facility that admits patients only after they are very sick. Eligibility requirements for case-control studies must, in any case, be carefully outlined in writing prior to the start of the study, just like for randomized trials.

- **Making Use of Incident or Common Cases:** Whether to include incident cases of a disease (newly diagnosed cases) or prevalent cases (people who may have had the disease for some time) is a crucial decision to make in case-control studies. The drawback of using incident cases is that we frequently have to wait for new cases to be diagnosed; in contrast, using prevalent cases, which have already received a diagnosis, frequently results in a higher number of cases that can be studied. In case-control studies of disease etiology, incident cases of the disease are typically preferred, despite the practical benefit of using prevalent cases. The rationale is that any risk factors that we might find in a study with a high incidence of the disease may be more closely associated with the disease's ability to survive than with its onset. For instance, if the majority of individuals with the disease pass away soon after diagnosis, these individuals will be underrepresented in a study using common cases, which is more likely to include survivors who have lived longer. This would be a very nonrepresentative set of cases, and any risk factors associated with this nonrepresentative set might only apply to survivors of the disease rather than all patients with the illness in general.

In a case-control study, we will inevitably be leaving out any patients who may have passed away prior to the diagnosis, even if we limit our inclusion to incident cases—that is, patients who have just received their diagnosis. While there isn't a simple answer for this or some other case selection problems, we must keep these things in mind when interpreting the data and drawing study conclusions. At that point, it is crucial to consider any selection biases that might have been brought about by the way the study was carried out and its design.

- **Selection of Controls:** A study was carried out in 1929 by Raymond Pearl, a biostatistics professor at Johns Hopkins University in Baltimore, Maryland, to investigate the theory that tuberculosis offered cancer prevention. At Johns Hopkins Hospital, Pearl identified 816 cases of cancer from 7,500 consecutive autopsies. Then, he chose a control group of 816 people from the other patients who had autopsies performed at Johns Hopkins, and he calculated the percentages of the cases and controls who had tuberculosis discovered during autopsy. In the 816 autopsies of cancer patients, 133 had tuberculosis (16.3%), compared to 54 (6.6%) in the 816 controls who did not have cancer. Based on the observation that the control group had a significantly higher prevalence of tuberculosis (no cancer findings) than the case group (diagnosed with cancer), Pearl deduced that tuberculosis had a protective or antagonistic effect on cancer.

The suitability of Pearl's control group will determine whether or not his conclusion was warranted. His conclusion would be sound if tuberculosis prevalence among non-cancer patients was comparable to that of all individuals without cancer. However, it wasn't the case. One of the main causes of hospitalization at Johns Hopkins Hospital at the time of the study was tuberculosis. Thus, Pearl had unintentionally selected a group in which many of the patients had received a tuberculosis diagnosis and had been admitted to the hospital when she chose the cancer-free control group. Because of how he chose the controls, the group's tuberculosis rate was heavily skewed toward tuberculosis patients, which did not accurately reflect the general population. Pearl had assumed that the rate of tuberculosis in the control group would be representative of the level of tuberculosis expected in the general population. He was effectively contrasting the incidence of tuberculosis in a cohort of cancer patients with that of a cohort of patients, many of whom had already received a tuberculosis diagnosis. It is obvious that these facts did not support his conclusion.

How might Pearl have solved this issue in his study? Perhaps he could have compared his cancer patients to a group of patients admitted for a particular diagnosis other than cancer (and not tuberculosis) rather than comparing his cancer patients with a group chosen from all other autopsied patients. In actuality, Carlson and Bell replicated Pearl's research, but they contrasted the Johns Hopkins cancer patients' deaths with those from heart disease. There was no discernible variation in the incidence of tuberculosis between the two groups at autopsy. Pearl's study had methodological limitations, but it's interesting to note that the tuberculosis vaccine, bacille Calmette-Guérin, or BCG, is still used today as an immunotherapy for a number of cancer types.).

Pearl's study presents an example of the difficulty in choosing suitable controls for case-control research. One of the trickiest epidemiological puzzles is this one. The problem is that, in a case-control study, we would like to be able to draw the conclusion that the disease under investigation and exposure are related if we find that the cases had greater exposure than the controls did. Whether or not such a conclusion is valid is largely dependent on how the controls are chosen (Table 3.2).

Table 3.2. Key Unanswered Questions Regarding Mycobacterium Tuberculosis Transmission

Unanswered Questions	**Insight from SARS-CoV-2 Research**
Are asymptomatic and/or subclinical tuberculosis cases infectious? Furthermore, if so, how infectious are they compared to those with clinically apparent disease and what is the combined contribution to epidemic spread?	Yes; people with asymptomatic SARS-CoV-2 infection shown to be infectious, albeit less infectious than symptomatic cases. However, symptomatic cases contribute a large proportion of population-level transmission

Are there strain related variability in transmission?	Yes; major differences demonstrated in different Variants of Concern (VoCs)
Is there a transmission fitness cost to tuberculosis drug-resistance?	No; little research on drug-resistance, less relevant. Some level of 'vaccine escape' associated with VoCs
In which community locations does transmission most commonly occur?	Yes; the vast majority of transmission shown to occur in crowded indoor settings with poor ventilation, including households, pubs and clubs, public transportation (e.g., buses and trains), hospitals, and elderly care settings.
What are the key variables associated with transmission heterogeneity, to close contacts and at population-level?	Yes; wide transmission heterogeneity was demonstrated, with consideration that asymptomatic spread makes a major contribution to population-level spread.
How frequently does superspreading occur and what factors are associated with superspreading?	Yes, a variety of factors have been described-mainly related to the infectiousness of the source case, their participation in large congregate settings and general mobility within the population.
To what extent do potential institutional amplifiers (e.g., prisons, mines, hospitals, churches, schools, etc.) contribute to community-wide tuberculosis transmission?	Not well characterized, but less relevant with extensive population spread.

Source: Coleman M, Martinez L, Theron G, Wood R, Marais B. Mycobacterium tuberculosis transmission in high-incidence settings—New paradigms and insights. Pathogens. 2022; 11(11):1228. https://doi.org/10.3390/pathogens11111228.

One of the basic conceptual questions in selecting controls is whether the controls should be representative of all individuals in the population from which the cases are selected or should they be identical to the cases in every other way except for having the disease in question. Although there has been a lot of discussion around this issue, the truth is that because the reference population may not be well defined, it is frequently unknown what traits the non-ill individuals in the population are from when the cases are chosen.

Take a case-control study with hospitalized cases as an example. In order to sample this reference population and choose controls, we need to determine which reference population is the source of the cases. Regretfully, identifying such a reference population for hospitalized patients is typically difficult or impossible. Patients admitted to a hospital may reside in the same city or in a nearby neighborhood, or they may travel from another city or nation via a referral process. It is nearly impossible to identify a precise reference population in these conditions from which the cases originated and from which we could choose controls. Sources of Controls. Controls may be selected from nonhospitalized persons living in the community or from hospitalized patients admitted for diseases other than that for which the cases were admitted.

Utilizing Non-Hospitalized Individuals as References. Nonhospitalized controls can be chosen from a variety of community resources. It would be ideal to choose a probability sample of the entire population, but in practice, this is rarely achievable. School rosters, insurance company lists, and selective service lists are additional sources. An additional choice would be to designate a resident of a specific area, like the case's neighborhood, as the control for every instance. Neighborhood controls like these have been in place for a long time. Using this method, interviewers are told to find the case's residence as a starting point, then proceed to walk past a predetermined number of homes in a predetermined direction in search of the first home that has an eligible control. However, many people are refusing to open their doors to interviewers due to growing security issues in American cities. Nevertheless, the door-to-door method of obtaining controls might be the best option in many other nations, especially developing nations.

Random-digit dialing is an alternative method for selecting neighborhood controls because door-to-door approaches to obtaining controls are often difficult in American cities. The seven-digit phone number of a case, of which the first three are the exchange, can be used to choose a control phone number, in which the terminal four digits of the phone number are chosen at random and the same three-digit exchange is used. This is because telephone exchanges typically correspond to neighborhood boundaries. This strategy is unworkable in many developing nations since only government buildings and commercial establishments are likely to have telephones. Using a best friend control is an additional method of control selection. By asking the name of a best friend who is also participating in the study, a person who has been chosen as a case may be more inclined to participate in the research. However, there are drawbacks to this approach to control selection as well. A best friend control acquired in this way could resemble the case in terms of age as well as numerous other demographic and social traits. The controls may be overly similar to the cases in terms of numerous variables, including the variables under investigation in the study, which could lead to issues. On occasion, though, it might be advantageous to designate a spouse or sibling as the control; a sibling could offer some influence over genetic variations between cases and controls. Use of Hospitalized Patients as Controls. Because hospital inpatients are frequently chosen as controls due to their status as a "captive population" and ease of identification, using them in a study should be comparatively more cost-effective. But as was just mentioned, they are merely a sample of a poorly defined reference population that is typically uncharacterizable. In addition, patients in hospitals are not the same as community members. For instance, it is well known that hospitalized patients smoke more frequently than community members do, and many diagnoses that lead to hospital admissions are related to smoking.

It is conceptually appealing to compare hospitalized cases to hospitalized controls from the same institution, who presumably would tend to come from the same reference population, given that we typically cannot characterize the reference population from which hospitalized cases originate; in other words, any referral system selection criteria that influenced a case's admission to a specific hospital would also apply to the controls. Such an assumption, however, might be dubious because referral patterns for different clinical services at the same hospital might vary (Figure 3.4).

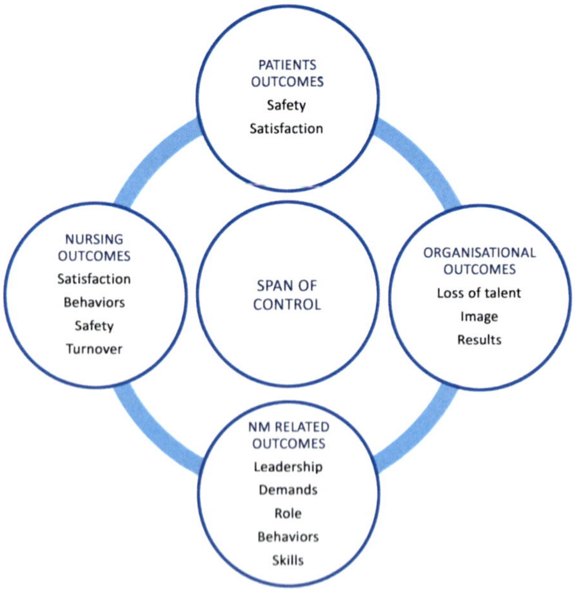

Figure 3.4. *Since both the cases and the hospital controls are selected from the defined population, any factors that affected the admission of cases to a certain hospital would also affect the admission of hospital controls.*

Source: Boned-Galán A, López-Ibort N, Gascón-Catalán A. Nurse manager span of control in hospital settings: an integrative review. Nursing Reports. 2023; 13(4):1577–1592. https://doi.org/10.3390/nursrep13040131.

The question of whether to choose a specific "other diagnosis" or to use a sample of all other hospitalized patients (apart from those with the case's diagnosis) emerges when using hospital controls. The problem is that although it is attractive to choose as hospitalized controls a disease group that is obviously unrelated to the putative causative factor under investigation, such controls are unlikely to be representative of the general reference population. Therefore, if we wish to choose specific diagnostic groups, on what basis do we select those groups, and on what basis do we exclude others? It won't be evident as a result who is different from the general population—the controls or the cases.

It is crucial to determine which diagnostic groups would be excluded from consideration for use as controls and which would be eligible. Consider the following scenario: we choose patients who have been hospitalized with lung cancer as cases and patients who have been hospitalized with emphyzema as controls for our case-control study on lung cancer and smoking. Given that smoking and emphyzema are strongly associated, what issue might this present? Our controls, the emphyzema patients, would include a large proportion of smokers. As a result, any link between smoking and lung cancer would be difficult to find in this study because we would have chosen a control group of people who smoke at a higher rate than would be predicted. Those with additional smoking-related diagnoses, such as emphyzema, bladder cancer, pancreatic cancer, or coronary heart disease, may therefore want to be excluded from our control group. These exclusions complicate the exclusion process and may result in a control group with a lower-than-expected smoking prevalence. An alternative approach would be to examine the study data independently for each of the diagnostic subgroups that make up the control group rather than eliminating any groups from selection as controls during the study's design.

MacÂ Mahon and coworkers published a case-control study on pancreatic cancer in 1981. Patients in 11 hospitals in Boston and Rhode Island between 1974 and 1979 who had a pancreatic cancer diagnosis verified by histopathology were considered cases. In addition to being chosen from among all patients admitted concurrently with the cases, controls were also chosen from among other inpatients admitted by the attending physicians who had admitted the cases. This study revealed a possible dose-response association between coffee consumption and pancreatic cancer, especially in women.

When this kind of correlation is seen, it can be challenging to determine whether coffee consumption or something closely associated with it is the cause of the illness. Acknowledging this issue, the authors stratified the data after analyzing for smoking history. Given that smoking is a known risk factor for pancreatic cancer and that coffee drinking is closely related to cigarette smoking (it is rare to find a smoker who does not drink coffee), did MacMahon and others observe an association between coffee drinking and pancreatic cancer because the coffee caused cancer, or because coffee drinking is related to cigarette smoking and cigarette smoking is known to be a risk factor for pancreatic cancer? Both current smokers and non-smokers showed the same association with coffee consumption.

The scientific and general public, especially coffee producers, were very interested in this report. As coffee is consumed by humans on a daily basis, if the link between the two were real, it would have a significant impact on public health.

Let's look at this study's design. The cases involved white patients from eleven hospitals in Boston and Rhode Island who had pancreatic cancer. The controls are especially interesting because they were patients treated by the same doctors who had admitted the cases but for different illnesses. In other words, after a case was identified, the attending physician was asked if a control patient could be interviewed who was also hospitalized at the same time but for a different ailment. This novel approach to control selection had a useful benefit: Getting hospital controls to participate in case-control studies is difficult because the attending physician must grant permission to contact the patient. Because the patients do not have the disease that is the subject of the study, the doctors are frequently not motivated to have them serve as controls. It was more likely that patients with other diseases would be allowed to participate as controls if doctors who had previously approved patients with pancreatic cancer to participate were asked to do so.

Was there anything wrong with that pragmatic choice? The main query the researchers aimed to address was whether patients with pancreatic cancer consumed more coffee than individuals in the same population who did not have pancreatic cancer (Table 3.3 below). The amount of coffee consumed in cases was higher than the level in controls, according to research by MacMahon and coworkers. In order to prove that cases show excessive coffee consumption, the investigators would like to be able to show that the level of coffee consumption seen in the controls is what would be expected in the general population without pancreatic cancer. Gastroenterologists are frequently the doctors who admit patients with pancreatic cancer to the hospital, but the issue is this: Which doctors are most likely to do so? Numerous other hospitalized patients (who functioned as controls) also experienced gastrointestinal issues, including peptic ulcers and esophagitis. Accordingly, it's possible that the individuals who participated in this study as controls cut back on their coffee consumption, either at the advice of a doctor or because they realized it might help them feel better. The controls may have an unusually low rate of coffee consumption, so we cannot assume that their levels are typical of what can be expected in the broader population. As a result, it's possible that the observed variation in coffee consumption between pancreatic cancer cases and controls was caused more by the controls' lower-than-expected coffee consumption.

Table 3.3. Studies, Designs, and Populations of Coffee and Cancer (References in Brackets)

Author, Journal, Year	City or Region, Country, Database Name (When Available), Period (Years)	Study Design, Study Population, Sampling Method	Patient Characteristics in NOD (Mean Age, Obesity, Smoking)	NOD Definition
Gupta et al., Clin Gastroenterol Hepatol, 2006	USA, VA National Patient Care database 1998–2004	Retrospective cohort, veterans, all without previous diagnosis of PDAC or DM were included, 36,631 developed NOD, of which 149 had PDAC	US veterans > 40 years, in NOD cohort 97% male, average age 64 years	1 year
Boursi et al., Gastroenterology, 2017	UK, THIN database 1995–2013	Retrospective cohort, all patients with incident DM were included: 109,385 patients with NOD, of which 390 had PDAC	All < 35 years were excluded	<3 years
Lee et al., Journal of Clinical Gastroenterology 2012	Seoul, Korea, 2003–2009	Retrospective case-control Cases: 151 NOD with PDAC, Controls: 302 NOD, no cancer 1:2 matched, randomly selected	Mean age 61 years (cases) and 56 years (controls) 58% male in cases, 66% in controls	<2 years
Ben et al., European Journal of Cancer 2011	Shanghai, China, Hospital Data 2000–2009	prospective case-control Cases: 1458 PDAC, of which 307 NOD Controls: 1:1 matched for time of admission, age, sex, sociodemographic variables, 1528 of which 88 NOD	Mean age 62 years 67% male	<2 years
Liao et al., Journal of Gastroenterology and Hepatology 2012	Taiwan, National Health Insurance 1998–2007	Retrospective cohort, entire population, nested case-control: Cases: all DM, of which 6911 had NOD, and 19 PDAC Controls: No DM, 1:4 matched for age and sex, randomly selected	Mean age of 55.9 years 54% male, Obesity 2.43%	<2 years
Tseng et al., Pancreas 2013	Taiwan, National Health Insurance 2005–2006	Retrospective cohort, general population, random sample including 29,236 NOD and of those 32 PDAC	48.5% male	Groups 1, 3 or >3 years

Lipworth et al., Diabetes/Metabolism Research and Reviews 2011	Milan, Italy 1983–1992; 1991–2008	Combined data from two prospective case-control studies, hospital population, convenience sample, including 51 PDAC/NOD cases and 39 NOD controls	Median age 55 years (controls), 63 years (cases) 63% resp. 53% male	Subgroup < 2 years
Lu et al., British Journal of Cancer 2015	UK, THIN Database 1996–2010	Two retrospective cohorts from the general population NOD cohort 44,373, of which 175 had PDAC Control-cohort: 188,734 had no diabetes, of which 354 had PDAC	Mean age ~70 years (age groups) 58% male, 35% obesity, 23% current smokers	Groups 1, 2, 5, and >5 years
Müller et al., Pancreatology 2019	Great Britain, Clinical Practice Research Datalink (CPRD) 2004–2013	retrospective case-control Cases: 588 PDAC and NOD Controls: 5486 NOD, 1:10, matched for age, sex, time DM diagnosis, follow up	Mean age ~70 years (age groups), 49.5% male, 28.7% BMI > 30, 18% current smokers	<2 years
Munigala et al., Clinical and Translational Gastroenterology 2015	St Louis, USA, Veterans' Health Administration national medical care data sets 1998–2007	Retrospective cohort, veterans, all without previous diagnosis of PDAC or DM, were included. 73,811 developed NOD, of which 183 had PDAC	Mean age 60.2 years, all < 40 years excluded by design 94% male, 74% white 46.8% obesity, 57% smoking	Groups 1, 2, 3, 4 years
Yuan et al., JAMA Oncology, 2020	USA Nurses' Health Study (NHS), baseline 1978, Health Professionals Follow-Up Study (HPFS), baseline 1988	Two retrospective cohorts, female nurses and male physicians, without previous diagnosis of PDAC or DM. Within the patients with NOD, 67 PDAC cases were observed.	Mean age 69 years White 93.3%, Black 3.5% Obesity 43% Ever-smokers 56%	<4 years
Bosetti et al., Annals of Oncology 2014	International, USA, Canada, Greece, Central Europe, Italy, Australia, 1983–2012	Combined data from 15 case-control studies Cases: PDAC Controls: hospital/ hospital visitors/ population NOD subgroup; including 525 NOD/PDAC cases	Not published for NOD subgroup	Groups < 1 years, 1–2, 2–5, >5
Illés et al., Pancreatology, 2016	Szeged, Hungary 2012–2014	Prospectively recruited, 108 patients with NOD, of which 3 had PDAC	Mean age 58 years 42.6% male, mean BMI 30.5, 29% ever smoker	<3 years

Chari et al., Gastroenterology 2005	Rochester, USA 1950–1994	Cohort of 2122 NOD including 18 PDAC with nested case-control: Cases: NOD with PDAC, 18 cases Controls: NOD, 1:4 matched for age, sex, time of diabetes diagnosis, 72 controls	All < 50 years excluded by design No demographic data on cohort	<3 years
Hart et al., Pancreas 2011	Rochester, USA 1981–2007	Retrospective case-control, 29 Cases: all NOD and PDAC in a 120-mile radius of Rochester 43 Controls: NOD matched for sex and age	Mean age 76 years cases, 72 years controls, 37% male cases, 56% controls	<3 years
Huang et al., Clinical Gastroenterology and Hepatology, 2020	Kaiser Permanente Southern California, USA (KPSC, Insurance) 2006–2016	Retrospective cohorts, all with sufficient data and without previous diagnosis of PDAC, were included. 110,699 NOD, of which 306 with PDAC	All < 45 years were excluded Mean age 59 years, Male 52% Whites (44%), Hispanics (37%), Asians (15%) Blacks (15%).	<3 years
Sharma et al., Gastroenterology 2018	Rochester, USA, Rochester Epidemiology Project (REP) 2000–2015	Retrospectively collected data from 4 independent cohorts, with 64 PDAC/NOD and 192 NOD-Controls in the discovery set, and a cohort of 1096 NOD, including 9 PDAC in the validation set	All < 50 years were excluded Mean age 65.6 years, 50% male	<3 years
Chen et al., Digestive Diseases and Sciences 2021	Kaiser Permanente Southern California, USA (KPSC, Insurance) 2010–2014	Retrospective cohort of all patients without previous diagnosis of PDAC, meeting NOD criteria during the enrollment period, 13,947 NOD including 99 PDAC	All < 50 years were excluded No PDAC: 64.1 years, 48% male, 91 kg, PDAC: 69.2 years, 57% male, 84.4 kg	<3 years
Molina-Montes et al., Gut, 2021	PanGenEU, Europe, 28 centers from Spain, Italy, UK, Ireland, Germany, Sweden 2007–2014	Retrospective case-control, we used only data from the subgroup with NOD, with general population as control. Data on long-standing diabetes was ignored. It included 200 cases of PDAC/NOD	63.4% male, mean age ~65 years (age groups), 30.5% obese	<2 years

Khan, Pancreatology, 2021	TrinetX—Validation of ENDPAC	Retrospective cohort of 15,539 NOD patients, of which 48 had PDAC	<50 years excluded by design PDAC 68 years, 54% male, 81% white, 39% smokers No PDAC, 67 years, 50% male, 76% white, 21% smokers	<3 years
Khan, Pancreas, 2021	TrinetX—validation of Boursi	Retrospective cohort of 27,893 NOD patients, of which 52 had PDAC	<35 years excluded by design PDAC 74 years, No PDAC 64 years	<3 years
Ullah, BMC Cancer, 2021	EL-PaC-Epidem London, UK 2008–2020	Case-Control study, 965 PDAC, 3963 Non-malignant pancreatic disease, 4355 Controls	Mean age 55.1, 51% male, 54.4% white	Groups 1,2,3 years

Source: Mellenthin C, Balaban VD, Dugic A, Cullati S. Risk factors for pancreatic cancer in patients with new-onset diabetes: a systematic review and meta-analysis. Cancers. 2022; 14(19):4684. https://doi.org/10.3390/cancers14194684.

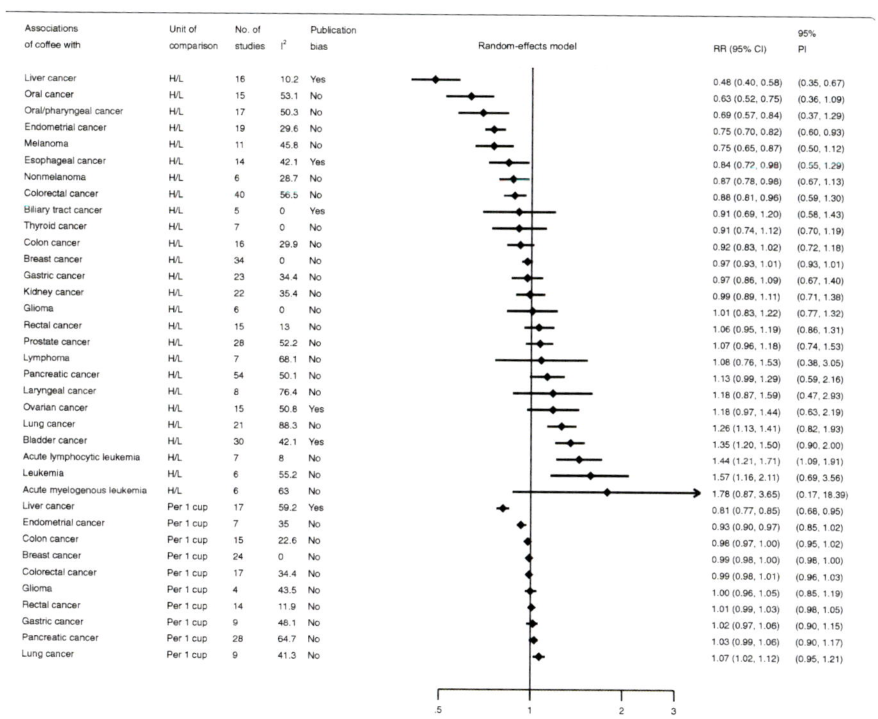

Figure 3.5. *Studies, designs, and populations of coffee and its link to cancer (References in brackets).*

Source: Zhao LG, Li ZY, Feng GS, Ji XW, Tan YT, Li HL, Gunter MJ, Xiang YB. Coffee drinking and cancer risk: an umbrella review of meta-analyses of observational studies. BMC Cancer. 2020 Feb 5;20(1):101.

Later, MacMahon and associates conducted the same analysis again, separating controls suffering from gastrointestinal disorders from controls suffering from other ailments. They discovered that while the risk of coffee consumption was higher when compared to controls with gastrointestinal disorders, the association between coffee consumption and pancreatic cancer remained, albeit to a reduced degree, when compared to controls with other illnesses. A new study that attempted to replicate these results was reported by Hsieh and coworkers a few years later; however, the results did not corroborate the initial findings.

3.3.3. Other Issues in Case-Control Studies

3.3.3.1. Matching

When doing a case-control study, one of the main concerns is that the exposures or characteristics of the cases and controls might not match the exposure that is being studied. The question of whether the observed association could be caused by variations in factors other than the exposure under investigation between the cases and controls may arise if it is discovered that more cases than controls have been exposed. For instance, we would not be able to determine whether exposure to the factor under study or another trait linked to having low income is the factor influencing the development of disease if it were discovered that more cases than controls had been exposed, and if the majority of the cases had low incomes while the majority of the controls had high incomes. So that a difference in exposure will probably constitute the critical difference and the presence or absence of disease is unlikely to be attributable to a difference in socioeconomic status, we would like to make sure that the distribution of the cases and controls by socioeconomic status is similar to prevent such a situation.

Matching the cases and controlling for variables that we might be concerned about, like income, as in the previous example, is one way to address this issue in the design and execution of the study. The process of choosing the controls so that they share certain traits—such as age, race, sex, socioeconomic status, and occupation—with the cases is known as matching. There are two different kinds of matching: (1) group matching and (2) individual matching.

- **Group Matching:** The process of choosing the controls so that the proportion of controls with a given characteristic is the same as the proportion of cases with the same characteristic is known as group matching or frequency matching. As a result, the controls will be chosen so that 25% of them are married if 25% of the cases are married. Usually, this kind of selection necessitates choosing every case first. A control group is chosen in which the same characteristics occur in the same proportions as the cases after calculations of the proportions of specific characteristics in the group of cases are completed.
- **Individual Matching:** Individual matching, also known as matched pairs, is a second kind of matching. According to this method, a control is chosen for every case chosen for the study that is comparable to the case in terms of the particular variable or variables of interest. For instance, we will look for a 45-year-old white female control if the 45-year-old case in our study is a white woman. We will choose a control who is also a 24-year-old black man if the second case involves a 24-year-old black man. With this kind of control selection, every case is matched to a control on

an individual basis, producing matched case-control pairs.

When conducting case-control studies with hospital controls, individual matching is frequently employed. This is due to a more pragmatic than philosophical reason. Assume for the moment that age and sex are significant variables. It is deemed critical that the cases and controls have similar attributes to each other. In most cases, it is not feasible to randomly choose a group of hospital patients based on specific age and sex characteristics. Instead, it is simpler to recognize a case and then select the subsequent hospital admission whose age and sex match the case. Individual matching is therefore most practical when research employs hospital controls.

What are the problems with matching? The problems with matching are of two types: practical and conceptual.

1. **Practical Problems with Matching:** If an attempt is made to match according to too many characteristics, it may prove difficult or impossible to identify an appropriate control. For example, suppose that it is decided to match each case for race, sex, age, marital status, number of children, zip code of residence, and occupation. If the case is a 48-year-old black woman who is married, has four children, lives in zip code 21209, and works in a photo-processing plant, it may prove difficult or impossible to find a control who is similar to the case in all of these characteristics. Therefore, the more variables on which we choose to match, the more difficult it will be to find a suitable control.
2. **Conceptual Problems with Matching:** Perhaps a more important problem is the conceptual one: Once we have matched controls to cases according to a given characteristic, we cannot study that characteristic. For example, suppose we are interested in studying marital status as a risk factor for breast cancer. If we match the cases (breast cancer) and the controls (no breast cancer) for marital status, we can no longer study whether or not marital status is a risk factor for breast cancer. Why not? Because in matching according to marital status, we have artificially established an identical proportion in cases and controls: if 35% of the cases are married, and through matching we create a control group in which 35% are also married, we have artificially ensured that the proportion of married subjects will be identical in both groups. By using matching to impose comparability for a certain factor, we ensure the same prevalence of that factor in the cases and the controls. We will not be able to ask whether cases differ from controls in the prevalence of that factor. We would therefore not want to match the variable of marital status in this study. Indeed, we do not want to match any variable that we may wish to explore in our study.

Recognizing that unintentional matching might happen in case-control studies is also crucial. When neighborhood controls are used, for instance, we are effectively matching not only for cultural and other neighborhood characteristics but also for socioeconomic status. Using best friend controls, we can infer that the case and his or her best friend have a lot of lifestyle traits in common, which results in a match for these traits. For instance, there was worry that if the case used oral contraceptives, it was possible that her best friend would also likely use oral contraceptives if best-friend controls were taken into account in a study of oral contraceptive use and cancer. This would lead to an unintentional matching in the use of oral contraceptives, making it impossible to continue investigating this variable in this study.

Therefore, when conducting a case-control study, we only match on variables that we are certain are risk factors for the disease; we are not interested in examining these variables in this study. Overmatching refers to matching on variables other than these, whether done intentionally or accidentally.

3.3.3.2. Use of Multiple Controls

Such controls may be either (1) controls of the same type, or (2) controls of different types, such as hospital and neighborhood controls, or controls with different diseases.

- **Controls of the Same Type:** To boost the study's power, multiple controls of the same kind—two or three controls for each case, for example—are employed. In practical terms, the power gain is only appreciable up to a ratio of roughly one case to four controls. For many of the relatively uncommon diseases we study, there may be a limit to the number of potential cases available for study. This raises the question, "Why use multiple controls for each case? Why not just increase the number of cases and keep the ratio of controls to cases at 1:1?" Only a specific number of patients with a particular cancer or connective tissue disorder may be seen annually by a clinic. The option of increasing the number of controls per case is frequently selected because increasing the number of cases is not possible without either developing a collaborative multicentered study or extending the study in time to enroll more cases. The only difference between these controls and cases is the proportion of controls to cases (Figure 3.6).

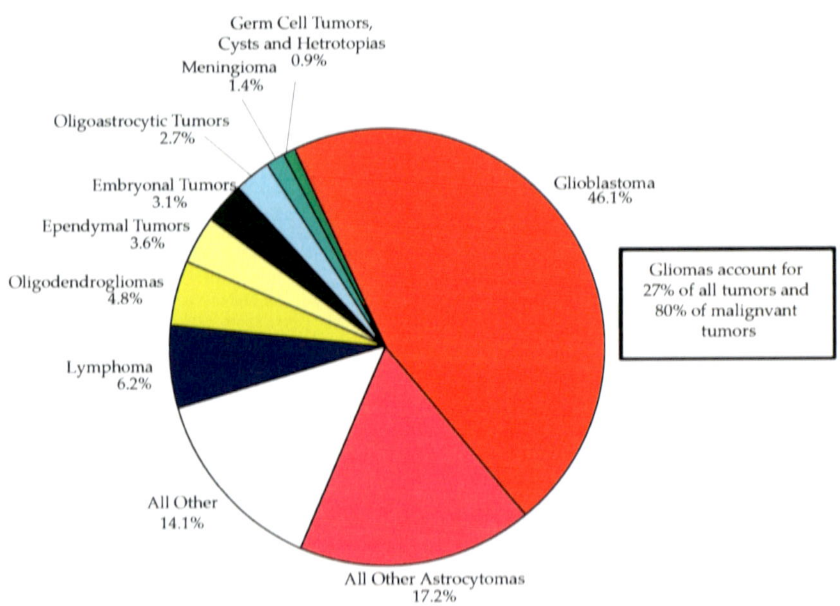

Figure 3.6. *Brain tumors in children.*

Source: Persaud-Sharma D, Burns J, Trangle J, Moulik S. Disparities in brain cancer in the United States: A literature review of gliomas. Medical Sciences. 2017; 5(3):16. https://doi.org/10.3390/medsci5030016.

- **Multiple Controls of Different Types:** On the other hand, we might decide to employ several distinct kinds of controls. For instance, we might be worried that the hospital controls we used in our research might not have had the same exposure experience as what is "expected" in a population of people without illnesses; in other words, the controls might have been a carefully chosen subset of people without illnesses and might not have had the same exposure. Hospitalized patients smoke more than the general population. This raises concerns because we are unsure of the prevalence level of smoking among hospitalized controls or how to interpret differences in smoking rates between them and the cases. We might decide to employ a second control group, like neighborhood controls, to solve this issue. It is anticipated that the outcomes of case comparisons with hospital controls will resemble those of case comparisons with neighborhood controls. If the results are different, it is important to determine why. The investigator should ideally choose which comparison will be the "gold standard of truth" before starting the actual study if they plan to use multiple controls of various kinds.

A case-control study of pediatric brain tumors was published in 1979 by Gold and coworkers. Two groups of controls were employed: children without cancer (referred to as normal controls) and children with cancers other than brain tumors (referred to as cancer controls). Why were these two control groups chosen? Let's ask: "Did mothers of children with brain tumors receive more radiation exposure during pregnancy than control mothers?" (Figure 3.7).

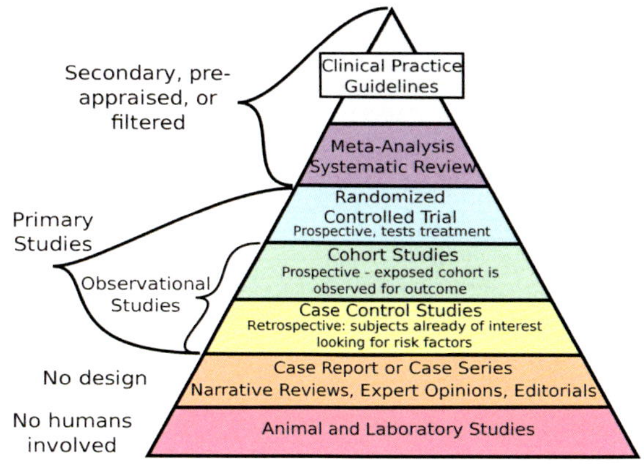

Figure 3.7. *Control groups.*

Source: Rationale for using two c.

What are the possible explanations for the findings that the radiation exposure of mothers of children with brain tumors is higher than that of mothers of normal controls, and that the radiation exposure of mothers of children with other cancers is also higher than that of mothers of normal children? One possibility is that prenatal radiation acts as a non-site-specific carcinogen, which increases the risk of both brain tumors and other cancers. Alternatively, mothers of children with cancer of any kind may have remembered prenatal radiation exposure better than mothers of healthy children, which could account for the findings due to recall bias.

Either results may indicate that prenatal radiation is a particular brain carcinogen if moms of children with brain tumors have a higher history of radiation exposure than do mothers of normal controls and mothers of children with other cancers. Given that it would seem improbable that mothers of children with brain tumors would remember prenatal radiation better than mothers of children with other cancers, these findings would also lessen the possibility that recall bias is at play. Therefore, it can be beneficial to examine alternative hypotheses and account for potential biases like recall bias by using multiple controls of different kinds.

3.3.4. When is a Case-Control Study Warranted?

When attempting to identify the cause of a negative health outcome, a case-control study can be helpful as an initial step. When we first start looking for an explanation, we might suspect one or more exposures, but we might not have any evidence—certainly not any solid evidence—that links any of the potential exposures to the illness in question. We compare individuals with the disease (cases) and those without it (controls) using the case-control design. Next, we can investigate the potential contributions of various exposures or traits to the development of the illness. The proportion of cases who have been exposed should be higher than the proportion of controls who have been exposed if the exposure is linked to the illness. Upon the identification of such a correlation in a case-control study, a cohort study is frequently conducted to provide additional insight into the relationship. Case-control studies are frequently the first step in establishing whether an exposure is linked to an increased risk of disease because they can be conducted more quickly and are generally less expensive than cohort studies (Figure 3.8).

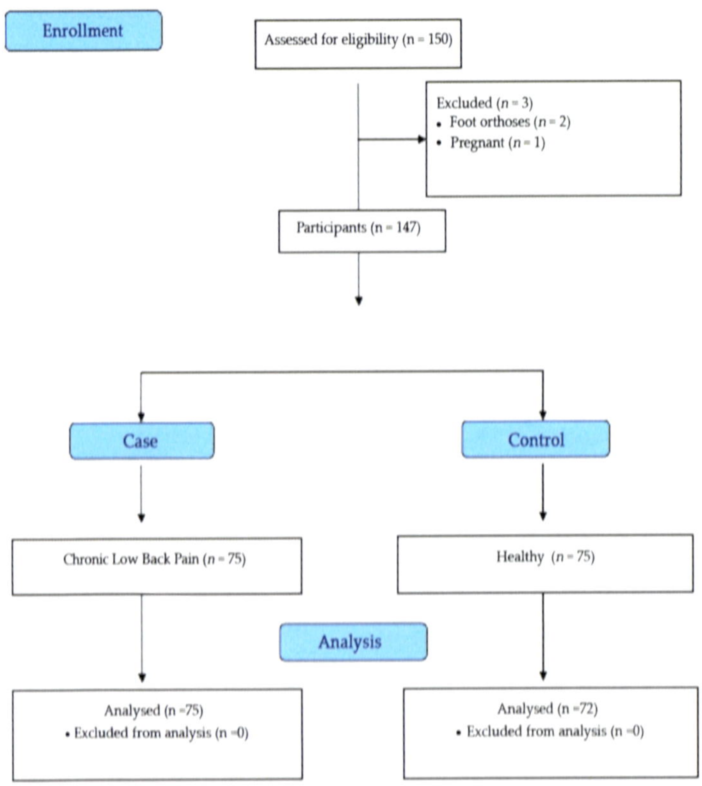

Figure 3.8. *CONSORT flow diagram..*

Source: Castro-Méndez A, Requelo-Rodríguez I, Pabón-Carrasco M, González-Elena ML, Ponce-Blandón JA, Palomo-Toucedo IC. A case–Control study of the effects of chronic low back pain in spatiotemporal gait parameters. Sensors. 2021; 21(15):5247. https://doi.org/10.3390/s21155247

If the disease under investigation is uncommon, case-control studies are especially helpful. From disease registries, hospital records, and other sources, cases can frequently be found for investigation.

On the other hand, in the event that a cohort study is carried out for a rare disease, a substantial study population might be required to ensure that a suitable proportion of the cohort members experience the disease in question. Moreover, a cohort design may require many years of cohort follow-up in addition to significant logistical challenges and costs in order to maintain and follow the cohort throughout the study period, depending on the duration of time between exposure and development of disease.

3.3.5. Case-Control Studies Based in a Defined Cohort

The characteristics of these two categories of research designs have been covered in these talks. Whether it is possible to combine some aspects of the cohort and case-control approaches into a single study in order to benefit from both types of studies' advantages has received a lot of attention in recent years. The resultant combined study starts a case-control study inside a cohort study, creating a hybrid design.

A population is recognized and tracked through time. Baseline data are gathered from documents or interviews, blood or urine tests, and other sources at the time the population is identified. After that, the population is monitored for a number of years. A small proportion of research participants exhibit the disease for the majority of the diseases that are studied, while the majority do not. The next step is to conduct a case-control study, utilizing a sample of people who did not develop the disease as controls and those who developed the disease as cases.

Such cohort-based case-control studies can be divided into two types largely on the basis of the approach used for selecting the controls. These two types of studies are called nested case-control studies and case-cohort studies.

3.3.5.1. Nested Case-Control Studies

A sample of people who are at risk for the disease at the time each case of the disease arises serves as the control in nested case-control studies. While some of them get the aforementioned illness, the majority do not. The cohort in this fictitious example is tracked for a duration of five years. Five cases arise during this period: one after one year, two after two years, two after four years, and one after five years.

At the time each case or cases develop, the same number of controls is selected. The solid arrows on the left side of the figure denote the appearance of cases of the disease, and the dotted arrows on the right side denote the selection of controls who are disease-free but who are at risk of developing the disease in question at the time the case develops the disease. Five years later, there have been five cases, and during that time, five controls have been chosen for the study. In this sense, the calendar time and duration of follow-up for the cases and controls are effectively matched. Since a control is chosen every time a case manifests itself, a control chosen early in the investigation may subsequently contract the illness and turn into a case in the same investigation.

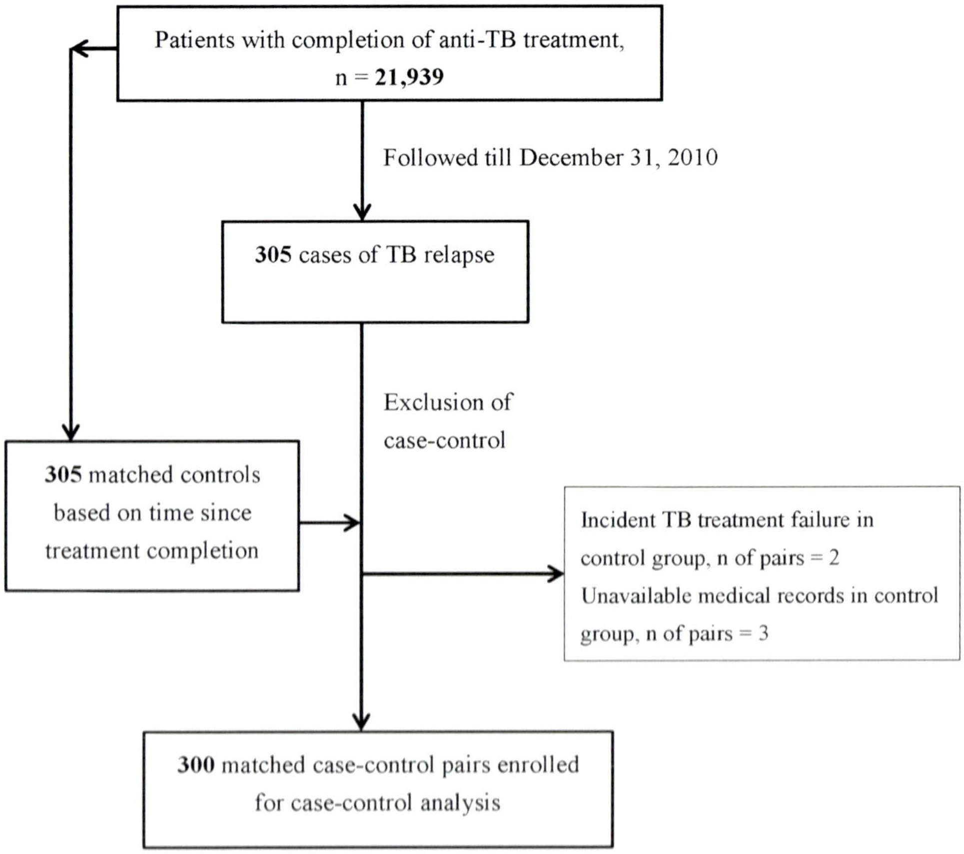

Figure 3.9. *Example of a hypothetical nested case-control study: Steps in selecting cases and controls.*

Source: Lee P-H, Lin H-C, Huang AS-E, Wei S-H, Lai M-S, Lin H-H (2014) Diabetes and risk of tuberculosis relapse: nationwide nested case-control study. PLoS One 9(3): e92623. https://doi.org/10.1371/journal.pone.0092623.

3.3.5.2. Case-Cohort Studies

The case-cohort design shown in Figure 3.10 represents the second kind of cohort-based case-control study. While the controls are selected at random from the defined cohort that the study started, cases in the hypothetical case-cohort study unfold at the same intervals as those observed in the just-discussed nested case-control design. The term "subcohort" refers to this portion of the entire cohort. One benefit of this design is that it allows different diseases (or sets of cases) to be studied in the same case-cohort study using the same cohort for controls, since controls are not matched to each case individually. Unlike the nested case-control design, exposure is characterized for the subcohort in this design, rather than cases and controls being matched on calendar time and follow-up duration. When analyzing the study results, it is important to consider this variation in study design (Figure 3.10).

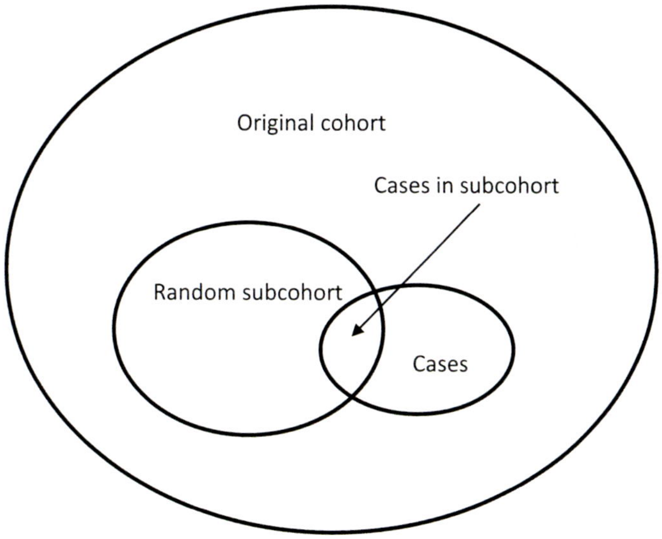

Figure 3.10. *Design of a hypothetical case-cohort study: Steps in selecting cases and controls.*

Source: Sharp SJ, Poulaliou M, Thompson SG, White IR, Wood AM (2014) A review of published analyzes of case-cohort studies and recommendations for future reporting. PLoS ONE 9(6): e101176. https://doi.org/10.1371/journal.pone.0101176.

3.3.6. Advantages and Disadvantages of Case-Control Studies

We will explore the advantages and disadvantages of case-control studies, shedding light on their utility and limitations in epidemiological research.

1. **Advantages:**

   i. **Efficiency:** Case-control studies are particularly efficient for investigating rare diseases or outcomes. By starting with a group of individuals who already have the outcome of interest (cases) and comparing them to a group without the outcome (controls), researchers can efficiently explore potential risk factors without the need to follow a large cohort over an extended period.

   ii. **Cost-Effectiveness:** Compared to cohort studies or randomized controlled trials, case-control studies are generally less resource-intensive and time-consuming. They require smaller sample sizes since only a subset of the population with the outcome is needed. This makes them a cost-effective option, especially when financial or logistical constraints are present.

   iii. **Suitability for Rare Outcomes:** When studying diseases with low prevalence, case-control studies provide a viable option for gathering data. Since cases are selected based on the presence of the outcome, researchers can still obtain sufficient information to analyze potential risk factors, even if the disease is rare in the general population.

   iv. **Temporal Relationship Assessment:** Case-control studies allow researchers to investigate exposures that occurred before the development of the outcome. By collecting information on past exposures from both cases and controls, temporal relationships between exposure and outcome can be inferred, providing valuable insights into potential causal relationships.

v. **Ethical Considerations:** In some cases, it may be unethical or impractical to conduct randomized controlled trials due to the nature of the exposure being studied. Case-control studies offer a way to investigate these exposures without subjecting participants to potentially harmful interventions, making them ethically sound alternatives in certain scenarios.

vi. **Flexibility in Study Design:** Case-control studies can be adapted to suit various research questions and settings. They can incorporate multiple controls per case, matching techniques to control for potential confounders, and stratification analyzes to explore subgroup differences. This flexibility enhances the study's ability to account for various factors influencing the association under investigation.

2. **Disadvantages**

i. **Susceptible to Bias:** One of the primary limitations of case-control studies is their susceptibility to selection bias and recall bias. Selection bias may arise if the selection of cases and controls is not adequately representative of the target population, leading to distorted associations. Similarly, recall bias occurs when cases are more likely to recall past exposures accurately compared to controls, leading to an overestimation or underestimation of the true association.

ii. **Inability to Establish Temporality:** While case-control studies allow researchers to assess temporal relationships between exposure and outcome, they cannot definitively establish causality. Unlike randomized controlled trials, which can demonstrate causality through random allocation of interventions, case-control studies can only infer associations based on observed relationships, leaving room for alternative explanations and confounding variables.

iii. **Limited to Exploring a Single Outcome:** Case-control studies are inherently focused on a specific outcome or disease, limiting their ability to investigate multiple outcomes simultaneously. This narrow focus may overlook potential associations with other health outcomes or fail to capture the broader impact of certain exposures on overall health.

iv. **Dependence on Recall and Documentation:** Since case-control studies rely on participants' self-reported exposure histories, they are vulnerable to inaccuracies stemming from recall errors or incomplete documentation. Participants may have difficulty remembering past exposures accurately, leading to misclassification of exposure status and potentially biased results.

v. **Difficulty in Establishing Prevalence Rates:** Unlike cohort studies, which provide information on both exposure and outcome prevalence rates, case-control studies only provide data on exposure prevalence among cases and controls. This limitation makes it challenging to calculate incidence rates or assess the overall burden of disease in the population accurately.

vi. **Limited Generalizability:** The findings of case-control studies may not always be generalizable to the broader population due to the specific selection criteria used for cases and controls. If the study sample is not representative of the target population, the results may not accurately reflect the true association between exposure and outcome in the larger community.

3.4. Cohort Studies

In epidemiology and medical research, cohort studies are a kind of observational study design that's used to look into the causes and risk factors of various diseases. A cohort study tracks a group of people over time to see how particular outcomes or diseases develop. These people share a common characteristic or experience, such as being exposed to a specific risk factor or having a specific disease.

3.4.1. Sampling and Cohort Formation Options

Cohort studies vary from one another, despite having some characteristics in common, like measuring exposure prior to disease onset and involving at least two periods of observation. The sampling techniques used to define the cohort—exposure-based samples and population-based samples—are one of the distinctions. Because these variations affect the measures of association that we'll learn to compute using the data produced in a later chapter, we take note of them now. These correlation measurements are referred to as effect measures. A quantity that gauges how a factor affects the likelihood or frequency of a health outcome is called an effect measure. The idea here is that, in contrast to some cohorts that are put together based only on exposures, population-based cohort studies allow for the estimation of a greater number of measures of association.

3.4.1.1. Population-Based Cohort Studies

In population-based cohort studies, the cohort includes either an entire population or a representative sample of the population. As illustrated in Figure 3.11 a population-based cohort study starts with N; the total of exposed (A + B) and nonexposed (C + D) subjects is determined as part of the research process. Population-based cohorts have been used in studies of coronary heart disease (CHD). Perhaps the best-known cohort study of CHD was initiated in 1948 in Framingham, Massachusetts. When the study commenced, the town had a population of 28,000; the study design called for a random sample of 6,500 from the targeted age range of 30 to 59 years. This sample, representative of the population, was followed subsequently for changes in risk factors and incidence of disease. Tecumseh, Michigan, a city chosen to investigate the role of environmental and constitutional factors in maintaining health and the causes of illness, provides an example of a cohort based on a whole population. The Tecumseh study, which was started in 1959–1960, successfully enrolled 8,641 participants—88% of the community's inhabitants. Cohort studies might cover more territory than a specific community in some situations. A random sample of 41,837 women in the state between the ages of 55 and 69 in 1986 was included in the Iowa Women's Health Study. It's crucial to keep in mind that none of the cohorts—Iowa, Tecumseh, and Framingham—were chosen due to a specific disease exposure or risk factor. Furthermore, it was anticipated that the cohort's exposure frequency would be typical of the parent population from which it was drawn. Therefore, the percentage of the population exposed in a population-based cohort study can be ascertained either directly (if the entire population is chosen) or indirectly (if a predetermined portion of the population is chosen). Exposures with a population-based cohort are not known until exposure data is gathered during the first observation period. The cohort may be split into two or more exposure categories, for instance, based on information gleaned from the subjects following the administration of questionnaires, the gathering of biological samples, clinical examinations, or physiologic testing. For a basic binary (i.e., exposed against nonexposed), with the nonexposed subjects serve as an internal reference point. To test for antibodies to the human papilloma virus (HPV), for instance, one could take blood samples from a sample of male college students; some would be exposed (test positive for the antibodies), while the others would not be exposed (no detectable antibodies). Exposition can occasionally be mapped onto a continuum and referred to as a continuous variable, a kind of variable with an infinite range of possible values. (The designation of exposed/nonexposed creates a dichotomy that denotes a discrete variable, while blood pressure measurements represent a continuous variable).

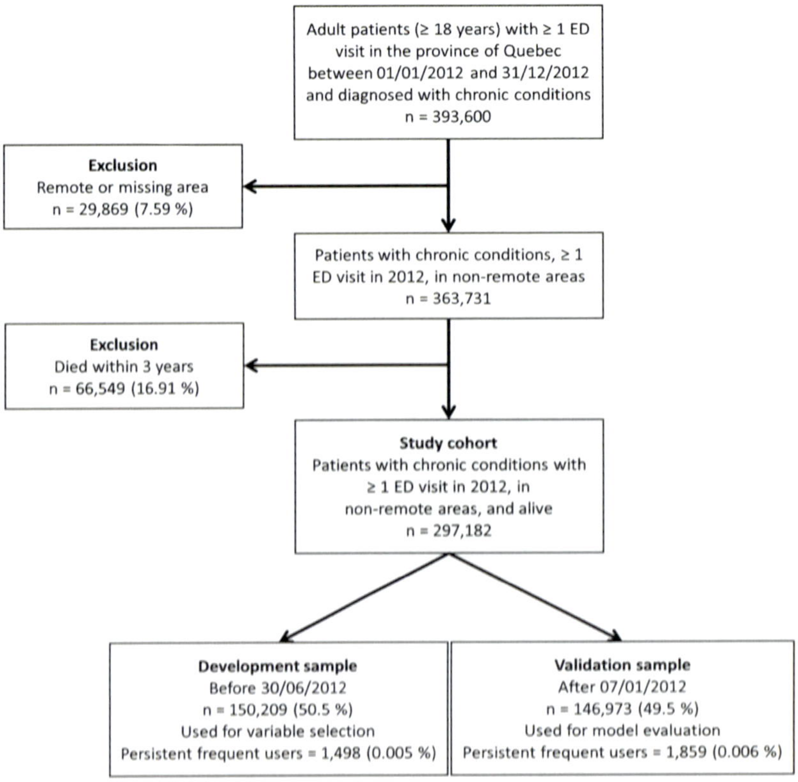

Figure 3.11. *Illustration of sample selection in a cohort study.*

Source: Chiu YM, Vanasse A, Courteau J, Chouinard MC, Dubois MF, Dubuc N, et al. (2020) Persistent frequent emergency department users with chronic conditions: A population-based cohort study. PLoS ONE 15(2): e0229022. https://doi.org/10.1371/journal.pone.0229022.

Usually, one constructs multiple levels of exposure for a continuous variable, like blood pressure or certain dietary intake measures. The exposure variable is divided using a statistical process into quantiles, which are divisions of distribution into equal, ordered subgroups 1 (e.g., both quintiles and quartiles). The exposure levels are then specified using these subdivisions. The comparison (or referent) category is made up of subjects that fall into one of the extreme categories, such as the upper or lower quintile. The anticipated rate of disease occurrence is determined by the incidence rate within this referent category.

Population-based cohort studies have the advantage of having broadly applicable results. This kind of cohort study, by definition, makes use of a random sample or the entire population. As a result, the parent population used in the study's demographics and other features can be defined. Hence, the study's conclusions can be more broadly applied to populations or groups that were not involved in the research.

3.4.1.2. Exposure-Based Cohort Studies

Cohort studies based on exposure allow for the examination of unusual exposures. They are a good substitute for population-based cohort studies, which are ineffective for infrequent exposures (or for case-control studies, either). The best way to demonstrate this claim is with an example. Assume that evidence from animal experiments showed that lead exposure results in long-term neurologic toxicity. The amounts of lead used were significantly higher than what is typically found in human exposures. However, some occupational groups—like those engaged in the production of batteries—may be exposed to enough workplace hazards to seriously jeopardize their health. Although a case-control study might be used, there probably wouldn't be many cases or controls with exposure in the study sample due to the low percentage of the population employed in the battery manufacturing industry. Creating an exposure-based cohort of workers in battery manufacturing facilities, measuring exposure levels with job titles and assignments, and calculating neurotoxicity incidence rates could be an alternate strategy. This design limits the public health inferences (generalization to a larger population or to other groups) because, except in specific cases, the use of special exposure groups to form study groups precludes the determination of the proportion of the target population exposed. Such designs usually include specific subgroups with known exposures, such as an exposed cohort (A + B) and a nonexposed, comparison cohort (C + D), possibly from a different industry. As a result, the cohort members are typically uniform in their level of exposure, and the selection process makes it impossible to ascertain the population's overall frequency of exposure.

• Sources of Exposure-Based Cohorts

Examples of exposure-based cohorts include:

- o Prepaid medical care plans, such as Kaiser Permanente or Group Health of Puget Sound, keep detailed medical information about a potentially large number of readily accessible subjects and maintain regular contact for follow-up information. In this case, the cohort is defined by insurance membership and the exposure of interest may be some medical condition or test recorded in the medical record.
- o Physicians, nurses, and other health professionals have been the focus of several cohort studies. Because these individuals typically belong to national organizations (e.g., the American Medical Association), they are often easier to follow over the long term than other occupational groups because they need to retain their association with the organization and they can be contacted through it. Their knowledge of disease makes them good respondents for surveys; they can be expected to report previous medical conditions and recent diagnoses reliably.
- o Childhood cancer survivors are becoming increasingly common, due mainly to remarkable improvements in therapy. The Childhood Cancer Survivor Study 14 represents the largest (> 14,000 five-year survivors initially

diagnosed between 1970 and 1986 from 25 centers) and most extensively characterized cohort of childhood and adolescent cancer survivors in North America. It serves as a resource for addressing important issues, such as the risk of second malignancies, endocrine and reproductive outcomes, cardiopulmonary complications, and psychosocial implications, among this unique and ever-growing population.

- Veterans, because of the benefits they receive from the U.S. government, usually remain in contact with the relevant agency, making long-term follow-up feasible.
- College graduates are a final example of special resource groups that have been investigated in several noteworthy epidemiologic studies.

• Comparison (nonexposed) Groups for Use in Exposure-Based Cohort Studies

Disease rates in exposed and nonexposed groups are compared in exposure-based cohort studies. There are basically three ways to define the comparison group, using the example of neurotoxicity and lead exposure among workers in the battery manufacturing industry from earlier. First, it's possible that some employees in the sector aren't exposed to lead. Sales personnel, secretaries, and managers, for instance, might be considerably less (or more) exposed to lead than workers in factories. Therefore, within the factory or factories under investigation, an internal comparison (exposed versus nonexposed) would be possible. But take into account the scenario where no one in the industry or factory is spared lead exposure and no one can pinpoint the nonexposed group. Therefore, the second option would be to create a nonexposed group from a different industrial cohort that is similar to the battery factory's demographics and geographic location but does not involve lead exposure. A third choice would be to contrast the disease rates among industry workers who produce batteries with the current population rates. However, because population rates are summary rates and may only be applicable to subgroups defined by age, sex, or race, their usefulness may be restricted in some circumstances.

Consider a cohort study on lung cancer in miners of uranium ore. Data on other exposures, such as diet and tobacco product use, that raise the risk of lung cancer are carefully gathered. In actuality, a sizable portion of the cohort in this population currently smokes.

Lung cancer population rates, however, are derived from the total population. Neither are they status-specific rates nor are they adjusted for smoking. Comparing the lung cancer rates among miners with the lung cancer rates in the general population would be meaningless in this case due to the high smoking rates.

3.4.1.3. Outcome Measures in Cohort Studies

While many cohort studies use the incidence of disease as their primary outcome measure, we pointed out that a variety of other outcomes could also be evaluated. Table 3.4 lists three categories of outcomes: levels of disease markers, changes in disease markers, and discrete events. It also illustrates the types of outcomes used for cohort studies. Both single events and multiple occurrences are considered discrete events. Examples of the former include death and the initial occurrence of a disease like cancer, while the latter refers to recurrent diseases like strokes or heart attacks. The age-standardized annual death rate, the age-specific annual death rate, and the cumulative incidence of disease over predetermined time intervals (e.g., 5 years).

Table 3.4. Difference in Serum Biomarkers Between the Control Group and Study Group

Parameter	Control Group	Study Group
Age (years)	65.16 ± 2.8	68.32 ± 7.34
BMI	34.90 ± 1.18	38.32 ± 1.86
Melatonin (pmol/L)	51.79 ± 7.52	61.41 ± 8.86 **
Ghrelin (pmol/L)	302.23 ± 18.85	269.56 ± 37.23 **
GABA (µmol/L)	0.51 ± 0.11	0.29 ± 0.13 ***
Dopamine (pmol/L)	190.37 ± 17.82	108.81 ± 19.19 ***
Serotonin (pmol/L)	0.52 ± 0.15	0.37 ± 0.13 ***
Epinephrine (pmol/L)	245.93 ± 21.70	302.85 ± 10.48 ***

All values are the mean ± SD, ** $p < 0.01$, *** $p < 0.001$ compared to study group.

Source: *Ahmed Abdelsalam KE, Asad M, Ahmed MAI, Asdaq SMB, Mohzari Y, Alrashed A, Alghamdi N, Alrami KN, Alharbi WA. A case control study on serum levels of potential biomarkers in male breast cancer patients. International Journal of Environmental Research and Public Health. 2021; 18(9):4852. https://doi.org/10.3390/ijerph18094852.*

The repeated evaluation of these outcomes over time is a requirement of cohort studies with multiple occurrences as outcomes. Discrete events such as recurrent heart attacks or modifications in the status of outcome markers may be involved in the multiple occurrences. Research topics could include the relationship between health status and changes in risk markers over time, studies of how aging affects the natural history of disease, and changes in health status, such as the transition for some elderly people from functional disability to disability.

3.4.2. Temporal Differences in Cohort Designs

Cohort designs vary depending on when exposure and outcome data are collected, even though measuring exposure and monitoring for disease are the fundamental components of all cohort studies. These are cohort studies that are both prospective and retrospective.

3.4.2.1. Prospective Cohort Studies

Determining exposure levels at baseline (the present) and monitoring for the possibility of disease development at a later date are characteristics of a prospective cohort study, which is wholly prospective in nature. A unique exposure of interest may serve as the basis for the sampling strategy, or it may be population-based.

There are numerous advantages to prospective studies:

- Prospective cohort studies enable the investigator to collect data on exposures. The collection of exposure information at baseline may result in the most direct and specific test of the study hypothesis. Examples include assessment of diet, physical activity, alcohol use, occupation, coping skills, and quality of life, each of which can be assessed with a few specific items or a comprehensive battery of items.

- The size of the cohort to be recruited is under greater control by the investigators than is the size of a retrospective cohort. Cohort studies that rely on historical records are sometimes fixed in size.
- Biological and physiological assays can be performed with decreased concern that the outcome will be affected by the underlying disease process. Examples include measures of serum factors or nutrient levels and medical examinations (e.g., specific functional tests, antibody titers, or cholesterol levels).
- Direct measures of the environment (e.g., indoor radon levels, electromagnetic field radiation, cigarette smoke concentration, or chlorination byproducts in the water supply) can be made in order to define exposures precisely.

3.4.2.2. Retrospective Cohort Studies

Prospective cohort studies have many advantages, but in order to carry them out, researchers must wait for cases to accumulate. A number of years may pass before conducting useful analyzes, depending on the cohort's size and the disease's prevalence in the community. A retrospective cohort study is an alternative that uses historical data to estimate exposure levels at a baseline in the past. It then conducts "follow-up" for any subsequent disease occurrences between the baseline and the present. The historical prospective cohort study, also referred to as an ambispective cohort study, is a design that uses both retrospective (to determine baseline exposure) and prospective (to determine disease incidence in the future) features.

There are several advantages to retrospective cohort studies:

- In a relatively short period of time, a significant amount of follow-up data may be accrued. For example, Sellers et al. performed a follow-up beginning in 1991 of a cohort of 426 families originally ascertained between 1944 and 1952 at the Dight Institute of Genetics at the University of Minnesota. Three-generation pedigrees were constructed at baseline with data collected from mothers, aunts, sisters, and daughters of breast cancer patients. Records of breastfeeding, reproductive history, and validated occurrences of cancer were stored. Thus, when the family members were recontacted and interviewed regarding subsequent occurrences of cancer, almost 50 years of follow-up were completed during a 5-year period of funding.
- The amount of exposure data collected can be quite extensive and can be available to the investigator at minimal cost. For example, Hartmann and colleagues at the Mayo Clinic, using an index of surgical procedures, were able to construct a cohort of women who received prophylactic mastectomy between 1963 and 1986. Details were available in the medical record on the type of surgery, age at surgery, family history of cancer, and complications following surgery. Follow-up through 1997 was performed to identify subsequent occurrences of breast cancer. Analyzes based on a median of 14 years of follow-up were possible, even though the actual study took less than 5 years to complete.

It can be challenging for many first-year epidemiology students to understand the difference between retrospective cohort studies and case-control studies. Even though they are subtle, the nuances are important. Remember that the initial step in conducting a case-control study is to determine the study subjects' disease status. Then, information about exposures that took place before the onset of the disease is gathered. Disease rates cannot be calculated because there is only one-time point of observation, meaning there is no longitudinal component. Even though these measurements were taken in the past, exposure is the first step in retrospective cohort studies. The main focus of research activity is the subsequent occurrence of disease, possibly supplemented with additional exposure assessments. Whereas a case-control study only includes identified cases and controls, a retrospective cohort study includes the entire cohort of study participants.

3.4.3. Practical Considerations

Cohort studies have many advantages over other observational study designs, so some readers might be wondering why they're not the only design used. We address this in a nutshell under the overarching heading of practical considerations. These factors include follow-up concerns, the adequacy of the scientific rationale, the size and cost of the cohort employed, the availability of exposure data, and data collection and management.

3.4.3.1. Availability of Exposure Data

The quality and quantity of historical exposure data are vitally important for retrospective cohort studies, even though the development of prospective cohort studies may make use of data gathered for purposes other than the cohort study itself. Most of the time, researchers will have to choose between the advantages of a retrospective study design, which provides more immediate follow-up, and the advantages of a prospective cohort design, which collects primary exposure data in the best possible way. There are no clear guidelines to follow when making this choice; instead, each unique research question must be carefully considered.

3.4.3.2. Size and Cost of the Cohort

From a scientific perspective, it is undeniable that the larger the cohort size, the higher the likelihood of receiving answers quickly. The only way to increase the number of cases during an interval for a fixed rate of disease or outcome is to increase the denominator. Let's take an example where the incidence rate of a certain type of cancer is 10 cases per 100,000 people annually. Out of a cohort of 50,000 individuals, only 50 cases would be anticipated over the course of a 10-year observation period. One would anticipate 100 cases if the cohort's size was doubled to 100,000. This higher figure may be more suitable for certain kinds of statistical analysis. Naturally, cost and size go hand in hand, and design decisions are usually influenced by available resources. Designing cohorts with the highest potential for future value can involve concentrating first on gathering biological samples and risk factor data, then pursuing grants for sample analyzes in the future or concurrently through nested studies.

3.4.3.3. Data Collection and Data Management

One of the tenets of epidemiologic research design is that, in terms of the difficulties in gathering and managing data, larger studies are inevitably more demanding than smaller ones. Organizing fieldwork becomes particularly intricate when recruiting takes place at several locations. Data entry could present additional difficulties, particularly if different sites input their own information to be sent to the coordinating center. In these circumstances, clear procedures for quality assurance (e.g., duplicate data entry, and scannable forms) ought to be taken into account during the planning and execution phase. Multiple levels of data collection (e.g., telephone interviews, mail-out questionnaires, consent forms to access medical records, and biological sample collection) at multiple time periods (especially when active follow-up is needed) increase the organizational and administrative burdens even more. Complex data-management systems may be needed for cohort study research protocols in order to track the progress of the various data collection components. These management systems assist researchers and study managers who keep an eye on overall progress, as well as field personnel responsible for the various components. When defining staffing needs, it is important to take into account the tremendous challenges associated with managing data from cohort studies. Data gathered from various sources, file mergers, and "cleaning" of data files present challenges. Cleaning is required when there are inconsistencies, out-of-range entries, and missing values (e.g., someone answers that they never smoke but then admits to having a habit of smoking two packs a day). These problems are not specific to cohort studies; they can also arise in large-scale cross-sectional surveys and case-control studies. Cohort studies are often larger than other designs due to their relative inefficiency when investigating rare diseases.

3.4.3.4. Follow-up Issues

Cohort studies have value, but only if a reliable mechanism is put in place to monitor the cohort for subsequent disease occurrence or other outcomes. At this point, it could be useful to differentiate between active and passive follow-up. Active follow-up refers to the circumstance where the researcher needs to collect information on the outcome's subsequent incidence (disease, altered risk factor, or altered biological marker) directly from the cohort. Follow-up letters, phone calls, or written invitations to return to study sites/centers for further medical evaluation and, in certain situations, biospecimen collection can all be used to establish such contact. It takes a lot of work to follow up, particularly with large cohorts. The Minnesota Breast Cancer Family Study, for example, contacted study participants by phone, mailed a survey, and sent a reminder postcard thirty days later. A second survey was then sent to those who did not respond. Active follow-up is getting more and more time-consuming and frustrating in the current era of telephone technology, with caller identification, automated telemarketing solicitations, answering machines, and the widespread use of cellular phones. This is especially true in our mobile society where addresses change frequently. However, for some cohort studies, the only way to follow up is through a continuous and labor-intensive effort. Compare that to passive follow-up, which doesn't involve speaking with cohort members directly. When databases containing the relevant outcomes are gathered and kept up to date by entities other than the investigative team, passive follow-up becomes feasible. Occasionally, record linkage between databases and the study cohort can be accomplished by epidemiologists. Cancer is a great example that can benefit from passive follow-up, and reporting on it is required by the federal and many state governments. In this way, the Iowa Women's Health Study is able to monitor the state's cancer incidence. It is evident that for many diseases, passive follow-up is not an option. Death is the only endpoint for which there is universal coverage; the National Center for Health Statistics gathers mortality data, which is then disseminated to researchers via the National Death Index (NDI). The degree of participant demographic data collection determines the success of linkage to the NDI. The best data element for linking is Social Security numbers. It is occasionally possible to link records for people with unusual last names even in the absence of Social Security numbers.

3.4.3.5. Sufficiency of Scientific Justification

The sections that came before this one stressed how much money, time, and effort must be invested in order to establish a cohort study. A cohort study should therefore have strong scientific justification. This justification ought to be based on earlier research conducted from a variety of angles, including study designs other than cohort studies, multiple investigators, and multiple study populations. Research on animals or in lab settings may provide more support for cohort studies. Moreover, one of the strongest arguments for a cohort study comes from the circumstance where researchers wish to investigate multiple outcomes from a specific exposure. Due to the design of case-control studies, one outcome can only be looked into at a time. The only type of observational research design that allows for the analysis of several individual-level outcomes in a single study is the cohort study design. Take the complicated topic of hormone replacement therapy (HRT) as an illustration. Many epidemiologic studies have found a small but discernible increase in the risk of breast cancer with hormone replacement therapy (HRT). As a matter of fact, prominent medical journals have issued guidelines advising women who have a family history of breast cancer to avoid using hormone replacement therapy. The finding from other epidemiologic studies that have linked HRT to several health advantages, such as decreased risks of CHD, osteoporosis, and Alzheimer's disease (AD), complicates such a recommendation. An appropriately designed cohort study 27 can investigate the benefits and drawbacks of HRT use by gathering baseline data on HRT measures and designing a follow-up protocol to gather information on various outcomes of interest.

3.5. Experimental Studies

The goal of intervention or experimentation is to try and alter a variable in one or more groups of individuals.

Table 3.5. Different Observational Study Designs

Bias domain	*Study design*	*Signalling question*
Confounding	Any	What are the important variables that might confound the effect of the exposure?
	Any	Were these variables measured with precision and at appropriate points in time?
	Any	Did the authors use an appropriate analysis method or design that adjusted for all of the important confounding variables?
Selection bias	Cohort studies/cross-sectional studies	Was selection into the study unrelated to both the exposure and outcomes?
	Cohort studies/cross-sectional studies	Were the reasons for missing data unrelated to the exposure and outcomes?
	Case-control studies	Were the controls sampled from the population that gave rise to the cases?
	Case-control studies	Were the reasons for missing data related to case or control status?
Information bias	Cohort studies/cross-sectional studies	Were outcome assessors unaware of the exposure status of study participants?
	Cohort studies/cross-sectional studies	Were the methods of outcome assessment comparable across exposure groups?
	Case-control studies	Was the definition of case status/control status applied without knowledge of exposure status?
	Case-control studies	Was data collection on exposure status unaffected by knowledge of the outcome or risk of the outcome?

Source: Dekkers OM, Vandenbroucke JP, Cevallos M, Renehan AG, Altman DG, Egger M (2019) COSMOS-E: Guidance on conducting systematic reviews and meta-analyzes of observational studies of etiology. PLoS Med 16(2): e1002742. https://doi.org/10.1371/journal.pmed.1002742.

This could entail testing a novel treatment on a specific patient population or removing a dietary component assumed to be the cause of allergy.

By contrasting the results of the experimental group with those of the control group, the effects of an intervention are quantified. Ethical considerations play a crucial role in the design of these studies because the study protocol strictly dictates the interventions. For instance, no patient should be excluded from receiving necessary treatment because they are taking part in an experiment; additionally, the treatment under test must be appropriate given the state of the art. In nearly all cases, study participants must give their informed consent (Table 3.5).

An interventional study is usually designed as a randomized controlled trial, a field trial, or a community trial.

3.5.1. Randomized Controlled Trials

A randomized controlled trial is an epidemiological experiment designed to study the effects of a particular intervention. Subjects in the study population are randomly allocated to intervention and control groups, and the results are assessed by comparing outcomes.

Figure 3.12 illustrates the design of a randomized controlled trial. Patients are assigned to the groups at random to guarantee that they are equivalent, i.e., by accident. The control and treatment groups will be comparable at the beginning of the investigation if the initial selection and randomization are done correctly; any differences between groups are the result of chance events unaffected by the investigators' conscious or unconscious biases.

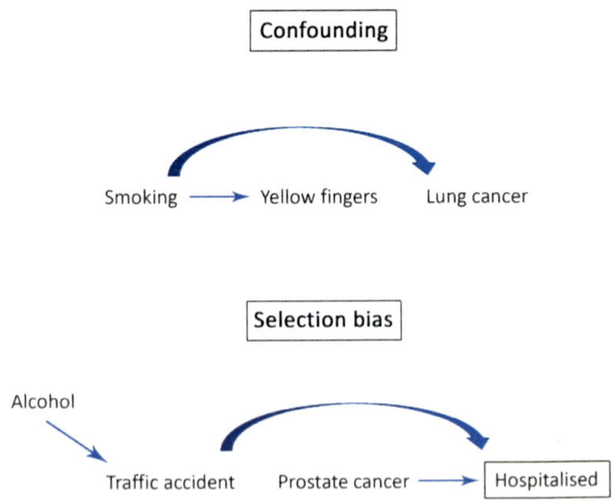

Figure 3.12. *Design of a randomized controlled trial.*

Source: Dekkers OM, Vandenbroucke JP, Cevallos M, Renehan AG, Altman DG, Egger M (2019) COSMOS-E: Guidance on conducting systematic reviews and meta-analyzes of observational studies of etiology. PLoS Med 16(2): e1002742. https://doi.org/10.1371/journal.pmed.1002742.

3.5.2. Field Trials

Contrary to clinical trials, field trials involve participants who are thought to be at risk but are otherwise healthy; data collection occurs "in the field," typically among non-institutionalized members of the general public. Field trials are frequently costly and logistically challenging projects because the goal is to prevent diseases that may occur with relatively low frequency and the subjects are disease-free. Over a million children participated in one of the biggest field trials to test the Salk vaccine for poliomyelitis prevention. Interventions targeted at lowering exposure can be assessed through field trials without having to track the occurrence of adverse health effects. For example, this approach has been used to test various protective strategies against pesticide exposure, and blood lead levels measured in children have demonstrated the protection afforded by getting rid of lead paint in the home. Because these intervention studies do not require long-term follow-up or measurement of disease outcomes, they can be conducted on a smaller scale and at a lower cost.

3.5.3. Community Trials

Instead of using individuals as treatment groups, this type of experiment uses communities. This is especially suitable for diseases whose prevention efforts focus on group behavior and which are influenced by social conditions. Although large-scale community intervention trials may encounter unforeseen methodological issues, cardiovascular disease is an excellent example of a condition suitable for community trials.

3.5.3.1. Limitations of Community Trials

Such studies are limited in that they can only include a small number of communities, and random community allocation is typically impractical. To ensure that any differences found at the end of the study can be attributed to the intervention rather than to intrinsic community differences, alternative methods are needed. Moreover, it is challenging to keep the communities receiving intervention apart from broader societal shifts that might be happening. It is difficult to overcome design constraints, particularly when confronted with unforeseen large, favorable changes in risk factors in control sites. Consequently, it is not always possible to draw firm conclusions regarding the overall efficacy of community-wide initiatives.

A community trial was done of a tuberculosis outreach program in rural Ethiopia communities – with a combined population of 350 000 people – were randomly allocated to intervention and control groups. The study showed that community outreach improved the speed of case-finding for smear-positive tuberculosis.

3.5.4. Potential Errors in Epidemiological Studies

The goal of epidemiological research is to accurately quantify the prevalence of disease (or other outcomes). Nonetheless, there are numerous ways for measurements to be off. Epidemiologists focus a lot of effort on reducing errors and evaluating the effects of errors that are unavoidable. Error sources can be systematic or random.

3.5.4.1. Random Error

A sample measurement's random error occurs when its value deviates from the true population value solely by chance. Measures of association are erroneous due to random error. Three main factors can lead to random error:

- Individual biological variation;
- Sampling error; and
- Measurement error.

It is impossible to totally eradicate random error because we can only examine a sample of the population. The majority of the time, sampling error results from a small sample that is not representative of all the variables in the population. Growing the study's sample size is the most effective strategy to lower sampling error. There is always going to be individual variation, and no measurement is exact. Strict protocols and optimal individual measurement precision can help minimize measurement error. The study's measurement techniques and the potential for error are important concepts for investigators to grasp. By using systematic quality control procedures, laboratories should ideally be able to document the precision and accuracy of their measurements.

3.5.4.2. Sample Size

The sample size must be large enough for the study to have sufficient statistical power to detect the differences deemed important. The following information is needed before the calculation can be done:

- Required level of statistical significance of the ability to detect a difference
- Acceptable error, or chance of missing a real effect
- The magnitude of the effect under investigation
- Amount of disease in the population
- Relative sizes of the groups being compared.

In actuality, logistical and financial factors frequently influence sample size, and sample size and costs must always be balanced. The World Health Organization has released a useful guide on how to calculate sample sizes for health research.

Making sure the groups are the right relative sizes can also increase a study's precision. In case-control studies, this is frequently a cause for concern when determining how many controls to select for each case. Since this depends on the relative costs of accumulating cases and controls, it is impossible to determine the ideal ratio of controls to cases. It makes sense to raise the controls-to-cases ratio when there are more controls than cases. For instance, afflicted children and 300 normal children were compared in the case-control study on the effects of thalidomide. Having more than four controls for every case may not be very beneficial in general. When data are to be analyzed by, say, age group or social class, it is crucial to make sure that there is enough similarity between cases and controls; otherwise, the study would not be able to account for the confounding factor of age. If the majority of cases and the majority of controls were in the older age groups.

3.5.4.3. Systematic Error

In epidemiology, systematic error, also known as bias, happens when findings methodically deviate from true values. A high-accuracy study is one that has a small systematic error. Sample size has little bearing on accuracy. Over thirty distinct types of bias have been identified as potential sources of systematic error in epidemiology. These are the main biases.

- Selection bias
- Measurement (or classification) bias.

1. **Selection Bias:** When there is a consistent discrepancy between the traits of individuals chosen for a study and those of those who are not, selection bias arises. When participants choose to participate in a study because they are ill or because they are especially concerned about an exposure, this is a clear example of selection bias. For instance, it is commonly known that individuals who accept an invitation to take part in research on the health effects of smoking have different smoking behaviors than those who do not; the latter group typically smokes more heavily. Selection bias can also arise in child health studies where parental cooperation is necessary. Successful 12-month follow-ups varied depending on the parents' income level in a cohort study of newborns. A biased estimate of the relationship between exposure and outcome results when participants in a study are either initially or later selected differently from those who withdraw before the study is finished.

   When an individual's illness or other research-related factor prevents them from participating in the study, this introduces a significant selection bias. For instance, employees who experience the most eye irritation in a factory setting where formaldehyde is present are more likely to quit. A prevalence study of the relationship between formaldehyde exposure and ocular irritation conducted solely in the workplace may be highly deceptive, as the remaining employees are less affected.

This significant selection bias in occupational epidemiology studies is known as the "healthy worker effect." Employees must be well enough to carry out their responsibilities; those who are gravely ill or disabled are typically not allowed to work. In a similar vein, results from studies based on exams conducted in health centers that do not include participants who do not show up may be skewed, with sick patients potentially lying in bed at home or in a hospital. Selection bias must be taken into account in all epidemiological study designs.

2. **Measurement Bias:** Measurement bias arises when specific assessments or categorizations of illness or exposure are imprecise – in other words, they fail to accurately gauge the intended outcome. The causes of measurement bias are numerous, and the consequences they have differ in significance. For example, it is rarely possible to obtain exact results from biochemical or physiological measurements, and different laboratories frequently yield disparate findings on the same specimen. There is less potential for systematic measurement bias when specimens from the exposed and control groups are randomly analyzed by separate laboratories as opposed to when all specimens from the exposed group are analyzed in one laboratory and all specimens from the control group are analyzed in another.

Recall bias is a type of measurement bias that is particularly significant in retrospective case-control studies. This happens when cases and controls recall information differently. For example, cases may remember past exposure more frequently, particularly if it is well-known to be linked to the disease being studied, such as heart disease and inactivity. Recall bias can either overstate or underestimate the degree of effect associated with the exposure, depending on whether cases are more likely than controls to deny past exposure, such as in the case of heart disease patients who are more likely to admit to a history of inactivity.

The true strength of the relationship is almost always underestimated when measurement bias affects the groups being compared equally. Such non-differential bias could explain the seemingly disparate outcomes of various epidemiological investigations. Knowledge of the exposure status can affect measurements and lead to observer bias if it is known by the participant, the laboratory technician, or the investigator. Measurements can be conducted blindly or double-blindly to prevent this bias. In a blind study, the participants' classification is kept a secret from the researchers.

3.5.5. Confounding

Another significant problem in epidemiological studies is confounding. Confounding can happen when another exposure occurs in the study population and is linked to both the disease and the exposure under investigation in a study of the relationship between exposure to a cause (or risk factor) and the occurrence of disease. If this unrelated factor, which is also a determinant or risk factor for the health outcome, is distributed differently amongst the exposure subgroups, then there is a problem. When two exposures (risk factors) have their effects combined and the analysis determines that one variable is responsible for the effect rather than the other, this is known as confounding. Two requirements must be satisfied for a factor to be considered confounding (Figure 3.13).

Empty Cell	Item number	Recommendation
Title and Abstract	1	(a) Indicate the study's design with a commonly used term in the title or the abstract (b) Provide in the abstract an informative and balanced summary of what was done and what was found
Introduction		
Background/rational	2	Explain the scientific background and rationale for the investigation being reported
Objectives	3	State specific objectives, including any prespecified hypotheses
Methods		
Study design	4	Present key elements of study design early in the paper
Setting	5	Describe the setting, locations, and relevant dates, including periods of recruitment, exposure, follow-up, and data collection
Participants	6	(a) *Cohort study*—Give the eligibility criteria, and the sources and methods of selection of participants. Describe methods of follow-up *Case-control study*—Give the eligibility criteria, and the sources and methods of case ascertainment and control selection. Give the rationale for the choice of cases and controls *Cross-sectional study*—Give the eligibility criteria, and the sources and methods of selection of participants (b) *Cohort study*—For matched studies, give matching criteria and number of exposed and unexposed *Case-control study*—For matched studies, give matching criteria and the number of controls per case
Variables	7	Clearly define all outcomes, exposures, predictors, potential confounders, and effect modifiers. Give diagnostic criteria, if applicable
Data sources/ measurement	8[a]	For each variable of interest, give sources of data and details of methods of assessment (measurement). Describe comparability of assessment methods if there is more than one group
Bias	9	Describe any efforts to address potential sources of bias
Study size	10	Explain how the study size was arrived at
Quantitative variables	11	Explain how quantitative variables were handled in the analyses. If applicable, describe which groupings were chosen, and why

Statistical methods	12	(a) Describe all statistical methods, including those used to control for confounding (b) Describe any methods used to examine subgroups and interactions (c) Explain how missing data were addressed (d) *Cohort study*—If applicable, explain how loss to follow-up was addressed *Case-control study*—If applicable, explain how matching of cases and controls was addressed *Cross-sectional study*—If applicable, describe analytical methods taking account of sampling strategy (e) Describe any sensitivity analyses
Results		
Participants	13[a]	(a) Report the numbers of individuals at each stage of the study—e.g., numbers potentially eligible, examined for eligibility, confirmed eligible, included in the study, completing follow-up, and analysed (b) Give reasons for non-participation at each stage (c) Consider use of a flow diagram
Descriptive	14[a]	(a) Give characteristics of study participants (e.g., demographic, clinical, social) and information on exposures and potential data confounders (b) Indicate the number of participants with missing data for each variable of interest (c) *Cohort study*—Summarise follow-up time (e.g., average and total amount)
Outcome data	15[a]	*Cohort study*—Report numbers of outcome events or summary measures over time *Case-control study*—Report numbers in each exposure category, or summary measures of exposure *Cross-sectional study*—Report numbers of outcome events or summary measures
Main results	16	(a) Give unadjusted estimates and, if applicable, confounder-adjusted estimates and their precision (e.g., 95% confidence interval). Make clear which confounders were adjusted for and why they were included (b) Report category boundaries when continuous variables were categorized (c) If relevant, consider translating estimates of relative risk into absolute risk for a meaningful time period
Other analyses	17	Report other analyses done—e.g., analyses of subgroups and interactions, and sensitivity analyses

Discussion		
Key results	18	Summarise key results with reference to study objectives
Limitations	19	Discuss limitations of the study, taking into account sources of potential bias or imprecision. Discuss both direction and magnitude of any potential bias
Interpretation	20	Give a cautious overall interpretation of results considering objectives, limitations, multiplicity of analyses, results from similar studies, and other relevant evidence
Generalisability	21	Discuss the generalisability (external validity) of the study results.
Other information		
Funding	22	Give the source of funding and the role of the funders for the present study and, if applicable, for the original study on which the present article is based.

Figure 3.13. *Confounding: checklist.*

Source: Vandenbroucke JP, von Elm E, Altman DG, Gøtzsche PC, Mulrow CD, Pocock SJ, et al. (2007) Strengthening the reporting of observational studies in epidemiology (strobe): explanation and elaboration. PLoS Med 4(10): e297. https://doi.org/10.1371/journal.pmed.0040297.

Confounding occurs when risk factors that are not distributed randomly in the source population also occur in the study population, leading to inaccurate estimates of effect. In this way, it could seem biased, but systematic error in research design is not the cause of it.

In epidemiological studies, age and socioeconomic status frequently act as confounders. It is important to take into account the potential confounding effect of age when examining the relationship between high blood pressure and coronary heart disease. When this is done, it is evident that high blood pressure does, in fact, increase the risk of coronary heart disease.

Since it is well known that coffee consumption is linked to tobacco use—drinkers are more likely to smoke than non-drinkers—confounding may account for the relationship shown between coffee consumption and the risk of coronary heart disease.

The link between smoking cigarettes and coronary heart disease is also widely established. Therefore, the link between coffee consumption and coronary heart disease may be just a reflection of the established link between heart disease and tobacco use. In this case, smoking complicates the apparent link between coffee consumption and coronary heart disease because it is associated with coffee consumption and poses a risk even for non-drinkers.

3.5.5.1. The Control of Confounding

Several methods are available to control confounding, either through study design or during the analysis of results. The methods commonly used to control confounding in the design of an epidemiological study are:

- Randomization
- Restriction

- Matching.

At the analysis stage, confounding can be controlled by:

- Stratification
- Statistical modeling.

1. **Randomization:** Randomization is the best way to make sure that potential confounding variables are distributed evenly among the groups under comparison in experimental studies. The sample sizes must be high enough to prevent such variables from being randomly maldistributed. By using randomization, the exposure under consideration is kept separate from any potentially confounding variables.
2. **Restriction:** Restricting the study to participants with specific traits is one method of mitigating confounding. To eliminate the possibility of cigarette smoking confounding results, for instance, participation in a study on the effects of coffee on coronary heart disease could be limited to nonsmokers.
3. **Matching:** In order to guarantee that any confounding variables are dispersed equally across the two groups under comparison, matching is used to control confounding through participant selection. To guarantee that age and sex confounding does not happen, for instance, in a case-control study of exercise and coronary heart disease, each patient with heart disease can be matched with a control of the same age group and sex. In case-control studies, matching has been widely employed. However, if the matching criteria are overly stringent or numerous, it can cause issues with the selection of controls; this is known as overmatching. Matching is costly and time-consuming, but it is especially helpful when there is a risk that there won't be any overlap between the cases and controls, as in the case of cases that are probably older than the controls.
4. **Stratification and Statistical Modeling:** It is usually better to account for confounding during the analytical stage of a large study as opposed to the design stage. Stratification, which measures the strength of associations in distinct and uniform categories (strata) of the confounding variable, is a means of controlling confounding. If sex or ethnicity is a confounding factor, the association is measured separately in men and women or in the various ethnic groups. If age is a confounding factor, the association may be measured in, say, 10-year age groups. There are techniques for generating a weighted average of the estimates determined in each distinct stratum, which can be used to summarize the overall association.

Despite being conceptually straightforward and comparatively simple to implement, stratification is frequently constrained by the size of the study and is unable to assist in controlling multiple factors at once, as is frequently required. To estimate the strength of the associations while simultaneously controlling for multiple confounding variables in this scenario, multivariate statistical modeling is necessary; a variety of statistical techniques are available for these analyzes.

3.5.5.2. Validity

A test's validity can be defined as its ability to measure the things it is supposed to measure. If a study's findings are consistent with reality, with as little random error and no systematic error, it can be considered valid. The measured values are dispersed but the mean is near to the true value when there is low reliability but high validity. Conversely, a high degree of measurement repeatability (or reliability) does not guarantee validity because the results could all be off from the true value. Validity comes in two flavors: internal and external.

1. **Internal Validity:** The degree to which the findings of an observation are accurate for the specific population under study is known as internal validity. Blood hemoglobin measurements, for instance, must correctly identify study participants who have anemia. Systematic error could lead to different results from a different laboratory's analysis of the blood, but an internal validity assessment of the relationships with anemia as determined by one laboratory might still exist.

   A study needs to be internally valid in order to be useful, but even one that is entirely valid internally could be meaningless if its findings cannot be compared to those of other studies. Any source of systematic error has the potential to compromise internal validity, but careful planning and attention to detail can help.

2. **External Validity:** The degree to which a study's findings apply to individuals who were not involved in it (or, for example, to laboratories not involved in it) is known as external validity or generalizability. Although it is simpler to attain, internal validity is required for external validity but does not ensure it. External quality control of the measurements and assessments of the extent to which study results can be generalized are necessary for external validity. The study sample does not have to be representative of the reference population in order for this to occur. For instance, determining the external validity of research conducted on men is necessary to assess the relevance of evidence showing that lowering blood cholesterol in men also affects women. Study designs that investigate well-defined populations and clearly stated hypotheses contribute to external validity. If similar results are found in studies conducted in other populations, then the study's external validity is supported.

3.5.5.3. Ethical Issues

Concerning actions and policies that are right or wrong, fair or unfair, just or unjust, ethical issues fall into this category. The practice of epidemiology frequently presents ethical conundrums, and like all human endeavors, epidemiology is conducted under ethical guidelines. To make sure that public health interventions do not have major unintended and harmful consequences—as happened in Bangladesh after wells were installed—research and monitoring are crucial.

All epidemiological studies must be reviewed and approved by ethical review committees. The ethical principles that apply to epidemiologic practice and research include:

1 **Informed Consent:** Participants in epidemiological studies must give their free, informed consent and retain the option to withdraw at any time. Giving informed consent, however, might not be feasible when it comes to routine medical record access. In these situations, epidemiologists have an obligation to maintain confidentiality and personal privacy, just like in any other research study. They owe it to the communities they serve to explain to them what they are doing and why, as well as to share study findings and their implications. Before any

research is conducted, all proposals for epidemiological studies should be sent to institutional ethics committees that have been duly established.

2. **Confidentiality:** Epidemiologists are also required to maintain the privacy of any information they learn from their research. This includes the freedom to keep information from being disclosed to third parties. Epidemiologists must obtain permission before accessing medical records, case registers, and other data files and databases because the information contained within is typically confidential.
3. **Respect for Individual Rights:** In epidemiological studies, tensions between the interests of the individual and the group can frequently surface. Attempts to lessen the impact of HIV/AIDS on public health serve as one example. Cuba was able to stop the spread of HIV/AIDS by testing those who were at risk and separating those who were infected from the general public. Others contend that since denial of individual human rights contributed to the spread of disease—for instance, women in many affected countries are powerless to refuse demands for unprotected sex—individual human rights are essential to preventing infection. Furthermore, a large portion of the behavior that puts people at risk for HIV/AIDS takes place in secret, outside the purview of the government. Without guarantees that the interests of those who are vulnerable will be protected, public health initiatives to change their behavior are unlikely to be successful.
4. **Scientific Integrity:** Every scientist has the capacity to act unethically, maybe due in part to the pressure to be successful. Epidemiologists can still engage in unethical activity. Examples include the publication of falsified data and research findings that appear to have been influenced by conflicts of interest. Ethical review committees must be vigilant in minimizing unethical behavior, and peer review of publications must be closely monitored. Serious and frequent discussions of these issues are essential components of epidemiologists' training and mentorship programs.

A Closer Look

Case-Control Studies

Case-control studies are a fundamental research design within epidemiology that plays a crucial role in investigating the association between exposures and outcomes, particularly for rare diseases or conditions with long latency periods. In a case-control study, researchers start by identifying individuals with the outcome of interest (cases) and individuals without the outcome (controls), then compare their past exposures to various risk factors. This retrospective approach allows researchers to efficiently assess potential risk factors by examining differences in exposure prevalence between cases and controls.

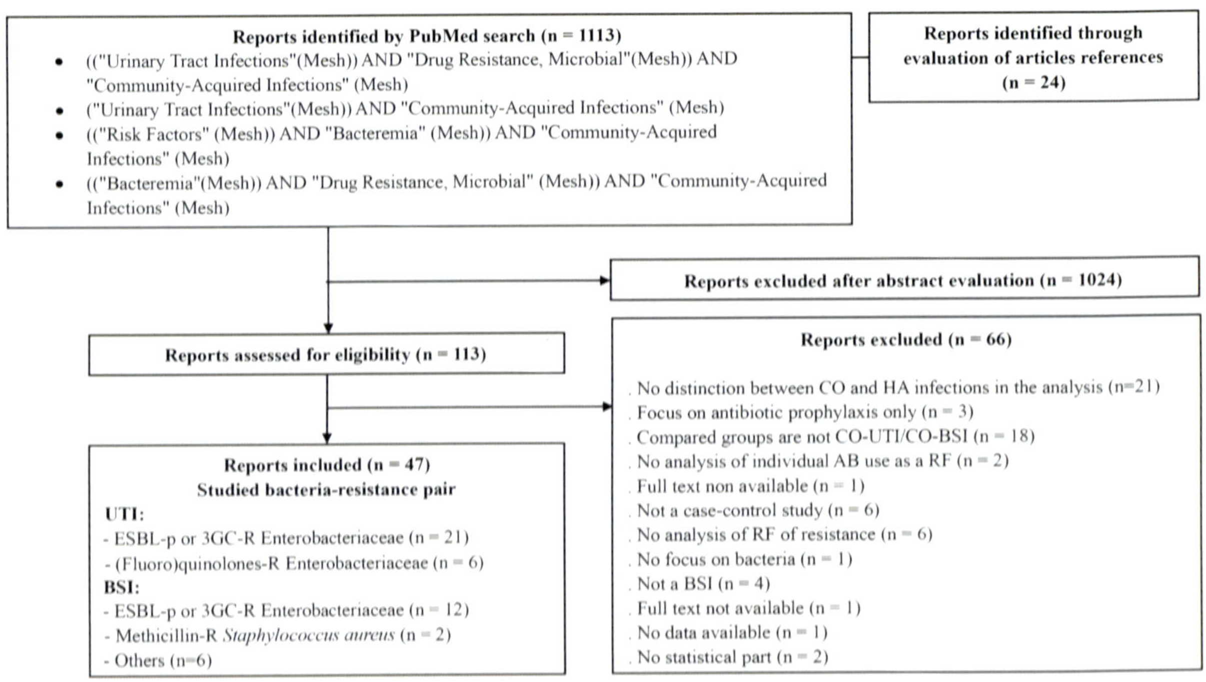

Source: Abbara S, Guillemot D, Brun-Buisson C, Watier L. From pathophysiological hypotheses to case–control study design: resistance from antibiotic exposure in community-onset infections. Antibiotics. 2022; 11(2):201. https://doi.org/10.3390/antibiotics11020201.

One of the key advantages of case-control studies is their efficiency in studying rare diseases or outcomes that have a low incidence rate. By selecting cases with the outcome of interest, researchers can achieve a sufficient sample size without having to follow a large cohort over an extended period. This makes case-control studies particularly valuable for investigating diseases with long latency periods, such as cancer or certain chronic conditions, where following a large cohort over time may be impractical or prohibitively expensive.

Additionally, case-control studies are well-suited for studying diseases with complex or multifactorial etiologies, where multiple risk factors may contribute to disease development. By comparing the exposure history of cases and controls, researchers can identify potential risk factors and evaluate their association with the outcome of interest. This allows for the investigation of interactions between different exposures and the identification of high-risk populations that may benefit from targeted interventions.

However, case-control studies also have limitations that need to be considered. One potential limitation is recall bias, where cases may recall past exposures differently than controls due to their knowledge of their disease status. To mitigate this bias, researchers often use standardized questionnaires and employ blinding techniques to minimize differential recall between cases and controls. Additionally, selection bias may occur if cases and controls are not adequately matched or if controls are not representative of the population from which the cases arose.

SUMMARY

- Epidemiology, as a field of public health, employs a range of study designs to examine patterns of disease occurrence and the factors that influence them within populations. These designs serve as the framework for systematically gathering and analyzing data to understand the distribution, determinants, and outcomes of health-related events. One of the fundamental study designs in epidemiology is observational studies, which include cross-sectional, case-control, and cohort studies.
- Cross-sectional studies are typically descriptive in nature. Primarily, they yield quantitative estimates of the magnitude of a problem but do not measure the temporal ordering of cause and effect.
- A probability sample has the characteristic that every element in the population has a nonzero probability of being included in the sample. A nonprobability sample is one based on a sampling plan that does not have that feature.
- Autism spectrum disorder (ASD) is a set of complex neurodevelopment disorders characterized by mild to severe problems in social interaction and communication along with restricted repetitive behavior patterns. ASD symptoms begin before age 3 years and last into adulthood, although symptoms may improve over time.
- Case-control studies are used to determine if there is an association between an exposure and a specific health outcome. These studies proceed from effect (e.g. health outcome, condition, disease) to cause (exposure). Case-control studies assess whether exposure is disproportionately distributed between the cases and controls, which may indicate that the exposure is a risk factor for the health outcome under study.
- In a case-control study, cases can be selected from a variety of sources, including hospital patients, patients in physicians' practices, or clinic patients. Many communities maintain registries of patients with certain diseases, such as cancer, and such registries can serve as valuable sources of cases for such studies.
- Group matching (or frequency matching) consists of selecting the controls in such a manner that the proportion of controls with a certain characteristic is identical to the proportion of cases with the same characteristic.
- Case-control studies are also valuable when the disease being investigated is rare. It is often possible to identify cases for study from disease registries, hospital records, or other sources. In contrast, if we conduct a cohort study for a rare disease, an extremely large study population may be needed in order to observe a sufficient number of individuals in the cohort develop the disease in question.
- Cohort studies are a type of observational study design used in epidemiology and medical research to investigate the causes and risk factors of diseases. In a cohort study, a group of individuals who share a common characteristic or experience (such as exposure to a particular risk factor or having a specific disease) are followed over time to observe the development of outcomes or diseases of interest.

References

1. Anderson, J. E., Warner, L., Jamieson, D. J., et al. (2010). Contraceptive sterilization use among married men in the United States: Results from the male sample of the National Survey of Family Growth. *Contraception, 82*(3), 230–235.
2. Brenner, H., & Savitz, D. A. (1990). The effects of sensitivity and specificity of case selection on validity, sample size, precision, and power in hospital-based case-control studies. *American Journal of Epidemiology, 132*, 181–192.
3. Brinton, L. A., Schairer, C., Haenszel, W., et al. (1986). Cigarette smoking and invasive cervical cancer. *JAMA, 255*, 3265–3269.
4. Buckley, H. L., Day, N. J., Lear, G., & Case, B. S. (2021). Changes in the analysis of temporal community dynamics data: A 29-year literature review. *PeerJ, 9*, e11250.
5. Carroll, K. K. (1975). Experimental evidence of dietary factors and hormone dependent cancers. *Cancer Research, 35*, 3374–3383.
6. Chatburn, R. L. (2017). Basics of study design: Practical considerations (From the "Biostatistics and Epidemiology Lecture Series, Part 1"). *Cleveland Clinic Journal of Medicine, 84*(9 Suppl 2), e10–e19.
7. Chernick, M. R., & Friis, R. H. (2003). *Introductory Biostatistics for the Health Sciences: Modern*
8. Ciruzzi, M., Pramparo, P., Esteban, O., et al. (1998). Case-control study of passive smoking at home and risk of acute myocardial infarction. *Journal of the American College of Cardiology, 31*, 797–803.
9. Comstock, G. W. (1994). Evaluating vaccination effectiveness and vaccine efficacy by means of case-control studies. *Epidemiologic Reviews, 16*, 77–79.
10. Dillon, C. F., Gu, Q., Hoffman, H., & Ko, C. W. (2010). Vision, hearing, balance, and sensory impairment in Americans aged 70 years and over: United States, 1999–2006. *NCHS Data Brief, no 31*. Hyattsville, MD: National Center for Health Statistics.
11. DiPietro, N. A. (2010). Methods in epidemiology: Observational study designs. *Pharmacotherapy, 30*(10), 973–984.
12. Diwan, S., & Moriarty, D. (1995). A conceptual framework for identifying unmet healthcare needs of community-dwelling elderly. *Journal of Applied Gerontology, 14*, 47–63.
13. Dwyer, D. M., Strickler, H., Goodman, R. A., & Armenian, H. K. (1994). Use of case-control studies in outbreak investigations. *Epidemiologic Reviews, 16*, 109–123.
14. Friis, R. H., Garrido-Ortega, C., Safer, A. M., et al. (2012). Socioepidemiology of cigarette smoking among Cambodian Americans in Long Beach, California. *Journal of Immigrant and Minority Health, 14*(2), 272–280.
15. Gallus, S., Altieri, A., Bosetti, C., et al. (2003). Cigarette tar yield and upper digestive tract cancers: Case-control studies from Italy and Switzerland. *Annals of Oncology, 14*, 209–213.
16. Garrard, J., Chen, V., & Dowd, B. (1995). The impact of the 1987 federal regulations on the use of psychotropic drugs in Minnesota nursing homes. *American Journal of Public Health, 85*, 771–776.
17. Gyawali, B., de Vries, E. G. E., Dafni, U., Amaral, T., Barriuso, J., Bogaerts, J., Calles, A., Curigliano, G., Gomez-Roca, C., Kiesewetter, B., Oosting, S., Passaro, A., Pentheroudakis, G., Piccart, M.,

Roitberg, F., Tabernero, J., Tarazona, N., Trapani, D., Wester, R., Zarkavelis, G., Zielinski, C., Zygoura, P., & Cherny, N. I. (2021). Biases in study design, implementation, and data analysis that distort the appraisal of clinical benefit and ESMO-Magnitude of Clinical Benefit Scale (ESMO-MCBS) scoring. *ESMO Open, 6*(3), 100117.

18. Hartge, P., Brinton, L. A., Rosenthal, J. F., et al. (1984). Random digit dialing in selecting a population-based control group. *American Journal of Epidemiology, 120*, 825–833.

19. Herbst, A. L., & Scully, R. E. (1970). Adenocarcinoma of the vagina in adolescence. *Cancer, 25*, 745–757.

20. Hiebert, R., & Nordin, M. (2006). Methodological aspects of outcomes research. *European Spine Journal, 15* (Suppl 1), S4–16.

21. Jacobsen, S. J., O'Fallon, W. M., & Melton, L. J. III. (1993). Hip fracture incidence before and after the fluoridation of the public water supply, Rochester, Minnesota. *American Journal of Public Health, 83*, 743–745.

22. Jones, S., & Silman, A. J. (1991). Re: "Problems ascertaining friend controls in a case-control study of lung cancer." *American Journal of Epidemiology, 134*, 673–674.

23. Kallen, B., & Mazze, R. I. (1990). Neural tube defects and first trimester operations. *Teratology, 41*, 717–720.

24. Kwan-Gett, T. S., Davis, R. L., Shay, D. K., et al. (2002). Is household antibiotic use a risk factor for antibiotic-resistant pneumococcal infection? *Epidemiology and Infection, 129*, 499–505.

25. Lasky, T., & Stolley, P. D. (1994). Selection of cases and controls. *Epidemiologic Reviews, 16*, 6–17.

26. Levy, P. S., & Lemeshow, S. (1980). *Sampling for Health Professionals.* Belmont, CA: Lifetime

27. Lilli, C., Biggeri, A., Zingaretti, C., Vertogen, B., Frassineti, V., Vespignani, R., Grossi, V., Florescu, C., Matteucci, L., Pazzi, C., Bongiovanni, A., Limarzi, F., Fausti, V., Bertoni, L., Donati, C., Galardi, F., Gentili, N., Mazza, F., Martinelli, G., Nanni, O. (2021). Is it possible to conduct clinical trials during a pandemic? The example of a trial of hydroxychloroquine. *Epidemiologia e Prevenzione, 45*(1–2), 28–36.

28. Linet, M. S., & Brookmeyer, R. (1987). Use of cancer controls in case-control studies. *American Journal of Epidemiology, 125*, 1–11.

29. López-Carrillo, L., Avila, M. H., & Dubrow, R. (1994). Chili pepper consumption and gastric cancer in Mexico: A case-control study. *American Journal of Epidemiology, 139*, 263–271.

30. Mahendraratnam, N., Mercon, K., Gill, M., Benzing, L., & McClellan, M. B. (2022). Understanding use of real-world data and real-world evidence to support regulatory decisions on medical product effectiveness. *Clinical Pharmacology and Therapeutics, 111*(1), 150–154.

31. Menotti, A., Blackburn, H., Kromhout, D., et al. (1997). The inverse relation of average population blood pressure and stroke mortality rates in the seven countries study: A paradox. *European Journal of Epidemiology, 13*, 379–386.

32. Murray, D. M., Roche, L. M., Goldman, A. I., & Whitbeck, J. (1988). Smokeless tobacco use among ninth graders in a North-Central metropolitan population: Cross-sectional and prospective associations with age, gender, race, family structure, and other drug use. *Preventive Medicine, 17*, 449–460.

33. Myers, S. M., & Johnson, C. P. (2007). Management of children with autism spectrum disorders. *Pediatrics, 120*(5), 1162–1182.

34. Nelson, D. E., Giovino, G. A., Shopland, D. R., Mowery, P. D., Mills, S. L., & Eriksen, M. P. (1995). Trends in cigarette smoking among U.S. adolescents, 1974 through 1991. *American Journal of Public Health, 85*, 34–40.

35. Niv, Y., Dickman, R., Figer, A., et al. (2003). Case-control study of screening colonoscopy in relatives of patients with colorectal cancer. *American Journal of Gastroenterology, 98*, 486–489.

36. Noordzij, M., Dekker, F. W., Zoccali, C., & Jager, K. J. (2009). Study designs in clinical research. *Nephron Clinical Practice, 113*(3), c218–c221.

37. Olson, S. H., & Kelsey, J. L., Pearson, T. A., et al. (1992). Evaluation of random digit dialing as a method of control selection in case-control studies. *American Journal of Epidemiology, 135*, 210–222.

38. Pang, D., McNally, R., & Birch, J. M. (2003). Parental smoking and childhood cancer: Results from the United Kingdom Childhood Cancer Study. *British Journal of Cancer, 88*, 373–381.

39. Peres, A. F. T., de Almeida, J. F., Vicentin, D., et al. (2011). Fall in homicides in the city of São Paulo: An exploratory analysis of possible determinants. *Revista Brasileira de Epidemiologia, 14*(4), 709–721.

40. Pickett, K. E., & Pearl, M. (2001). Multilevel analyses of neighbourhood socioeconomic context and health outcomes: A critical review. *Journal of Epidemiology and Community Health, 55*, 111–122.

41. Pringle, B. A., Colpe, L. J., Blumberg, S. J., et al. (2012). Diagnostic history and treatment of school-aged children with autism spectrum disorder and special healthcare needs. *NCHS Data Brief, no 97*. Hyattsville, MD: National Center for Health Statistics.

42. Röhrig, B., du Prel, J. B., Wachtlin, D., & Blettner, M. (2009). Types of study in medical research: Part 3 of a series on evaluation of scientific publications. *Deutsches Ärzteblatt International, 106*(15), 262–268.

43. Sargent, J. D., Brown, M. J., Freeman, J. L., Bailey, A., Goodman, D., & Freeman, D. H. (1995). Childhood lead poisoning in Massachusetts communities: Its association with sociodemographic and housing characteristics. *American Journal of Public Health, 85*, 528–534.

44. Schlesselman, J. J. (1982). *Case-Control Studies: Design, Conduct, Analysis*. New York, NY: Oxford University Press.

45. Selby, J. V. (1994). Case-control evaluations of treatment and program efficacy. *Epidemiologic Reviews, 16*, 90–101.

46. Shaw, G. L., Tucker, M. A., Kase, R. G., et al. (1991). Problems ascertaining friend controls in a case-control study of lung cancer. *American Journal of Epidemiology, 133*, 63–66.

47. Steiner, G. G. (2002). Cancer incidence rates and environmental factors: An ecological study. *Journal of Environmental Pathology, Toxicology and Oncology, 21*, 205–212.

48. Sylvester, G. C., Khoury, M. J., Lu, X., & Erickson, J. D. (1994). First-trimester anesthesia exposure and the risk of central nervous system defects: A population-based case-control study. *American Journal of Public Health, 84*, 1757–1760.

49. Valls, V., Lozano, M. S., Yanez, R., et al. (2007). Use of safety devices and the prevention of

percutaneous injuries among healthcare workers. *Infection Control & Hospital Epidemiology, 28*, 1352–1360.

50. Weiss, N. S. (1994). Application of the case-control method in the evaluation of screening. *Epidemiologic Reviews, 16*, 102–108.
51. Yang, W., Zilov, A., Soewondo, P., Bech, O. M., Sekkal, F., & Home, P. D. (2010). Observational studies: Going beyond the boundaries of randomized controlled trials. *Diabetes Research and Clinical Practice, 88* (Suppl 1), S3–S9.
52. Zhong, L., Goldberg, M. S., Gao, Y. T., et al. (2001). A population-based case-control study of lung cancer and green tea consumption among women living in Shanghai, China. *Epidemiology, 12*, 695–700.

Chapter

INFECTIOUS DISEASE EPIDEMIOLOGY

4

Contents

Introduction

Infectious Disease Epidemiology is a branch of epidemiology concerned with the study of the patterns, causes, and effects of infectious diseases within populations. It aims to understand how diseases spread, the factors influencing their transmission, and how they can be controlled and prevented. Infectious disease epidemiology investigates the dynamics of disease transmission, including the identification of risk factors, modes of transmission, and the impact of interventions.

One of the fundamental concepts in infectious disease epidemiology is the transmission dynamics of pathogens. This includes understanding how infectious agents such as bacteria, viruses, parasites, and fungi are transmitted from one host to another. Transmission routes can vary widely depending on the specific pathogen, ranging from direct person-to-person contact, through respiratory droplets, contaminated food or water, or via vectors such as mosquitoes or ticks.

Moreover, infectious disease epidemiology investigates the factors influencing disease spread within populations. These factors encompass a wide range of biological, environmental, social, and behavioral determinants. Biological factors may include characteristics of the pathogen itself, such as its virulence and ability to survive outside the host. Environmental factors encompass conditions that affect the survival and transmission of pathogens, such as temperature, humidity, and sanitation practices. Social and behavioral factors, including population density, travel patterns, and healthcare-seeking behaviors, also play crucial roles in disease transmission.

Infectious disease epidemiology also emphasizes the importance of surveillance and monitoring systems to track the occurrence and spread of diseases. Surveillance allows public health authorities to detect outbreaks, identify trends, and implement timely interventions to control and prevent further transmission. This may involve the collection and analysis of data from various sources, including laboratory reports, clinical diagnoses, hospital admissions, and population-based surveys.

Additionally, infectious disease epidemiologists play a key role in the development and evaluation of interventions to prevent and control infectious diseases. This includes strategies such as vaccination programs, vector control measures, antimicrobial stewardship, and public health education campaigns. Epidemiological studies are essential for assessing the effectiveness of these interventions, guiding public health policies, and improving our understanding of disease dynamics.

Orientation and Directional Terms

Term	Definition	Illustration
Bladder Cancer	Bladder cancer is a relatively rare form of cancer that starts in the lining of your bladder. There are many ways to treat bladder cancer, including surgery that removes bladder cancer.	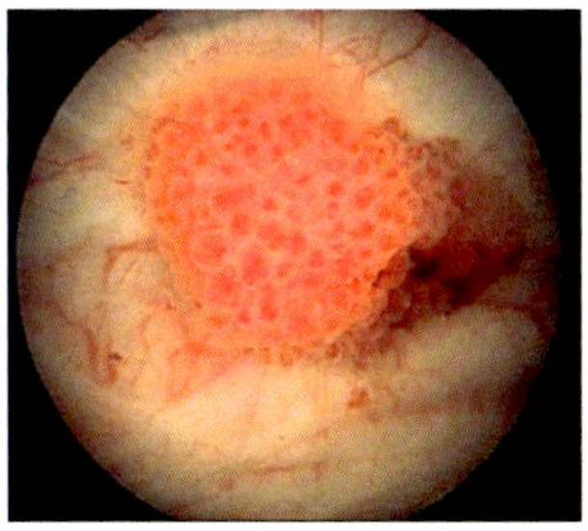
Infectious Diseases	Infectious diseases are disorders that are caused by organisms, usually microscopic in size, such as bacteria, viruses, fungi, or parasites that are passed, directly or indirectly, from one person to another.	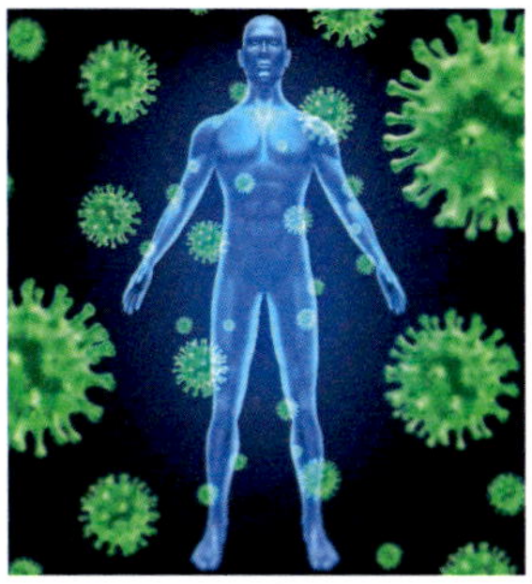
Epidemiologic Triangle	Epidemiologic triangle is a model for explaining the organism causing the disease and the conditions that allow it to reproduce and spread.	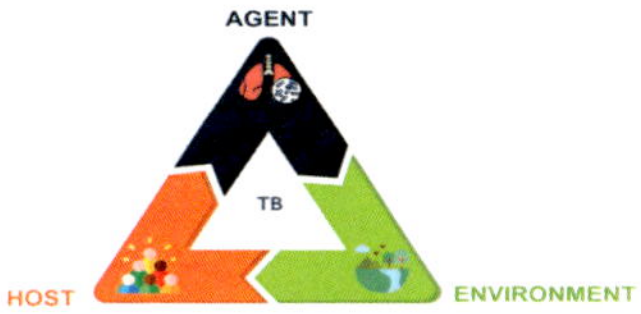
Rickettsial Infections	Rickettsial infections are caused by a variety of obligate intracellular bacteria in the genus Rickettsia and are grouped into one of four categories: spotted fever group, typhus group, ancestral group, and transitional group.	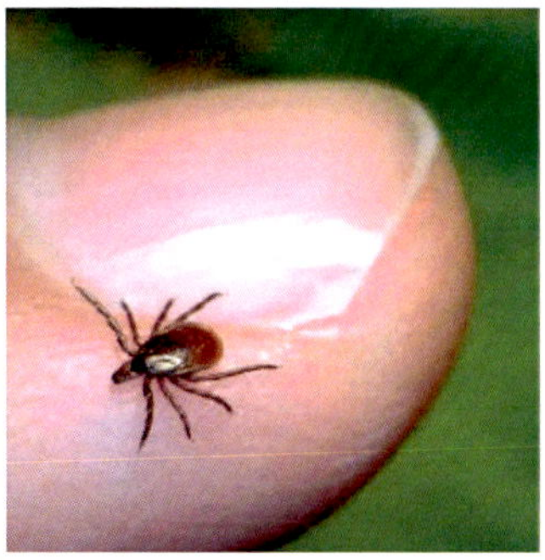
Case Fatality Rate (CFR)	Case Fatality Rate (CFR) measures the severity of disease by defining the total number of deaths as a proportion of reported cases at a specific time.	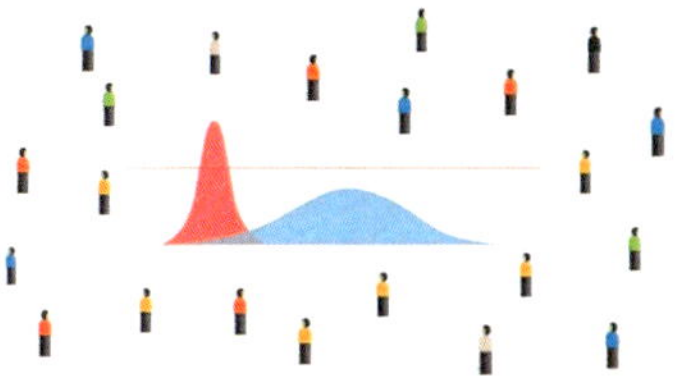

4.1. Epidemiology of Infectious Diseases

One of the most well-known uses of epidemiology in the workplace is the management of infectious diseases. In spite of numerous advancements in the prevention and treatment of infectious diseases, these illnesses continue to be major global causes of morbidity and mortality for both developed and developing nations. Pneumonia and influenza combined ranked as the eighth most common cause of death in the U.S. in 2008. Infections are the primary cause of death for children and young adults worldwide. Furthermore, illnesses like cancer (e.g., bladder cancer, certain types of liver cancer, and cervical cancer) are linked to infectious agents. As a result of increased international travel, a passenger carrying a communicable disease that is hazardous or uncommon can spread the illness over the course of a long-haul flight from a remote location in the world to a busy metropolis. The 2011 film Contagion presented a fictitious story of a mysterious and deadly infectious disease that spread across international borders and posed a threat to the entire world. Contagion depicted events that were compelling due to their realism in the modern global village era.

Institutional settings (e.g., hospitals, day care centers, and facilities for the developmentally dizabled) are important venues for infectious disease outbreaks. Estimates from 2002 indicated that approximately 4.5 per 100 patients admitted to U.S. hospitals experienced nosocomial (hospital- or healthcare unit-acquired) infections, which ranged from wound infections to pneumonia to bloodstream infections. About 100,000 of the estimated 1.7 million hospital-acquired infections were fatal. An example of an infectious disease that affects children in child care centers is giardiasis, a gastrointestinal illness. In addition, outbreaks of hepatitis B occur in children's day care centers and residential settings for the developmentally disabled. Also commanding the attention of public health practitioners is the spread of hospital-acquired antibiotic-resistant bacterial infections into the community.

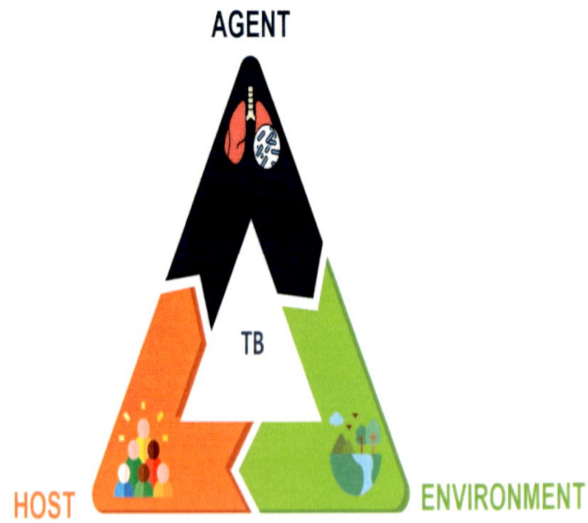

Figure 4.1. *Epidemiologic triangle.*

Source: https://courses.lumenlearning.com/suny-buffalo-environmentalhealth/chapter/application-to-chronic-disease/.

We'll look at the epidemiologic triangle, one of the models that helps explain why disease outbreaks happen, including those that affect entire communities and institutional settings. The three main components of the pathophysiology of disease—agent, environment, and host—are acknowledged by the epidemiologic triangle. Throughout many decades, epidemiologists have relied on this respected model, which they often cite. The epidemiologic triangle (Figure 4.1) offers a basic understanding of disease causation in public health.

Although more complex multivariate causality is also believed to play a role in the etiology of infectious diseases, the three-factor epidemiologic triangle is a particularly good fit for explaining this process. Examining agent, host, and environmental factors is another method for investigating and controlling epidemics. Figure 4.2 illustrates one method of grouping the various infectious diseases.

Rank	Infectious Disease/Pathogen	YLL	YERF	HALY	% of total HALYs
1	Hepatitis C virus	8823	983	9807	11.02%
2	*Streptococcus pneumoniae*	6669	1601	8270	9.30%
3	*Escherichia coli*	7485	341	7826	8.80%
4	Human papillomavirus	6191	1418	7609	8.55%
5	Hepatitis B virus	6918	86	7004	7.87%
6	Human immunodeficiency virus	5036	1312	6349	7.14%
7	*Staphylococcus aureus*	3740	400	4140	4.65%
8	Influenza virus	2482	1076	3558	4.00%
9	*Clostridium difficile*	3216	107	3323	3.74%
10	Rhinoviruses	125	1615	1740	1.96%
11	Respiratory syncytial virus	968	397	1364	1.53%
12	Parainfluenza virus	601	259	861	0.97%
13	Group A streptococcus	598	216	814	0.92%
14	*Haemophilus influenzae*	649	125	774	0.87%
15	Group B streptococcus	603	123	725	0.82%
16	Tuberculosis	675	16	691	0.78%
17	Legionellosis	588	40	628	0.71%
18	Chlamydia	19	442	461	0.52%
19	Varicella	150	303	453	0.51%
20	Adenovirus	301	150	451	0.51%
21	Coronaviruses	28	369	397	0.45%
22	Gonorrhea	17	371	388	0.44%
23	*Neisseria meningitidis*	177	152	329	0.37%
24	Herpes simplex virus	117	138	256	0.29%
25	Pertussis	0	220	220	0.25%
26	*Candida spp.*	126	92	218	0.24%
27	*Campylobacter spp.*	26	144	170	0.19%
28	*Blastomyces*	135	2	137	0.15%
29	*Pneumocystis jiroveci*	103	2	105	0.12%
30	Poliomyelitis	102	0	101	0.11%
31	*Aspergillus*	70	31	100	0.11%
32	*Salmonella spp. (excluding typhi/ paratyphi)*	40	42	81	0.09%

33	West Nile virus	45	16	61	0.07%
34	*Giardia lamblia*	0	52	52	0.06%
35	*Listeria monocytogenes*	36	1	36	0.04%
36	*E. coli* O157	14	17	31	0.03%
37	Syphilis	13	18	31	0.03%
38	Hepatitis A	4	22	26	0.03%
39	Malaria	6	0	6	0.01%
40	*Histoplasma*	0	6	6	0.01%
41	*Shigella*	0	4	4	0.00%
42	Rubella virus	0	2	2	0.00%
43	*Yersinia enterocolitica* (not *Yersinia pestis*)	0	1	1	0.00%
44	Typhoid/Paratyphoid fever	0	1	1	0.00%
45	*Cryptosporidium*	0	1	0	0.00%
46	*Cyclospora cayetensis*	0	0	0	0.00%
47	Dengue	0	0	0	0.00%
48	Tetanus	0	0	0	0.00%
49	Mumps virus	0	0	0	0.00%
50	Measles virus	0	0	0	0.00%
51	Diphtheria	0	0	0	0.00%
	Syndromes due to other pathogens	17401	1957	19348	21.75%
	Top 5 pathogens	36087	4429	40516	45.55%
	Top 10 pathogens	50686	8940	59626	67.03%
	Top 20 pathogens	55837	11010	66848	75.15%
	Total	74297	14668	88956	100.0%

Figure 4.2. *Number and proportion of average annual HALYs by infectious disease or pathogen, 2005–07, Ontario, Canada.*

Source: Kwong JC, Ratnasingham S, Campitelli MA, Daneman N, Deeks SL, Manuel DG, et al. (2012) The impact of infection on population health: Results of the ontario burden of infectious diseases study. PLoS ONE 7(9): e44103. https://doi.org/10.1371/journal.pone.0044103.

4.1.1. Agents of Infectious Disease

The first component of the epidemiologic triangle is an agent, which must be present for an infection to occur. Microbial agents include the following:

- **Bacteria:** In the United States and Europe, bacterial diseases were among the leading killers during the 19th century. Antibiotics and improvements in medical care have helped to control some of these killers. Nevertheless, bacteria remain a significant cause of human illness. Examples of diseases caused by bacteria are tuberculosis (TB), salmonellosis, and streptococcal infections (e.g., strep throat and flesheating disease–necrotizing fasciitis). Of particular concern is the growing emergence of bacterial strains that are resistant to antibiotics (e.g., methicillin-resistant Staphylococcus aureus–MRSA).
- **Viruses:** A virus is "[a] microorganism composed of a piece of genetic material (RNA or DNA) surrounded by a protein coat. To replicate, a virus must infect a living cell." Examples of diseases caused by viruses include viral hepatitis A, herpes simplex, influenza, and viral meningitis (aseptic meningitis). A family of RNA viruses is known as retroviruses. The human immunodeficiency virus (HIV) is a retrovirus.
- **Rickettsia:** Rickettsia is a genus of bacteria that can grow within cells. Ectoparasites (e.g., fleas, lice, and ticks) transmit the majority of rickettsial agents, which cause a variety of diseases. These include typhus fever, Q fever, Rocky Mountain spotted fever, and rickettsialpox.
- **Fungi:** An example of a fungal disease is coccidioidomycosis (also called San Joaquin Valley fever), which is an endemic mycosis; the term mycosis refers to a disease caused by fungi. Other examples are blastomycosis, ringworm (tinea capitis), and athlete's foot (tinea pedis). Opportunistic mycoses, which impose an increasing threat to immunocompromised patients, include candidiasis, cryptococcosis, and aspergillosis. During the fall of 2012, a major outbreak of fungal meningitis was associated with a contaminated steroid medication shipped by a Massachusetts compounding pharmacy. More than 400 cases and 30 deaths in at least 19 states were linked to injections of the medication.
- **Protozoa:** These are microscopic single-cell organisms, which are responsible for diseases such as malaria, amebiasis, babesiosis, cryptosporidiosis, and giardiasis. For example, malaria is transmitted by mosquitoes in endemic areas; one of the modes for acquiring giardiasis is through ingestion of contaminated water that contains cysts of the protozoa *Giardia lamblia*.
- **Helminths:** These organisms (found most frequently in moist, tropical areas) include intestinal parasites—roundworms (which cause ascariasis), pinworms, and tapeworms—as well as the organisms that cause trichinellosis (trichinosis; infectious agent *Trichinella spiralis*). Another well-known helminth, *Schistosoma mansoni* (and several other species), is responsible for schistosomiasis, sometimes known as snail fever, which occurs in Africa (e.g., along the Nile River) and in South America (Brazil, Surinam, and Venezuela), China, Japan, and many other areas. The infectious agents responsible for schistosomiasis are not indigenous to North America
- **Arthropods:** One of the largest classes of living things, arthropods act as insect vectors that carry a disease agent from its reservoir to humans.

Mosquitoes, ticks, flies, mites, and other insects of this type are examples of arthropod vectors that transmit a number of significant human diseases, such as Dengue fever, Lyme disease, viral encephalitis, Rocky Mountain spotted fever, trypanosomiasis, and leishmaniasis.

4.1.2. Characteristics of Infectious Disease Agents

The following traits affect an infectious disease agent's ability to spread to a host, as well as the likelihood that the disease will manifest, how severe it will be, and how the infection will turn out.

- The ability of an agent to infect or cause disease in a susceptible host by entering and multiplying there is referred to as infectiousness. Both measles and polio have a high contagiousness. Infectivity is quantified using the secondary attack rate.
- The ability of an agent to manifest disease in the infected host is referred to as pathogenicity. Polio is a disease of low pathogenicity (the majority of cases are subclinical), while measles is a disease of high pathogenicity (few subclinical cases). The ratio of people with clinically evident disease to those exposed to an infection is a measure of pathogenicity.
- The ability of an agent to cause illness in the host is referred to as virulence. Pathogenicity and virulence are sometimes used interchangeably. The ratio created by dividing the total number of cases with overt infection by the total number of infected cases is a measure of virulence. If the illness is lethal, the case fatality rate (CFR) can be used to gauge virulence. The rabies virus is a highly virulent agent with a high CFR that nearly always causes fatal disease in humans.
- The term "toxicogenicity" describes an agent's ability to create a toxin or poison. The toxin that the microbe produces, rather than the microbe itself, is what causes the pathologic effects of agents for diseases like botulism and shellfish poisoning.
- Resistance (of agent) refers to the ability of the agent to survive adverse environmental conditions. Some agents are remarkably resistant (e.g., the agents responsible for coccidioidomycosis and hepatitis) and others are extremely fragile (e.g., the gonococcus and influenza viruses). Note: The term resistance also is applied to the host.
- The term "antigenicity" describes an agent's capacity to stimulate the production of antibodies in the host. Immunogenicity is a term that describes the capacity of an infection to elicit a particular type of immunity. Long-term immunity against infection may or may not be induced by agents. For instance, recurrent reinfection with gonococci is typical, but recurrent infection with the measles virus is regarded as uncommon.

4.1.3. Host

Even though it was previously mentioned, the presence of an agent is not a sufficient cause for the development of an infectious disease. In other words, the agent needs to be able to infect a host. Following exposure to an infectious agent, the host may go through a series of steps that eventually result in an active case of the disease from a subclinical (inapparent) infection. The outcome could be total recuperation, irreversible impairment, deformity, or even death. For instance, the common cold typically resolves on its own and requires no further treatment. A great deal of fear once surrounded smallpox due to its high morbidity and mortality rate. Rheumatic fever and nephritis are the debilitating consequences of an untreated group A streptococcal infection (Β hemolytic), which can occur in a tiny percentage of cases. In further variations in the degree of illness, research shows that the majority of tuberculosis cases are non-fatal, with a tiny percentage being fatal. Compared to tuberculosis, a higher percentage of cases of the measles virus result in moderately severe illness and a small number of fatalities. Certain highly contagious and virulent agents, like the rabies virus, almost always result in death.

A variety of factors, some of which are host-specific, influence the capacity to cause infection. The host's capacity to resist the infectious agent plays a significant role in determining the extent of infection and the severity of the ensuing disease. There are two main types of defense mechanisms in this ability: general defense mechanisms and disease-specific defense mechanisms.

4.1.3.1. Nonspecific Defense Mechanisms

The human body has several defense mechanisms in place to lessen the chance that an agent will get inside and cause illness. The majority of environmental agents are unable to penetrate the body due to the barrier that our skin provides. In a similar vein, the mucosal surfaces offer defense against external invaders. Saliva and tears can be considered ways to wash away potential infectious agents. Many substances that can enter the body through ingestion are fatally affected by the high pH of our gastric juices. The immune system is also well-developed to absorb infectious agents through the action of phagocytes and macrophages.

The nonspecific mechanisms mentioned above play a significant role in determining host susceptibility, but there are several other factors that also affect how the host reacts to infectious agents. The capacity of nonspecific defense mechanisms to fight agents may decline with age (e.g., using weakened immunity). The host's nutritional state may also be crucial since malnourished people may be less able to fight off infections than those who eat a healthy diet. There are genetic factors at play as well, as demonstrated by the pronounced variations in people's responses, for instance, to mosquito bites. While some people might react minimally or not at all, others might get a significant welt at the location.

4.1.3.2. Disease-Specific Defense Mechanisms

Disease-specific defenses include immunity against a particular agent. Immunity refers to the resistance of the host to a disease agent. Immunity to a disease may be either natural or artificial and active or passive:

- **Active:** A pathogenic organism stimulates the potential host's immune system to create antibodies against the disease. Active immunity is long-lasting but requires time to develop.
- **Passive:** A preformed antibody is administered to a recipient; the immunity is usually of short duration (half-life, 3–4 weeks) for immune globulin (gamma globulin) derived from the pooled plasma of adults.
- **Natural, Active:** This type of immunity, also called natural immunity, results from an infection by the agent. For example, a patient develops long-term immunity to measles because of a naturally acquired infection.
- **Artificial, Active:** This type of immunity, also called vaccine-induced

immunity, results from an injection with a vaccine that stimulates antibody production in the host. All or part of a microorganism or a modified part of that microorganism is administered to invoke an immunologic response. The response mimics the natural infection but presents little or no risk to the recipient.

- **Natural, Passive:** Preformed antibodies during pregnancy are transferred across the placenta to the fetal bloodstream to produce short-term immunity in the newborn.
- **Artificial, Passive:** Preformed antibodies against a specific disease are administered to an exposed individual to confer protection against a disease. An example is prophylaxis against hepatitis by administration of immune globulin to individuals who have been exposed.

4.1.4. The Environment

The domain in which the agent causing the disease may exist, persist, or have its origins is referred to as the environment. The physical, climatologic, biologic, social, and economic factors that are not a part of the host are collectively referred to as the external environment. The weather, humidity, temperature, geological formations, and other comparable physical characteristics make up the physical environment. The social environment, which is the sum of a group of the behavioral, psychological, attitudinal, and cultural traits of humans, is in contrast to the physical environment. Because the environment can either increase or decrease the survival of disease agents and can act to bring agents and hosts into contact, both of these aspects of the external environment have an effect on disease agents and potential hosts.

The environment can act as a niche or reservoir that helps agents of infectious diseases survive. The reservoir could live in the physical world, or it could be a part of other people—human reservoir hosts—or in animals, insects, or other vectors. Contaminated food and water sources can contain infectious disease agents that cause cholera, typhoid, and numerous other illnesses, making them an example of an environmental reservoir. San Joaquin Valley fever, also known as coccidioidomycosis, is caused by fungi that can live in the soil. There are vertebrate animal reservoirs for certain infectious diseases. Zoonoses are illnesses that have the potential to spread from human hosts to animal reservoirs in natural settings. Notable instances of zoonoses include plague and rabies. Certain diseases can only be contracted from humans; smallpox is one such illness that has been effectively eradicated because the virus doesn't seem to be able to survive outside of humans. Certain illnesses, like typhoid fever, can cause a chronic carrier state in certain people, even if they don't exhibit symptoms and can still spread the illness to other vulnerable people.

4.2. Means of Transmission: Directly or Indirectly from Reservoir

The stages of an infectious disease's transmission—which can occur either directly or indirectly—are shown in Figure 4.3. For instance, the transmission of disease requires portals for the entry and exit of infectious agents.

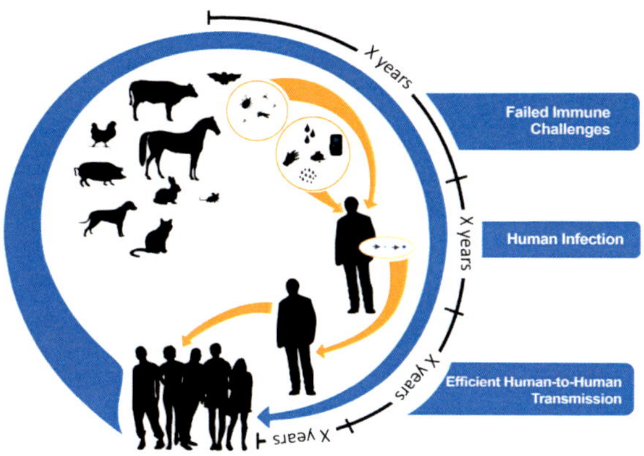

Figure 4.3. *The chain of infection.*

Source: Gray GC, Robie ER, Studstill CJ, Nunn CL. Mitigating future respiratory virus pandemics: new threats and approaches to consider. Viruses. 2021; 13(4):637. https://doi.org/10.3390/v13040637.

4.2.1. Direct Transmission

The term "direct transmission of diseases" describes the spread of an infection from person to person when there is no intermediary contaminated object contact. As in the case of the spread of sexually transmitted diseases, direct transmission can happen, for instance, through contact with the blood or bodily fluids of an infected individual.

4.2.2. Indirect Transmission

The spread of an infection via a middleman, such as a vehicle, a pest, or a vector, is known as indirect transmission. Contaminated water, contaminated blood on used hypodermic needles, and food are a few examples of vehicles that can be connected to the spread of infectious diseases. A fomite is an inanimate object that contains pathogens, like clothing or doorknobs. An inanimate object is said to be contaminated if it contains a live infectious agent. Inadequate sterilization of medical equipment, shared toys in a pediatric ward, unwashed hands of healthcare personnel, and patient-care items contaminated with microbes are additional indirect transmission routes.

An animated, living insect or animal that aids in the spread of the disease agent is called a vector. Sometimes, the disease agent's life cycle includes arthropod vectors like flies and mosquitoes. For instance, the Anopheles mosquito is necessary for the infectious agents that cause malaria to survive (e.g., *Plasmodium vivax*); the frequency of malaria cases decreases if the mosquito population is eliminated. Preventing the spread of diseases like malaria by controlling arthropod vectors can be a useful strategy.

4.2.3. Portals of Exit and Entry

The alimentary canal, skin lesions, genitourinary system openings, respiratory passages, and alimentary canal are examples of portals of exit, which are locations where infectious agents may leave the body. Additional exit points could be created by wounds, blood draws, insect bites, and surgical procedures. The portal of exit needs to be suitable for the specific agent in order for the chain of transmission to continue. In order to cause infection, the agent needs to leave the source in large enough quantities to endure in the surroundings and get past the barriers protecting the entry points in the new host.

An entry point, or portal of entry, is a location where an infectious agent can enter the human body and spread. The respiratory system is one example (e.g., for illnesses like the common cold and influenza); the oral and digestive tracts (e.g., for illnesses like staphylococcal food poisoning or hepatitis A); and the skin's mucous membranes or wounds (e.g., in the case of bacterial illnesses like staphylococcal infections).

4.2.4. Other Concepts Related to Disease Transmission

Other concepts related to disease transmission shown in the following are:

4.2.4.1. Inapparent Infection

An infection that has not yet crossed the clinical horizon is referred to as inapparent (subclinical) (i.e., lacks clinically evident symptoms). However, inapparent infections can have a significant epidemiologic impact because asymptomatic people have the potential to spread the illness to other vulnerable hosts, some of whom may become seriously ill. When the infectious disease is clinically evident, isolation of infected individuals is more likely to happen (i.e., when there is a high ratio of apparent to inapparent cases. Cholera, infectious tuberculosis, and the plague are a few examples of infectious diseases that need to be isolated. Immunoassay can be used to look for serologic evidence of infection in order to establish whether an infection has occurred in both symptomatic and asymptomatic individuals. An increased titer of blood antibodies indicates a history of infection and exposure to the pathogen. For instance, children in nursery school may carry the disease even though they do not exhibit clinical symptoms when they have hepatitis A (infectious hepatitis), which frequently presents as a subclinical infection. Blood antibody and enzyme responses to hepatitis A virus infection can be used to track the infectious process (HAV). After a suitable incubation period, the epidemiologist and clinician may note increases in hepatitis A antibodies and enzymes, leading them to conclude that infection has occurred.

4.2.4.2. Incubation Period

The amount of time that passes between being exposed to an infectious agent and the onset of the disease's initial signs and symptoms is known as the incubation period. For every disease agent, the incubation period—during which the infectious organism replicates inside the host—is typically set for a specific number of hours, days, or weeks. When trying to determine the origin of an infectious disease outbreak in relation to the time and circumstances of exposure as well as the type of agent, epidemiologists frequently consider the incubation period. For instance, the measles (rubeola) typically takes 10 days to incubate, but it can take anywhere between 7 and 18 days, and it takes roughly 2 weeks for a rash to develop. Finding the origins of foodborne illness outbreaks is another use for incubation periods; calculating the incubation period aids in eliminating potential etiologic agents, each of which has a distinct incubation period.

4.2.4.3. Herd Immunity

Herd immunity is the ability of a population, group, or community to fend off an infectious disease when a sizable portion of the population is immune (either from prior infections or vaccinations). Although not every member of the population is immune, herd immunity protects the population as a whole when immune individuals stop a disease from spreading to unimmunized people. For instance, herd immunity against rubella might need 85–90% of community members to be immune, whereas for diphtheria, that number might only be 70%.

4.2.4.4. Generation Time

The period of time between the arrival of an infectious agent in a host and the host's maximum communicability is referred to as the "generation time." It's possible that the incubation period and the generation time of an infectious disease are not equal. With certain illnesses (e.g., mumps), the peak contagious period occurs before the onset of clinical signs. The peak contagious period for mumps occurs approximately 48 hours before salivary gland enlargement. Between the generation time and the incubation period, there is an additional distinction. While the term "generation time" refers to both inapparent and apparent cases of disease, the term "incubation period" only refers to clinically apparent cases of disease.

4.2.4.5. Colonization and Infestation

It is crucial to stress that not every agent exposure results in disease. When an infectious agent spreads across the surface of the body without triggering a tissue or immune response, this is referred to as colonization. A living infectious agent that is present on the outside of the body and has the potential to trigger a local reaction is referred to as an infestation. Therefore, the community setting may encompass a much wider range of diseases than just those exhibiting clinical symptoms.

4.2.4.6. Iceberg Concept of Infection

According to the "iceberg" theory of infection, only a small percentage of infections and agent exposures in hosts are caused by the tip of the iceberg, or active clinical disease. As seen in Figure 4.4, a significant portion of infections are subclinical, and exposure to a pathogen may not result in infection or cell entry.

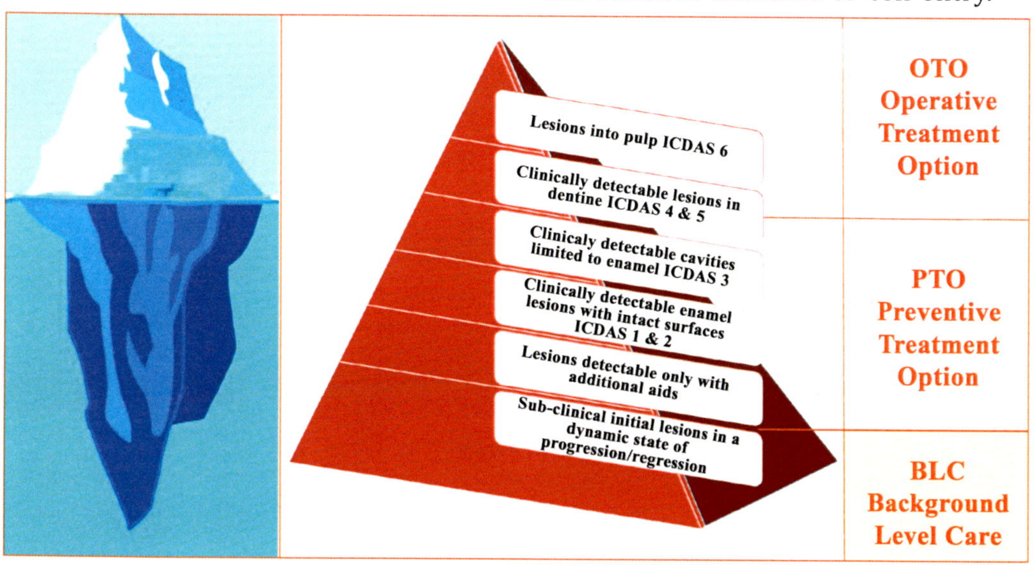

Figure 4.4. *Iceberg concept of infection.*

Source: Dobrzański LA, Dobrzański LB, Dobrzańska-Danikiewicz AD, Dobrzańska J. The concept of sustainable development of modern dentistry. Processes. 2020; 8(12):1605. https://doi.org/10.3390/pr8121605.

4.2.4.7. Inapparent/Apparent Case Ratio

There is a great range in viral infection clinical presentation. While the great majority of polio infections do not result in severe illness, this is not the case for rabies, where only a small number of infected cases have survived when rabies prophylaxis was not administered in a timely manner. The proportion of apparent clinical cases of hepatitis A rises as a person ages. Among adults, about half of cases of hepatitis B and rubella are clinically evident (Table 4.1).

Table 4.1. Variations in the Clinical Presentations of Viral Infections with Comparative Rank in H5N1 Cases

Signs and symptoms	At illness onset, no. (%)	At hospital admission, no. (%)
Fever	24 (92)	18 (69)
Chills	12 (46)	12 (46)
Malaise	10 (39)	12 (46)
Myalgia	11 (42)	8 (31)
Headache	4 (15)	4 (15)
Sore throat	2 (8)	4 (15)
Rhinorrhea	3 (12)	1 (4)
Cough	15 (58)	20 (77)
Sputum production	9 (35)	15 (58)
Tachypnea*	2 (8)	18 (69)
Dyspnea	0	6 (23)
Vomiting	2 (8)	3 (12)
Abdominal pain	1 (4)	1 (4)
Diarrhea	1 (4)	2 (8)

Source: Yu H, Gao Z, Feng Z, Shu Y, Xiang N, Zhou L, et al. (2008) Clinical characteristics of 26 Human cases of highly pathogenic avian influenza A (H5N1) Virus infection in China. PLoS ONE 3(8): e2985. https://doi.org/10.1371/journal.pone.0002985.

4.3. Measures of Disease Outbreaks

4.3.1. Attack Rate

An attack rate is "[t]he proportion of a group that experiences the outcome under study over a given period (e.g., the period of an epidemic)." An attack rate, a variant of an incidence rate, is used when the occurrence of disease among a population at risk increases greatly over a short period of time, often related to a specific exposure. In addition, the disease rapidly follows the exposure during a fixed time period because of the nature of the disease process. Thus, the term attack rate is frequently applied to the occurrence of acute infectious disease outbreaks (e.g., microbial foodborne illness and other acute infectious diseases) and also can be used for other acute health-related events (e.g., acute exposures of large groups to toxic agents). An attack rate is often expressed as a percentage.

The number of individuals who become ill as a result of being exposed to the suspected agent is the numerator, and all individuals who were exposed to the agent during a specific time period—whether healthy or not—make up the denominator. An attack rate is not a true rate because the time period in which exposure occurred is a crucial component of the definition, but it is frequently defined arbitrary or uncertainly.

A calculation example for attack rates related to a foodborne illness outbreak can be discussed. An example shows how food items that may have caused the outbreak were identified with the aid of attack rates; in the hypothetical outbreak, multiple foods were found to be implicated. Food X showed a 64% attack rate among those who refrained from eating and a 77% attack rate among those who did. The following process is advised to identify foods suspected of causing an outbreak.

First, compile a list of all foods consumed during the outbreak. Next, categorize the persons involved in the outbreak in two columns: A (ate the food) and B (did not eat the food). One calculates the attack rate among those in categories A and B by dividing the number of ill persons by the total number of persons and multiplying the result by 100. For example, the attack rate in column A is (10/13) × 100 = 77%. After calculating the attack rate, one finds the difference in attack rates (A – B) between those who ate and those who did not eat the food, in this case 13% (77% – 64%). One would repeat this process for each of the foods that were suspected in the outbreak of foodborne illness. Those foods that have the greatest difference in attack rates may be the foods that were responsible for illness. To complete the investigation, additional studies, including cultures and laboratory tests, might be required. In the foregoing situation, "time" is the estimated time interval during which the outbreak occurred—from exposure through appearance of all associated cases of disease.

Table 4.2. Data to Illustrate Calculation of Attack Rates for Food

A (eat the food)				B (did not eat the food)			
Ill	Not Ill	A total	Attack rate	Ill	Not Ill	B total	Attack rate
10	3	13	77%	7	4	11	64%

Source: http://repository.stikim.ac.id/file/22-02-25.pdf

4.3.2. Secondary Attack Rate

An indicator of the spread of a disease within a household or other similar confined unit is produced by the secondary attack rate (EXHIBIT 4–1). "[T]he number of cases of an infection among contacts within the incubation period following exposure to a primary case in relation to the total number of exposed contacts" is the definition of the secondary attack rate. The denominator is limited to susceptible contacts when these can be identified. Contagiousness is gauged by the secondary attack rate, which is helpful in assessing control strategies.

As a hypothetical example of a secondary attack rate, suppose measles spreads from two initial cases of measles brought into a barracks to other residents. Take the example of a secondary attack rate for the hypothetical spread of measles (rubeola) in a military barracks housing Reserve Officers' Training Corps summer cadets. The two initial cases occurred at the beginning of the military summer program and were presumed to have resulted from exposure outside the military base. Of the two initial cases, the case that came to the attention of public health authorities is called the index case. The other case could be considered a coprimary case. This term refers to a case that is related to the index case so closely in time that it is thought to belong to the same generation of cases as the index case. The eight secondary cases occurred approximately 10–12 days after measles symptoms were observed in the index cases. The total number of new cases (initial cases plus secondary cases) in the group was 10. The secondary attack rate was [(10 – 2)/(14 – 2)] × 100 = 66.7%.

Exhibit 4–1

Secondary Attack Rate

The secondary attack rate refers to the spread of disease in a family, household, dwelling unit, dormitory, or similar circumscribed group.

$$\text{Sec ondaryAttrack rate (\%)} = \frac{\text{Number of new cases in group} - \text{initial case(s)}}{\text{Number of susceptible persons in the group} - \text{initial case(s)}}$$

Initial case(s)	=	Index case(s) + coprimaries
Index case(s)	=	Case that first comes to the attention of public health authorities
Coprimaries	=	Cases related to index case so closely in time that they are considered to belong to the same generation of cases

Here is a second example of how to calculate a secondary attack rate:

"Seven cases of hepatitis A occurred among 70 children attending a child care center. Each infected child came from a different family. The total number of persons in the 7 affected families was 32. One incubation period later, 5 family members of the 7 infected children also developed hepatitis A." By applying the formula shown in Exhibit 2–1 to these data, we obtain the following information:

Numerator = 5 (number of cases of hepatitis A among family contacts with hepatitis)

Denominator = 25 = 32 – 7 (total number of family members minus children already infected)

The secondary attack rate is (5/25) × 100 = 20%.

For diseases such as measles, which confer prolonged immunity, the index cases (and coprimaries) are excluded (subtracted) from the denominator. If means are available to determine immune status, any other immune persons also would be excluded from the denominator (as implied by the definition). In addition to assessing the infectivity of an infectious disease agent, the secondary attack rate may be used to evaluate the efficacy of a prophylactic agent (e.g., a vaccine or gamma globulin). It also may be used to trace the secondary spread of a disease of unknown etiology to determine whether there is a transmissible agent.

Here is an example of a calculation of a secondary attack rate for an outbreak of pandemic influenza. Communicable disease experts estimated the secondary attack rate of pandemic influenza during a 2009 outbreak in Western Australian households. The researchers studied a total of 595 households in which pandemic influenza A (H1N1) 2009 had occurred. A household consisted of at least two people residing together in a home but excluded residential institutional settings. The definition of an index case was the first symptomatic case of influenza in a household. Anyone who developed influenza within 1–7 days following the index case's development of symptoms was called a secondary case. Among the 1,589 household contacts of the index cases, 231 persons developed influenza. The secondary attack rate was 14.5% [(231/1,589) × 100].

4.3.3. Case Fatality Rate

The term "case fatality rate" (CFR) describes a percentage that is derived from the total number of deaths among individuals with a disease (or, more broadly, a health condition) over a given period of time. (See Exhibit 4–2). An index of a disease's virulence within a given population is provided by the CFR.

There is occasionally misunderstanding about the difference between a cause-specific mortality rate and a CFR. One key distinction is that, depending on the denominator used, the CFR is not the same as a cause-specific death rate for a given disease. The number of cases of a particular disease serves as the denominator for a CFR for that disease. The size of the population where disease-related mortality occurs serves as the denominator for a cause-specific mortality rate.

Let us examine the types of data that the CFR and a cause-specific death rate yield. Human rabies mortality is extremely rare in the United States, according to recent epidemiologic surveillance. Because rabies is limited to wildlife (epizootic rabies) and is prevented in humans through post-exposure prophylaxis (passive immunization and vaccinations) for those who may have been exposed to rabies, it is uncommon in humans. As a result, the death rate from rabies in any given recent year would be low.

EXHIBIT 4–2

Case Fatality Rate (CFR)

$$\text{CFR } (\%) = \frac{\text{Number of deaths due to disease "X"}}{\text{Number of cases of disease "X"}} \times 100 \text{ during a time period}$$

Note that the numerator and denominator refer to the same time period.

Sample calculation: Assume that an outbreak of plague occurs in an Asian country during the month of January. Health authorities record 98 cases of the disease, all of whom are untreated. Among these, 60 deaths are reported.

CFR = (60/98) × 100 = 61.2%

Examples of diseases with a high CFR are rabies and untreated bubonic plague.

The population as a whole is used as the denominator in the CFR for this condition, which explains why it has a small numerator. As a result, the cause-specific mortality rate from rabies would be quite low. The CFR for rabies, on the other hand, would be high. The disease's fatal outcome, which is influenced by treatment efficacy, is reflected in the CFR. Mortality is still virtually a given in cases of human rabies that could arise from not receiving post-exposure prophylaxis, as has historically been the case.

4.3.4. Basic Reproductive Rate (R_0)

The basic reproductive rate (R_0) is "[a] measure of the number of infections produced on average by an infected individual in the early stages of an epidemic when virtually all contacts are susceptible." Among its possible applications, R0 can be used as a measure of the transmissibility of influenza. As an example, Kenah et al. developed a model to explain influenza transmission patterns during the 2009–2010 pandemic of influenza A (H1N1) 2009 and to project the possible future global pandemics. Their model included factors such as the cities where influenza originated, linkages among cities through air transportation networks, time of the year, and R_0. As a reflection of seasonality, the basic reproductive rate was hypothesized to be higher during the influenza season than at other times of the year.

4.3.5. Procedures Used in the Investigation of Infectious Disease Outbreaks

These include a plethora of methods that John Snow invented, such as case mapping and tabulation, agent identification, and clinical observation. Five fundamental steps can be logically separated out when conducting an outbreak investigation.

1. **Define the Problem:** It is important to determine from the outset whether the outbreak or epidemic is real. For example, suppose a restaurant patron claimed that a gastrointestinal illness she developed was caused by the food she ate in the restaurant. The epidemiologist would need to verify that this was a case of foodborne illness and not a sporadic case of stomach upset. Other cases of the same illness reported to the health department would increase the index of suspicion that the illness originated at the restaurant.
2. **Appraise Existing Data:** This step includes the evaluation of known distributions of cases with respect to person, place, and time. Examples of activities performed at this stage include case identification, making clinical observations, and generation of tables and spot maps.

a. **Case Identification**: This step includes tracking down all cases of disease potentially involved in the outbreak, for instance, in a mass occurrence of foodborne illness. Examples of foodborne illnesses include staphylococcal food poisoning and trichinosis. For communicable diseases, such as TB, contacts of cases need to be identified.

b. **Clinical Observations:** The epidemiologist records the number, types, and patterns of symptoms associated with the disease (e.g., whether the symptoms are primarily gastrointestinal, respiratory, or febrile). Additional clinical information may come from stool samples, cultures, or antibody assays.

c. **Tabulation and Spot Maps:** Cases of disease may be plotted on a map to show geographic clustering (as in an outbreak of TB in a high school). Cases may be tabulated by date or time of onset of symptoms, by demographic characteristics (i.e., age, sex, and race), or by risk categories (e.g., intravenous drug use or occupational exposure). This method is similar to Snow's mapping of cholera cases in the Broad Street district of London in the mid-1800s. It remains an important epidemiologic technique. Graphing cases according to time of onset helps determine the modal incubation period or other aspects of the outbreak.

3. **Identification of Responsible Agent:**

The epidemiologist may be able to determine the agent or other factors responsible for the disease outbreak by estimating the incubation period, by reviewing the specific symptoms, and by noting evidence from cultures and other laboratory tests. In some outbreaks of foodborne illness, it may be possible to link an etiologic agent to cultures of food specimens and stool samples.

4. **Test the Hypothesis:** Collect the data necessary to confirm or refute your initial suspicions. At this stage, it is important to continue to search for additional cases, evaluate alternative sources of data, and begin laboratory investigations to identify the causative agent.
5. **Draw Conclusions and Formulate Practical Applications:** Based on the results of your investigation, it is likely that programs, policies, or procedures will need to be implemented to facilitate long-term surveillance and ultimate prevention of the recurrence of similar outbreaks.

4.4. Epidemiologically Significant Infectious Diseases in the Community

The discussion that follows exemplifies significant infectious disease outbreaks and shows how the previously mentioned techniques are applied. Foodborne, waterborne, vaccine-preventable, sexually transmitted, person-to-person, arthropod-borne, zoonotic, and fungal diseases are among the general categories of these.

4.4.1. Foodborne Illness in the Community

One of the most prevalent infectious disease issues in the community is food contamination, which is linked to the diseases and agents listed in Table 4.4. Staphylococcus aureus is one of the foodborne illness agents listed in Table 4.4. When food is stored at the incorrect temperature, it can lead to outbreaks. A historical example that has been documented happened on February 3, 1975, while a jumbo jet was departing Japan. Nearly 200 passengers became ill when they were served omelets that had been prepared in Alaska and kept for the flight. This episode showed that food contamination can happen in any setting where food is produced. The food production chain's component parts are shown in Figure 4.6. Every location in the figure—from the farm to the house—offers a chance for the spread of contagious foodborne pathogens (Figure 4.5).

Table 4.3. Percent of Reported Food-Based Pathogens During the Study Period 2010–2018

Pathogen	Percent
Campylobacter	**15.5**
Escherichia coli O157:H7	0.9
Hepatitis A	0.4
Listeriosis	0.4
Non-O1 And Other *Vibrio spp.*	0.4
Salmonellosis	**80.1**
Shiga Toxin-producing *E. coli* (STEC)	**1.6**
Shigellosis	**9.35**
Vibrio parahemolyticus	0.2
Vibrio vulnificus	0.4

Disease/Agent	Usual Incubation Period and Syndrome	Mode of Transmission
Classic	12–36 hours,	Contaminated food containing

Source: Akil L. Trends of foodborne diseases in mississippi: Association with racial and economic disparities. Diseases. 2021; 9(4):83. https://doi.org/10.3390/diseases9040083.

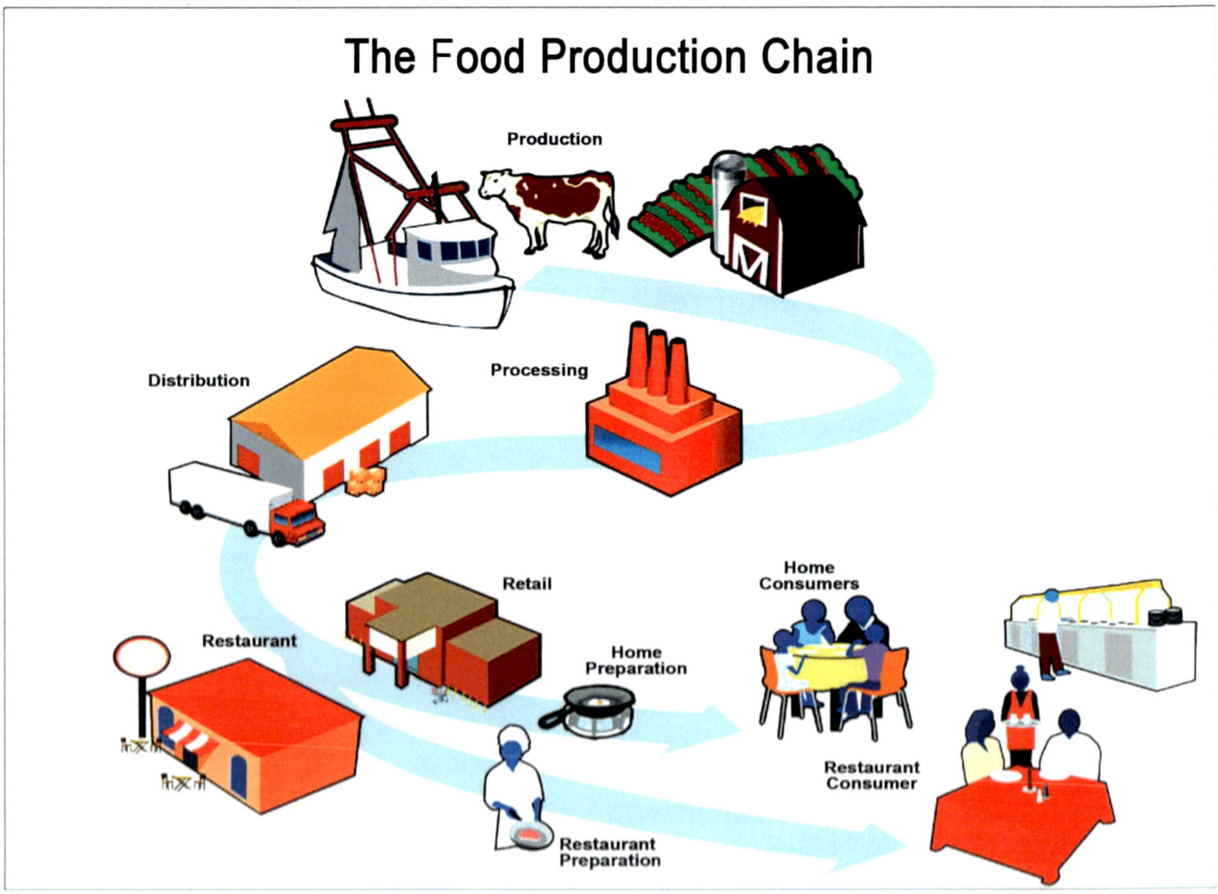

Figure 4.5. *The food production chain.*

Source: Reproduced from CDC. The food production chain—How food gets contaminated. Available at: http://www.cdc.gov/outbreaknet/investigations/figure_food_production.html Accessed: November 3, 2012.

4.4.2. Water- and Foodborne Diseases

Foodborne and waterborne illnesses include schistosomiasis, giardiasis, amebiasis, and legionellosis. In the places where they manifest, these illnesses carry a heavy burden of morbidity and mortality. Numerous human endeavors (e.g., leisure, personal hygiene duties, and disposing of sewage). Schistosomes, the parasitic worms that cause schistosomiasis, contaminate waterways when human wastes are deposited into them. People who come into contact with water run a higher risk of contracting schistosomiasis. Because of human interference in the schistosomiasis life cycle, rates of the disease rose following the construction of the Aswan Dam.

Figure 4.6 shows the schistosomiasis life cycle. The intermediate snail host for schistosomes, *Biomphalaria glabrata*, is necessary for the transmission of schistosomiasis. The three main human-infecting species are *S. mansoni*, *S. intercalulatum*, and *Schistosoma haematobium*. *S. mansoni* is the species that primarily causes schistosomiasis in Africa. Schistosomes have a complicated life cycle that includes switching between human and snail hosts. Please refer to the numbers in the figure:

1. Eggs are illuminated with feces or urine.
2. Under optimal conditions, the eggs hatch and release miracidia.
3. The miracidia swim and penetrate specific snail intermediate hosts.
4. This stage in the snail includes two generations of sporocysts.
5. The snails produce cercariae.
6. Upon release from the snail the infective cercariae swim and penetrate the skin of the human host.
7. In the human host, they shed their tails, becoming schistosomulae.
8. The schistosomulae migrate through several tissues and stages to their residence in the veins.
9. The schistosomulae migrate to the portal blood in the liver and mature into adults.
10. Paired adult worms migrate to mesenteric venules of bowel/rectum (laying eggs that circulate in the liver and shed in stools).

Another example of a food- or water-borne illness is cholera. It manifests as an acute enteric illness with abrupt onset, sporadic vomiting, severe dehydration, acidosis, and collapse of the circulatory system.

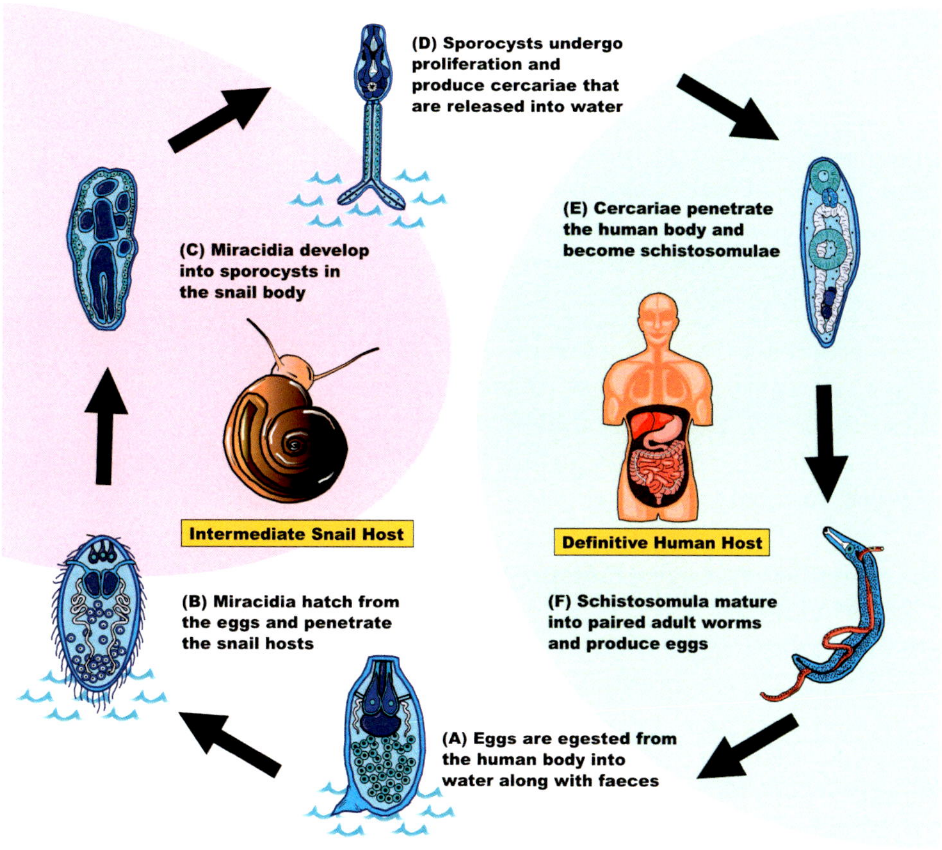

Figure 4.6. *Life cycle of Schistosoma mansoni.*

Source: Au MFF, Williams GA, Hui JHL. Status quo and future perspectives of molecular and genomic studies on the genus biomphalaria—The intermediate snail host of Schistosoma mansoni. International Journal of Molecular Sciences. 2023; 24(5):4895. https://doi.org/10.3390/ijms24054895.

This bacterial disease, which is still prevalent in many developing nations, is caused by Vibrio cholerae. Cholera epidemics struck South America in 1991 and 1992, eventually making their way to Mexico and Central America. In 21 western hemisphere countries, there were over 700,000 cases of cholera and 6,000 deaths from cholera-related causes recorded during this time. With 102 cases reported in the US in 1992, more cases than in any other year since cholera surveillance started in 1961 were recorded. As of December 2010, there had been 8 cases reported of cholera, making it an uncommon condition in the United States, with 5 to 10 cases reported annually between 2005 and 2009. Since 2000, there has been a rising trend in the number of cholera cases worldwide, with about 317,000 cases and 7,500 deaths. Endemic areas include developing nations in Asia and Africa; these nations are frequently populated, have subpar sanitation, and have tainted water supplies. In August of 2007, 30,000 people in Kirkuk, Iraq, were impacted by an outbreak.

A powerful earthquake that struck Haiti on January 12, 2010, severely damaged the country, including its drinking water treatment facilities. The Haitian Ministry of Public Health and Population was notified in October 2010 of multiple cases exhibiting cholera symptoms, which were later verified through laboratory testing. As of November 2010, 16,111 hospitalizations for cholera-related symptoms had occurred (e.g., severe diarrhea with water) had happened. Ten departments, or departments in French, serve as the administrative divisions of Haiti. Seven out of ten Haitian departments had hospitalizations. The department with the most cases reported was Artibonite (10,230). More than a century had passed since the last cholera outbreak in Haiti prior to the 2010 outbreak.

A third example of a water- or foodborne disease agent is *Entamoeba histolytica*, a fairly common parasitic organism associated with amebiasis, which in many cases manifests as intestinal disease. The following excerpt from a report by the Centers for Disease Control and Prevention demonstrates the transmission of *E. histolytica* through colonic irrigation:

The Colorado State Department of Health has reported an outbreak of amebiasis that occurred in the period December 1977–November 1980 and was associated with a chiropractic clinic. All of the cases had received colonic irrigation—a series of enemas performed by machine to "wash out" the colon—a practice that has been gaining popularity recently among some chiropractors, naturopaths, and nutritional counselors. Thirteen cases were confirmed by biopsy review or serologic tests. Seven cases were fatal.

Stool cultures, blood tests, and biopsy studies strongly suggested amoebas as the etiologic agent. Specimens from the colonic irrigation machine were heavily contaminated with fecal bacteria.

4.4.3. Sexually Transmitted Diseases

The HIV/AIDS epidemic, which has had significant domestic and international effects on economic activity and the use of health resources, is one of the category's most pressing public health issues. Descriptions of five cases of Pneumocystis carinii pneumonia among previously healthy men were published in the Morbidity and Mortality Weekly Report in 1981. Because of the human immunodeficiency virus (HIV), the illness was later termed acquired immune deficiency syndrome (AIDS).

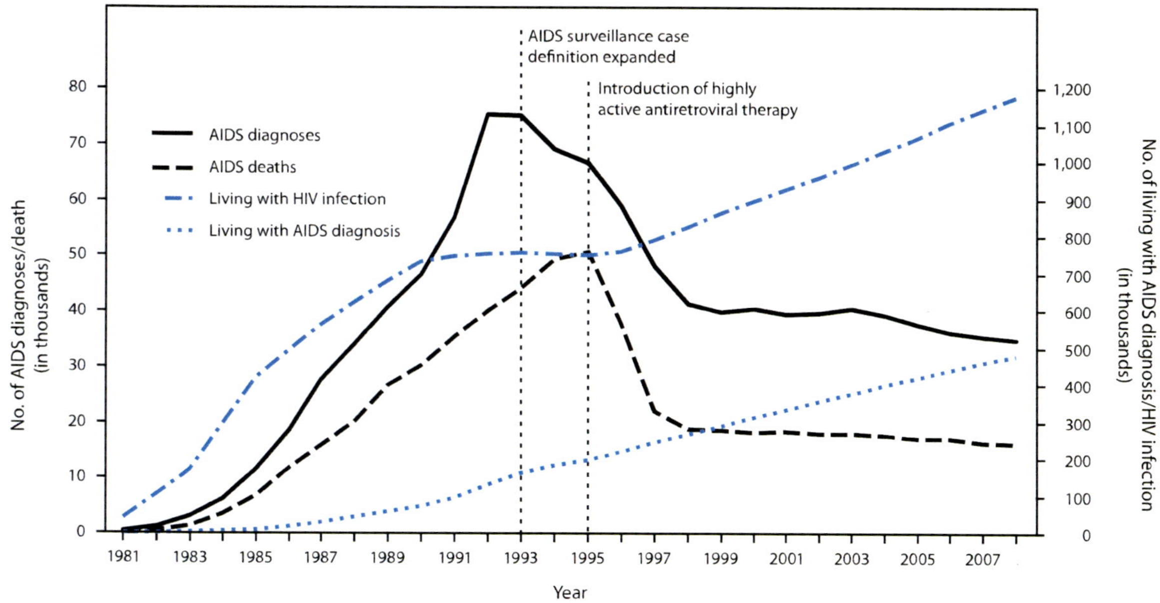

Figure 4.7. *Estimated number of AIDS diagnoses and deaths and estimated number of persons living with AIDS diagnosis and living with diagnosed or undiagnosed HIV infection among persons aged ≥3 years– United States, 1981–2008.*

Source: https://en.m.wikipedia.org/wiki/File:AIDS_diagnoses_and_deaths_in_the_U.S._1981%E2%80%932008.svg.

Following 1981, the number of AIDS cases diagnosed in people 13 years of age and older rose quickly, reaching a peak in 1992 with 75,457 cases. A total of 50,624 people died from AIDS in 1995. Both the number of AIDS diagnoses and deaths has significantly decreased in correlation with highly active antiretroviral therapy. According to CDC estimates, 1,178,350 people had HIV as of 2008; of those, about one-fifth were undiagnosed.

Most HIV infections (75.0%) occur among men. High-risk populations for HIV infection include men who have sex with men (MSN), African Americans, and Hispanics or Latinos. HIV infections are most likely to be undiagnosed among younger persons (13–34 years of age), males with high-risk heterosexual contacts, MSM, and certain ethnic and racial groups (e.g., Asian or Pacific Islanders; American Indians or Alaska natives). Refer to the text box for more information.

When looking at the global HIV epidemic, the situation appears especially dire. According to estimates from the World Health Organization, 34.2 million individuals worldwide were living with HIV in 2011. The estimated number of HIV-positive adults and children residing in the sub-Saharan region of Africa is 23.5 million. Other regions with high prevalence were Latin America and North America, each with 1.4 million people, East Europe/Central Asia, with 1.5 million people, and South/Southeast Asia, with 4.2 million people.

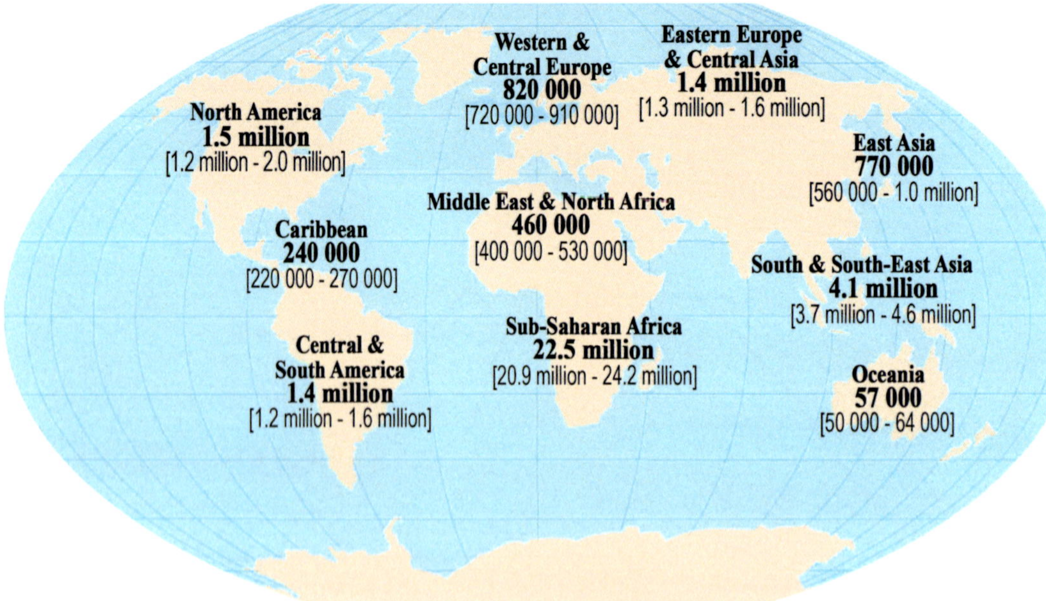

Figure 4.8. *Adults and children estimated to be living with HIV in 2011.*

Source: Courtesy of UNAIDS. Joint United Nations Program on HIV/AIDS (UNAIDS) and World Health Organization (WHO), July 2012 Core Epidemiology Slides, Slide #5.

4.4.4. Vaccine-Preventable Diseases

In the United States, healthcare providers administer routine vaccinations to children aged 0–6 years for the prevention of several diseases. Among these conditions are diphtheria, pertussis, tetanus, *Haemophilus influenzae* type B infections, hepatitis A, hepatitis B, measles, mumps, rubella, paralytic poliomyelitis, influenza, meningococcal meningitis, chicken pox, pneumococcal disease, and rotaviral enteritis. As a result of public health efforts and the availability of effective vaccines, many vaccine-preventable diseases have low incidence in the U.S. According to data reported by the CDC for 2010, the following are the reported numbers of cases of several vaccine-preventable conditions that reached very low frequency:

- Congenital rubella syndrome, 0
- Rubella, 6
- Diphtheria, 0
- Paralytic poliomyelitis, 0

Since the measles vaccine was approved in 1963, the incidence of the disease has generally remained low in the U.S. That being said, there was a significant measles resurgence from 1989 to the early 1990s. In that order, the figures were 2,231 (1992), 9,643 (1991), and 27,786 (1990). There were 138 confirmed cases of measles in 1997, which was a sharp decline from the early 1990s. The incidence was 61 cases in 2010, and the number of cases decreased further in the late 1990s and beyond. Figure 4.9 shows the total number of measles cases that were reported between 1950 and 2009. Part A (1950–1994) illustrates the sharp decline in cases following the measles vaccine's 1963 license. Since 1994, the measles incidence trend in Part B (1974–2009) has been stable.

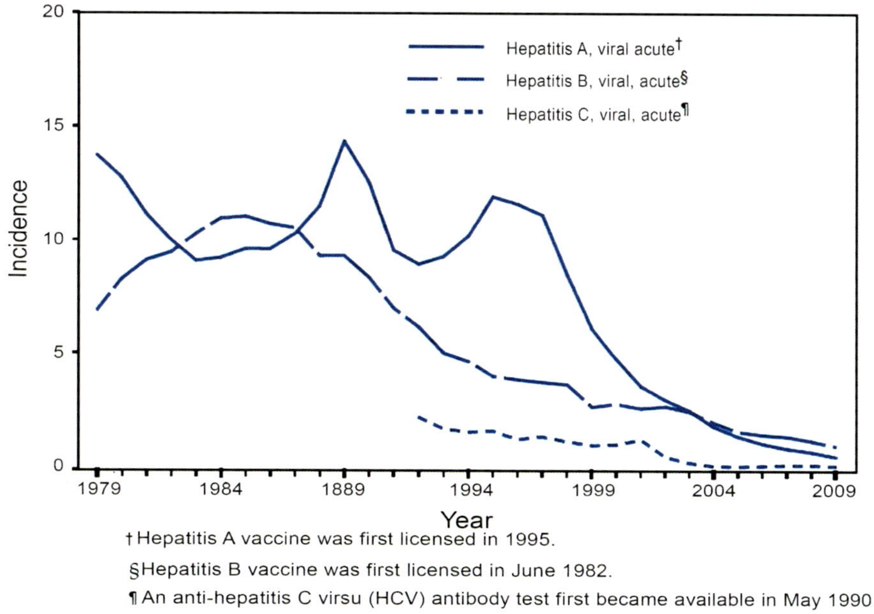

Figure 4.9. *Measles. (Part A) Reported measles cases, by year–United States, 1950–1997. (Part B) measles incidence (per 100,000 population), by year—United States, 1974–2009.*

Sources: (Part A) Reproduced from centers for disease control and prevention. Measles—United States, 1997, MMWR. 1998;47(14): 273. (Part B) reproduced from centers for disease control and prevention. Summary of notifiable diseases—United States, 2009, MMWR. Vol 58, p. 67, May 13, 2011.

In the past, measles outbreaks happened in institutional settings, like colleges or universities, as well as other locations where susceptible people gathered. These days, measles outbreaks are uncommon in the U.S. since the majority of people have received vaccinations. The conclusion that endemic transmission of the measles has been eradicated in the U.S is supported by the epidemiology of the disease. Recent years have seen an increase in sporadic cases that were imported from other nations. Due to the complete coverage of U.S. residents may never be attained, precise surveillance and prompt response to epidemics are crucial for halting the spread of imported measles. Public health professionals will need to keep pushing for high vaccination rates.

4.4.5. Diseases Spread by Person-to-Person Contact

Examples of infectious diseases in this category are aseptic meningitis, group A streptococcal diseases, and respiratory infections

4.4.5.1. Tuberculosis

Tuberculosis is a significant cause of morbidity and mortality throughout the world. However, TB was uncommon in many developed countries, including the United States. Beginning in the late 1980s, TB incidence increased greatly in the United States and then declined toward the end of the 20th century. Reasons for the resurgence of TB included the increasing prevalence of HIV infection, growing numbers of homeless persons, and the importation of cases from endemic areas. From 1984 to 1992, the number of reported TB cases trended upward from 22,201 to 26,673. During this time period 51,700 excess cases were reported, according to statistical models of expected cases in comparison with observed cases. (Figure 4.10 presents a historically important chart that shows this upward trend.) Between 1985 and 1992, the number of cases increased in all racial/ethnic groups except non-Hispanic whites and Native Americans.

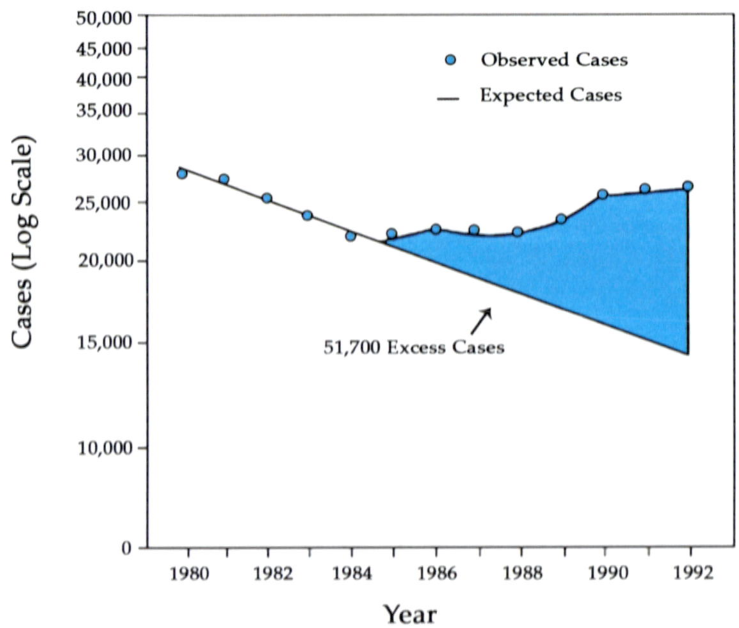

Figure 4.10. *Expected and observed number of tuberculosis cases— United States, 1980–1992.*

Source: Reprinted from Centers for Disease Control and Prevention. Tuberculosis morbidity—United States, 1992. MMWR, vol 42, p 696, September 17, 1993. All age groups except for the over-65 age group showed increases, with the largest increase occurring among the 25- to 44-year age group.

By 2010 TB incidence had declined to 11,181 cases (3.6 per 100,000 population). The most affected groups in the United States were foreign-born individuals and racial and ethnic minorities. At present, two high-risk populations are migrant farm workers and homeless persons. Even though the number of TB cases has declined over time, this communicable disease remains a significant public health threat. In 2007, a suspected case of extensively drug-resistant tuberculosis (XDR TB) commanded media attention.

4.4.5.2. Viral Hepatitis

There are various types of viral hepatitis and related viruses; these are covered in Table 4.4. Hepatitis A, B, and C are the three most prevalent types. Since the late 1980s, the incidence of both hepatitis A and hepatitis B has been progressively decreasing. Children in states with high rates of HAV infections receive vaccinations, which contributes to the decline in the incidence of these infections. Immunization of infants on a regular basis has been associated with a decrease in HBV infections (Figure 4.11) (Table 4.3).

Table 4.4. Five types of Viral Hepatitis

	Hepatitis A virus (HAV)	**Hepatitis B virus (HBV)**	**Hepatitis C virus (HCV)**	**Hepatitis D virus (HDV)**	**Hepatitis E virus (HEV)**
Viral Species	*Hepatovirus A*	*Hepatitis B virus*	*Hepacivirus C*	*Hepatitis delta virus*	*Orthohepevirus A*
Viral Family	*Picornaviridae*	*Hepadnaviridae*	*Flaviviridae*	*Incertae sedis*	*Hepeviridae*
Genome	(+)ssRNA	dsDNA-RT	(+)ssRNA	(−)ssRNA	(+)ssRNA
Antigens		HBsAg, HBeAg	Core antigen	Delta antigen	
Transmission	Enteral	Parenteral	Parenteral	Parenteral	Enteral
Incubation Period	20–40 days	45–160 days	15–150 days	30–60 days	15–60 days
Severity/ Chronicity (Kuo 2012)	Mild; acute	Occasionally severe; 5–10% chronic	Subclinical; 70% chronic	Exacerbates symptoms of HBV; chronic with HBV	Mild in normal patients; severe in pregnant women; acute
Vaccine	2 injections; at least 20 years of protection ("Hepatitis a Q&As for Health Professionals CDC". 9 April 2021.)	3 injections; lifetime protection	None available	None available, but not considered necessary; Hep B vaccine provides protection (Tayor JM (2009))	Investigational (approved in China

Source: https://en.wikipedia.org/wiki/Viral_hepatitis.

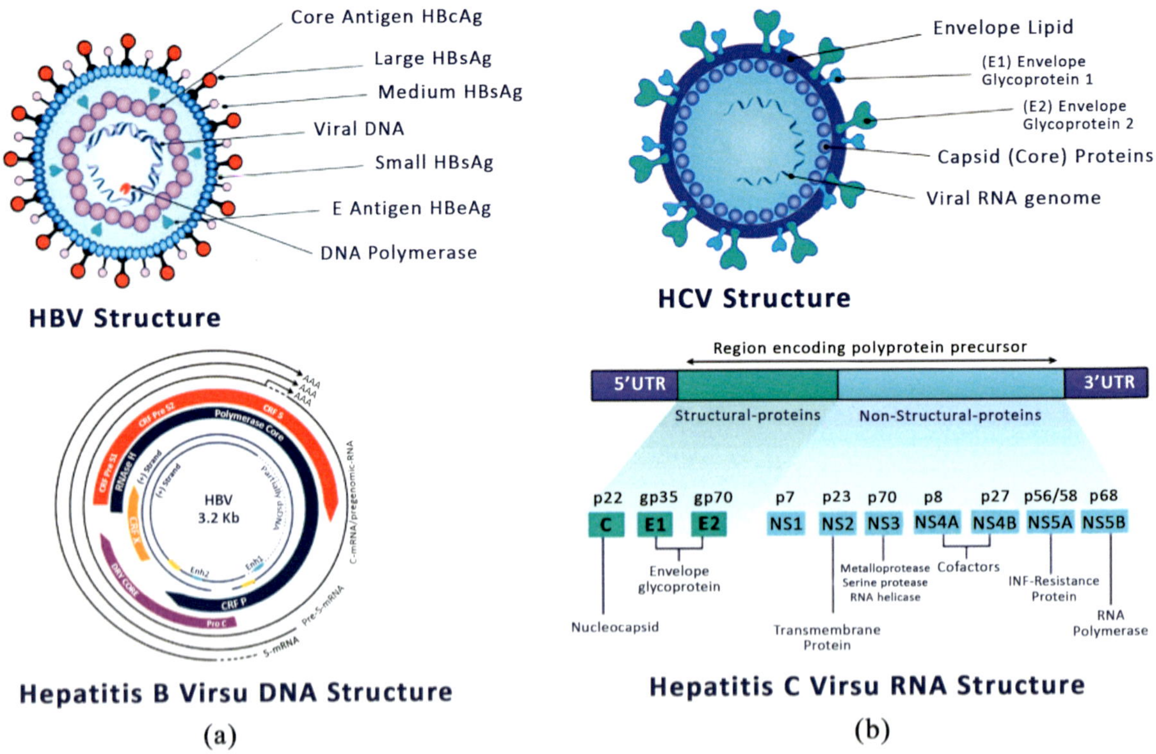

Figure 4.11. *Hepatitis B and C.*

Source: Zaki MYW, Fathi AM, Samir S, Eldafashi N, William KY, Nazmy MH, Fathy M, Gill US, Shetty S. Innate and adaptive immunopathogeneses in viral hepatitis; crucial determinants of hepatocellular carcinoma. Cancers. 2022; 14(5):1255. https://doi.org/10.3390/cancers14051255.

The hepatitis C virus is mainly carried in blood and can be spread through intercourse and injectable drug use. Additionally, the virus is passed from mother to child during the perinatal stage. HCV infection is the primary cause of liver transplantation; about 80% of cases are asymptomatic.

4.4.6. Zoonotic Diseases

An illness known as a zoonosis is one that can naturally travel from vertebrate animals to humans. Zoonotic diseases can be classified as either epizootic (like epidemic human diseases) or enzootic (like endemic human diseases).

Although anthrax (agent, *Bacillus anthracis*) is rare in industrialized nations, workers who handle wool, hair, or hides run the risk of contracting it; it has been purposefully disseminated through the U.S. mail system as a vehicle for bioterrorism. As a result of their exposure during a bioterrorism attack in 2001, several people died.

Brucellosis (undulant fever) is caused by *Brucella abortus*. Those primarily at risk are farmers and others who work with infected cattle, swine, goats, and sheep. Sometimes raw (unpasteurized) milk is a vehicle associated with outbreaks of brucellosis. Leptospirosis (agent [a type of spirochete] leptospira bacteria) is an infrequent condition that can occur among persons who swim in freshwater bodies of water (e.g., rivers and lakes), especially in tropical and sub-tropical regions. Also at risk are rice farmers, fish harvesters, and veterinarians. The bacteria can infect domestic and wild animals; sometimes urine from these infected animals finds its way into freshwater where the bacteria can be hazardous.

Q fever (agent, *Coxiella burnetii*) is a fourth example of a zoonosis. The reservoir for *C. burnetii* is infected livestock (cattle, sheep, and goats). The spectrum of infection in humans ranges from mild to severe, debilitating illness with symptoms similar to those of influenza or pneumonia. Those at high risk for infection include workers and others who come into contact with infected livestock: veterinarians, farmers, agricultural employees, and laboratory personnel. For example, Q fever occurred among laboratory personnel who used sheep in their research at a medical center in San Francisco, California. A more ordinary source of transmission is infected raw milk. See the figure below for data on the distribution of Q fever cases in the United States. A total of 131 cases were reported in 2010, with the greatest number occurring in California and Texas.

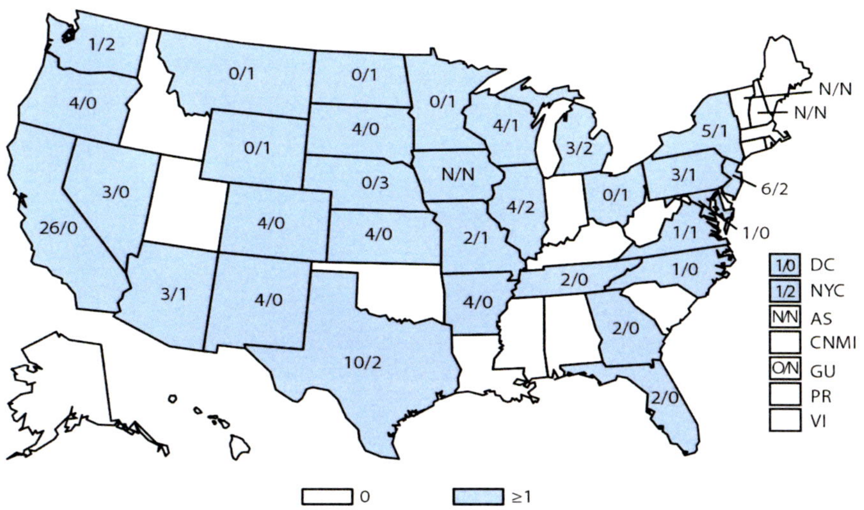

Figure 4.12. *Q fever, acute and chronic, number of reported cases– United States and U.S. territories, 2010.*

Source: Reproduced from Centers for Disease Control and Prevention, Summary of notifiable diseases—United States, 2010. MMWR. Vol 59, No 53, p. 77, 2012.

The disease known as rabies, caused by the rabies virus, affects the central nervous system and is extremely lethal. Most often, saliva from an infected animal's bite spreads the rabies virus. The main way that humans contract rabies is through dog bites. Because of animal control measures, public health laboratories for testing rabies, and vaccination programs for domestic animals, human cases of rabies are uncommon in the United States. The majority of cases of rabies are in wild animals, with bats and raccoons being the most frequently afflicted species. Examine the headline box pertaining to a male U.S. army soldier who became rabid while deployed overseas.

4.4.7. Fungal Diseases

The term "fungus diseases" (mycoses) refers to three main categories of infections: community-acquired infections, hospital-associated infections, and opportunistic infections in individuals with compromised immune systems. Coccidioidomycosis, also known as San Joaquin Valley fever, is an example of a third type of infection. It is primarily caused by the fungus *Coccidioides immitis* and frequently presents as a lung illness. The agent is native to the lower Sonoran life zone, which includes portions of Texas, Mexico, Arizona, and California, as well as the San Joaquin Valley in California. Infection cases have been linked to professions or pursuits that expose vulnerable individuals to contaminated soil (e.g., building, archaeology, and riding dirt bikes). Driving through an area where infection is endemic can lead to infection. At a naval air station in Lemoore, California (Kings County), exposure to a strong dust storm in December 1977 caused an epidemic of coccidioidomycosis. Williams along with others concluded that there was a temporal correlation between the dust storm and the noticeable rise in the number of cases of San Joaquin Valley fever. A coccidioidomycosis outbreak (1,208 cases) was documented in California in 1991. Since coccidioidomycosis is endemic in Kern County, the majority of cases—80%—occurred there.

The numbers of reported cases of coccidioidomycosis in the United States for the year 2009 are shown in Figure 4.13. California and Arizona reported the largest numbers of cases; the incidence of reported U.S. cases of coccidioidomycosis has shown an increasing trend during this century. The CDC estimates that about 60% of coccidioidomycosis cases occur in Arizona.

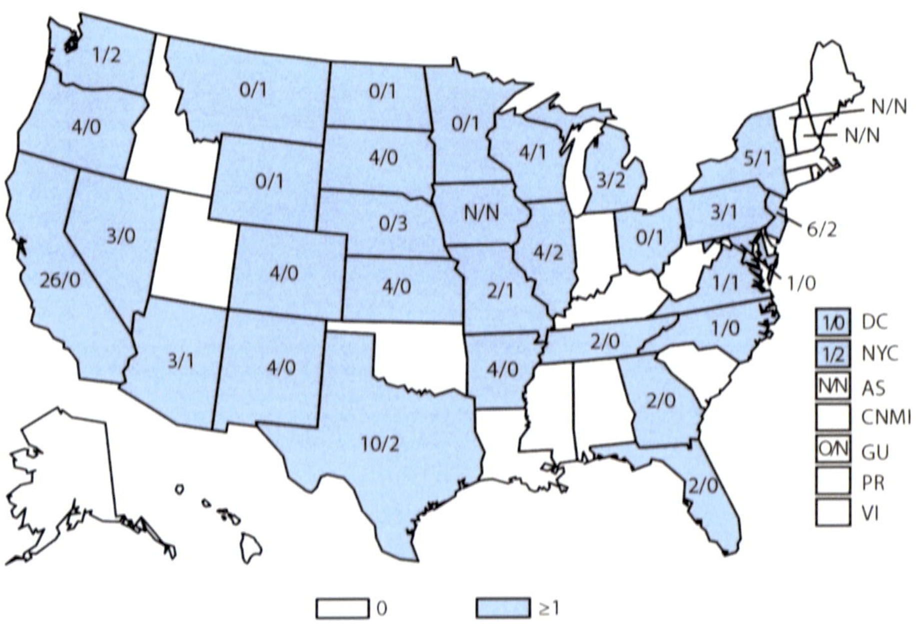

Figure 4.13. *Coccidioidomycosis. Number of reported cases—United States and U.S. territories, 2009.*

Source: Reproduced from Centers for Disease Control and Prevention. Summary of notifiable diseases—United States, 2009. MMWR. Vol 58, No 53, p. 52, May 13, 2011.

4.4.8. Arthropod-Borne Diseases

The term "arthropod-borne diseases" refers to illnesses spread by insect vectors like ticks, mosquitoes, and sand flies. Arboviral diseases are a subset of arthropod-borne illnesses. Arthropod-borne illnesses include West Nile virus, malaria, Lyme disease, Dengue fever, and viral encephalitis.

4.4.8.1. Arboviral Diseases

Arboviral diseases are a diverse group of diseases that involve the transmission of arboviruses (arthropod-borne viruses) between vertebrate hosts (e.g., from animal to animal or from animal to human) by blood-feeding arthropod vectors, the last of which are responsible for the transmission of the encephalitis virus. During 2010 (as of December 25, 2010), the following types and numbers of cases of encephalitis were reported: St. Louis encephalitis, 8 reported cases; California serogroup, 71 reported cases; Eastern equine encephalitis, 10 reported cases; and Western equine encephalitis, 0 reported cases. Enzootic arboviruses afflict animals in a particular locality. Viral isolates or antigens of arboviruses may be found in wild birds, sentinel birds, and captured mosquitoes. Transmission cycles involve interactions between arthropods and vertebrates (birds or small mammals); human beings are incidental or dead-end hosts.

4.4.8.2. Lyme Disease

Lyme disease, a second example of a vector-borne illness, is transmitted by ticks. The reservoir for Lyme disease consists of various species of vertebrate host animals (e.g., mice, squirrels, and shrews). Lyme disease cases are distributed across the United States and showed a steady increase from 1992 to 2006. During this period, the CDC received aggregate reports of 248,074 cases. In 1992 a total of 9,908 cases were reported; in 2006 the number of reported cases was 19,931—an increase of 101%. Figure 4.16 shows a map of the distribution of cases during 2009, with cases heavily concentrated in New England and the upper Midwest (Figure 4.14).

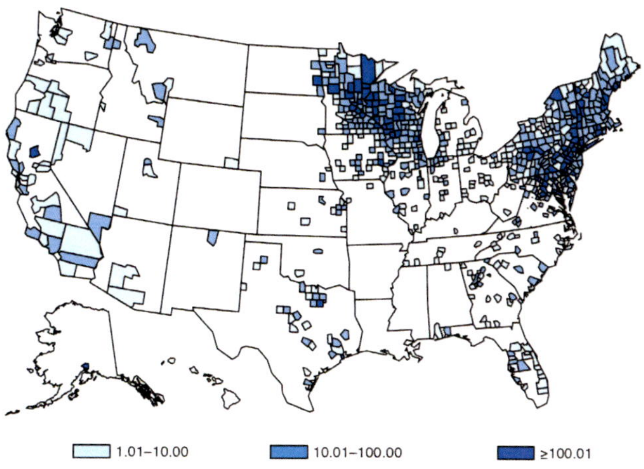

Figure 4.14. *Lyme disease. Incidence per 100,000 population of reported confirmed cases, by county—United States, 2009.*

Source: Reproduced from Centers for Disease Control and Prevention. Summary of notifiable diseases —United States, 2009. MMWR. Vol 58, No 53, p. 66, May 13, 2011.

A Closer Look

Epidemiologic Triangle

The epidemiologic triangle, also known as the epidemiologic triad, is a conceptual framework that illustrates the interplay between three essential components in the occurrence of disease: the host, the agent, and the environment. Understanding the dynamics of these three elements is fundamental to elucidating the complex pathways through which diseases develop and spread within populations.

At the center of the epidemiologic triangle is the host, which refers to the individual or population susceptible to a particular disease. Host factors such as age, sex, genetics, immune status, and underlying health conditions influence the likelihood of developing the disease and its severity. By studying characteristics of the host population, epidemiologists can identify risk factors and vulnerable groups, informing targeted interventions and preventive measures to protect public health.

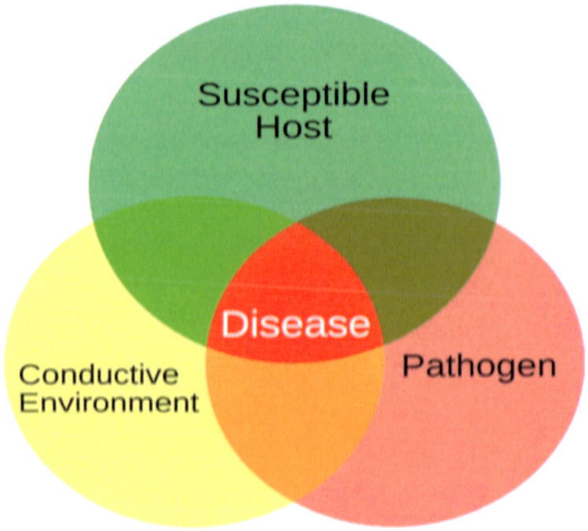

Source: By Johannes Rössel (talk) – Self-made, after Image: Plant Disease Triangle.png, CC BY-SA 3.0, https://commons.wikimedia.org/w/index.php?curid=4265044.

The second component of the epidemiologic triangle is the agent, which encompasses the biological, chemical, or physical factors that cause or contribute to the development of disease. Agents can include infectious pathogens such as bacteria, viruses, and parasites, as well as non-infectious factors like toxins, allergens, and carcinogens. Understanding the characteristics of the agent, including its mode of transmission, virulence, and environmental survival, is critical for designing effective control strategies and interventions to prevent disease transmission and mitigate its impact on the population.

The third component of the epidemiologic triangle is the environment, which encompasses the physical, social, economic, and cultural factors that surround the host and influence their exposure to disease agents. Environmental factors such as living conditions, sanitation, access to healthcare, socioeconomic status, and cultural practices shape the risk of disease transmission and impact the health outcomes of individuals and communities. Epidemiologists study the role of environmental factors in disease causation and transmission to inform policies and interventions aimed at addressing underlying social determinants of health and reducing health disparities.

By considering the interactions between the host, agent, and environment, the epidemiologic triangle provides a framework for understanding the multifactorial nature of disease causation and transmission. This holistic approach allows epidemiologists to identify modifiable risk factors, assess the impact of interventions, and develop comprehensive strategies for disease prevention and control. By addressing all components of the epidemiologic triangle, public health efforts can effectively reduce the burden of disease and improve the health and well-being of populations worldwide.

Summary

- Infectious disease epidemiology focuses on understanding the patterns and dynamics of infectious diseases within populations. Key aspects of infectious disease epidemiology include studying the transmission, distribution, and determinants of infections, as well as developing strategies for prevention and control.
- Infectious disease epidemiology investigates the factors influencing disease spread within populations. These factors encompass a wide range of biological, environmental, social, and behavioral determinants. Biological factors may include characteristics of the pathogen itself, such as its virulence and ability to survive outside the host. Environmental factors encompass conditions that affect the survival and transmission of pathogens, such as temperature, humidity, and sanitation practices. Social and behavioral factors, including population density, travel patterns, and healthcare-seeking behaviors, also play crucial roles in disease transmission.
- The term "direct transmission of diseases" describes the spread of an infection from person to person when there is no intermediary contaminated object contact. As in the case of the spread of sexually transmitted diseases, direct transmission can happen, for instance, through contact with the blood or bodily fluids of an infected individual.
- An infection that has not yet crossed the clinical horizon is referred to as inapparent (subclinical) (i.e. lacks symptoms that are clinically evident). However, inapparent infections can have a significant epidemiologic impact because asymptomatic people have the potential to spread the illness to other vulnerable hosts, some of whom may become seriously ill.
- Herd immunity is the ability of a population, group, or community to fend off an infectious disease when a sizable portion of the population is immune (either from prior infections or vaccinations). Although not every member of the population is immune, herd immunity protects the population as a whole when immune individuals stop a disease from spreading to unimmunized people.
- An attack rate, a variant of an incidence rate, is used when the occurrence of disease among a population at risk increases greatly over a short period of time, often related to a specific exposure.
- The term "case fatality rate" (CFR) describes a percentage that is derived from the total number of deaths among individuals with a disease (or, more broadly, a health condition) over a given period of time.

References

1. Armstrong, G. L., Hollingsworth, J., & Morris, J. G. (1996). Emerging foodborne pathogens: Escherichia coli 0157:H7 as a model of entry of a new pathogen into the food supply of the developed world. *Epidemiologic Reviews, 18*, 29–51.
2. Carcione, D., Giele, C. M., Goggin, L. S., et al. (2009). Secondary attack rate of pandemic influenza A(H1N1)2009 in Western Australian households. *Euro Surveillance, 29*, 1–8.

3. Centers for Disease Control and Prevention. (1981). Amebiasis associated with colonic irrigation—Colorado. *MMWR, 30*, 101–102.
4. Centers for Disease Control and Prevention. (1992). Measles surveillance—United States, 1991. *MMWR, 41*, 1–11.
5. Centers for Disease Control and Prevention. (1993). Coccidioidomycosis—United States, 1991–1992. *MMWR, 42*, 21–24.
6. Centers for Disease Control and Prevention. (1993). Tuberculosis morbidity—United States, 1992. *MMWR, 42*, 696–697, 703–704.
7. Centers for Disease Control and Prevention. (1993). Update: cholera—Western Hemisphere, 1992. *MMWR, 42*, 89–91.
8. Centers for Disease Control and Prevention. (2011). HIV surveillance—United States, 1981–2008. *MMWR, 60*, 689–693.
9. Centers for Disease Control and Prevention. (2011). Trends in tuberculosis—United States, 2010. *MMWR, 60*, 333–337.
10. Centers for Disease Control and Prevention. (2011). West Nile virus disease and other arboviral diseases—United States, 2010. *MMWR, 60*, 1009–1013.
11. Cutler, S. J., Fooks, A. R., & van der Poel, W. H. M. (2010). Public health threat of new, reemerging, and neglected zoonoses in the industrialized world. *Emerging Infectious Diseases, 16*(1), 1–7.
12. Heron, M. P. (2008). Deaths: Leading causes for 2008. *National Vital Statistics Reports, 60*(6). Hyattsville, MD: National Center for Health Statistics.
13. Kenah, E., Chao, D. L., Matrajt, L., et al. (2011). The global transmission and control of influenza. *PLOS ONE, 6*(5), e19515. doi: 10.1371/journal.pone.0019515.
14. Klevens, R. M., Edwards, J. R., Richards, C. L., Jr., et al. (2007). Estimating healthcare-associated infections and deaths in U.S. hospitals, 2002. *Public Health Reports, 122*, 160–166.
15. Morse, S. S. (1996). Patterns and predictability in emerging infections. *Hospital Practice, 31*, 85–91, 96–101, 104.
16. Williams, P. L., Mendez, P., & Smyth, L. T. (1979). Symptomatic coccidioidomycosis following a severe natural dust storm. *Chest, 76*, 566–569.
17. Yoder, J. S., & Beach, M. J. (2007). Giardiasis surveillance—United States, 2003–2005. *MMWR Surveillance Summaries, 56*(SS-7), 11–18.

Chapter 5

DESCRIPTIVE EPIDEMIOLOGY

Contents

Introduction

Descriptive epidemiology serves as a fundamental pillar in the field of public health, providing a comprehensive framework for understanding the distribution of diseases within populations. Descriptive epidemiology focuses on characterizing the patterns and trends of diseases based on factors such as time, place, and person. By systematically analyzing epidemiological data, researchers can uncover crucial insights into the burden of diseases, identify populations at higher risk, and inform targeted interventions and policy decisions.

One key aspect of descriptive epidemiology is the examination of disease occurrence over time. Temporal analysis allows epidemiologists to detect changes in disease incidence, prevalence, and mortality rates, providing essential information about disease trends and fluctuations. By identifying seasonal variations, secular trends, and epidemic outbreaks, temporal patterns help guide public health surveillance efforts and inform timely response strategies to mitigate the spread of infectious diseases and manage chronic conditions.

Furthermore, descriptive epidemiology explores the spatial distribution of diseases, examining geographical variations in disease occurrence and clustering. Through geographic mapping and spatial analysis techniques, researchers can identify hotspots of disease activity, spatial patterns of transmission, and disparities in healthcare access. Spatial epidemiology plays a crucial role in identifying environmental risk factors, understanding disease transmission dynamics, and targeting resources to areas with the greatest need, thereby supporting efforts to reduce health inequities and improve population health outcomes.

Moreover, descriptive epidemiology considers the characteristics of affected populations, including demographic factors such as age, sex, race/ethnicity, and socioeconomic status. By analyzing differences in disease burden across population subgroups, researchers can identify vulnerable populations and disparities in health outcomes. This information is essential for designing culturally sensitive interventions, addressing social determinants of health, and promoting health equity to ensure that all individuals have access to appropriate healthcare services and resources.

Orientation and Directional Terms

Term	Definition	Illustration
Coronary Heart Disease (CHD)	Coronary heart disease (CHD), also known as coronary artery disease (CAD), is a condition characterized by the narrowing or blockage of the coronary arteries, which supply oxygen-rich blood to the heart muscle.	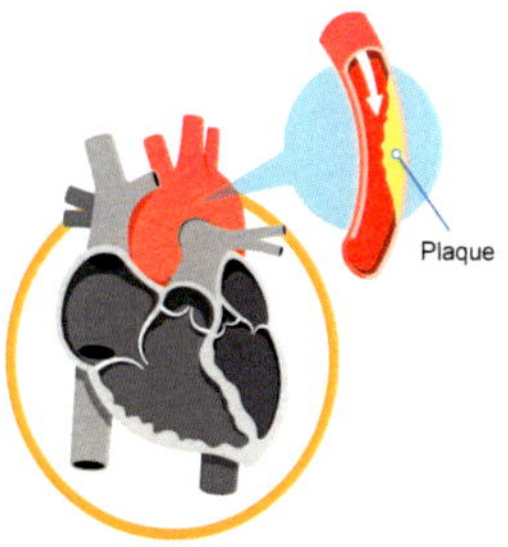
Legionnaires' Disease	Legionnaires' (LEE-juh-nares) disease is a serious type of pneumonia (lung infection) caused by Legionella (LEE-juh-nell-a) bacteria. People can get sick when they breathe in small droplets of water or accidently swallow water containing Legionella into the lungs.	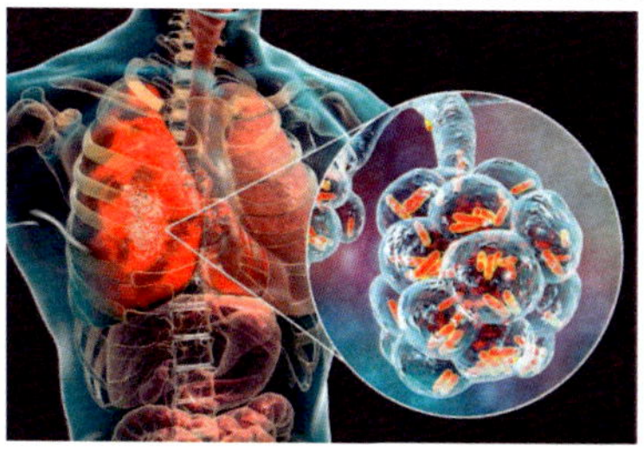
Hantavirus Pulmonary Syndrome (HPS)	Hantavirus Pulmonary Syndrome (HPS) Hantavirus Pulmonary Syndrome (HPS) is a severe, sometimes fatal, respiratory disease in humans caused by infection with hantaviruses. Anyone who comes into contact with rodents that carry hantaviruses is at risk of HPS.	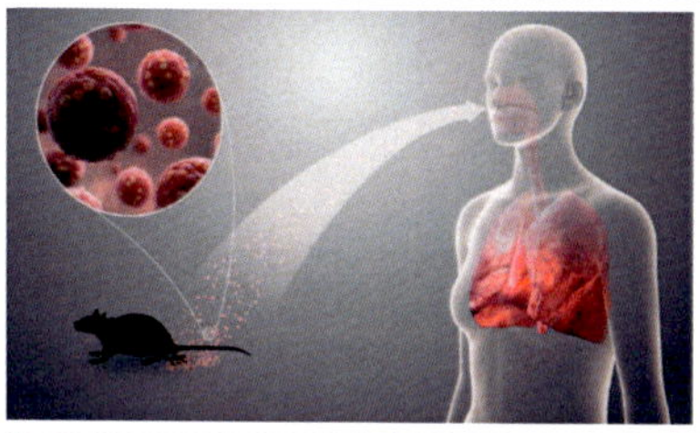
Analytic Epidemiologic	Analytic epidemiologic studies measure the association between a particular exposure and a disease, using information collected from individuals, rather than from the aggregate population.	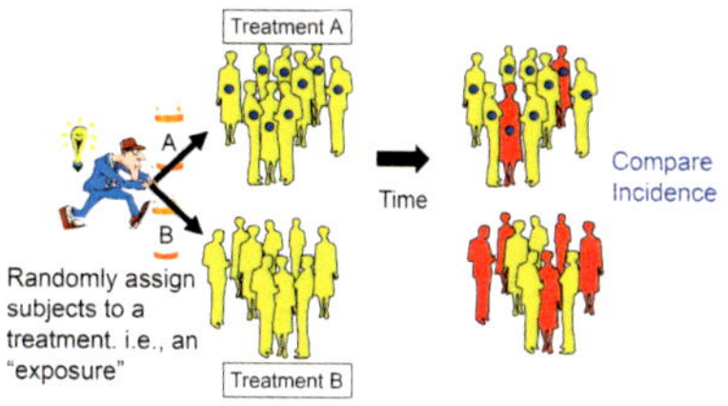
Disease Surveillance	Disease surveillance is an ongoing process that involves the systematic collection, analysis, interpretation, and dissemination of information regarding the occurrence of diseases in defined populations for public health action to reduce morbidity and mortality.	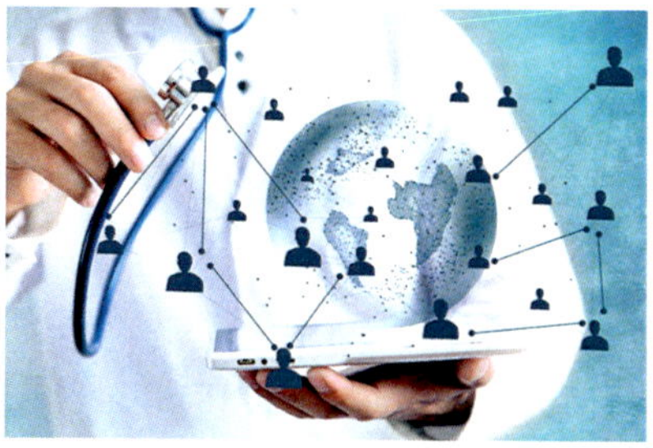

5.1. The Basics of Descriptive Epidemiology

The fundamental tenet of epidemiology is that illnesses don't just happen; rather, they follow patterns that are indicative of underlying causes. The approaches to characterizing disease patterns covered in this chapter generally fall into one of three categories: person, place, or time. The term "person" refers to the group of people who are impacted, such as young versus old, males versus females, rich versus poor, migrants versus nonmigrants, and more educated versus less educated. The term "place" refers to the location of the problem, such as cities versus rural areas, certain states versus others, the United States versus other counties, high altitudes versus low altitudes, areas with abundant or little rainfall, polluted areas versus uncontaminated areas, etc. Time describes when the problem first appeared, such as a sudden increase over a brief period of time, or does it gradually worsen over years or drastically increase in just a few years?

To find etiologic hints, epidemiologists must precisely and meticulously describe patterns of disease occurrence. The writers will list descriptive qualities (e.g., age, sex, and race—all individual characteristics)—that aid in the identification of disease patterns and the creation of theories about the underlying causes of those patterns. Person, place, and time are variables that impact a variety of exposures related to lifestyle, behavioral patterns, access to healthcare, and exposure to environmental hazards, among other things, and which either directly or indirectly relate to the occurrence of illnesses. For example, there is a higher likelihood of unintentional death or injury associated with male gender; behavior patterns typical of a specific racial or ethnic group may influence subcultural stress levels and coping strategies. Race and ethnicity are sometimes referred to as social group membership factors that influence how people perceive, understand, and respond to their social and physical surroundings. People's perceptions, interpretations, and reactions to health risks are influenced by their membership in particular social groups. We will also note that certain combinations of variables, like age and sex, are significant.

5.1.1. Objectives of Descriptive Epidemiology

There are three broad objectives of descriptive epidemiology; these are to:

1. permit evaluation of trends in health and disease and comparisons among countries and subgroups within countries; this objective includes monitoring of known diseases as well as the identification of emerging problems
2. provide a basis for planning, provision, and evaluation of health services; data needed for efficient allocation of resources often come from descriptive epidemiologic studies
3. identify problems to be studied by analytic methods and suggest areas that may be fruitful for investigation

The widespread AIDS epidemic serves as an example of how these goals are attained. The AIDS epidemic's emergence was indicated by descriptive data on the epidemiology of the disease (objective 1), which also helped with the allocation of hospital beds and treatment centers (objective 2) and sparked etiologic investigations into the reasons why gay and bisexual men and intravenous drug users were more likely to contract the disease than other groups (objective 3).

5.1.2. Mill's Canons

What is the source of hypotheses that guide

epidemiologic research? The logical processes for deriving hypotheses are patterned after John Stuart Mill's canons of inductive reasoning. The following are four of his canons:

1. The method of difference
2. The method of agreement
3. The method of concomitant variation
4. The method of residues

5.1.2.1. The Method of Difference

Except for one factor, every factor in two or more domains is the same. It is hypothesized that differences in the single causative factor account for the variation in the frequency of disease between the two settings. In epidemiologic research, the method of difference has been applied extensively. It bears a resemblance to traditional experimental design. An instance of its potential application could be observed in the investigation of how physical activity mitigates the morbidity associated with coronary heart disease (CHD). Assume that comparisons were made between groups of workers in the same factory with respect to age, diet, socioeconomic status, and other constants (equivalent for all groups). Employees in a given factory can have comparable lifestyles and sociodemographic traits but very different levels of physical activity at work. It is hypothesized that variations in CHD morbidity are caused by physical activity levels; sedentary workers are therefore more likely to experience a heart attack than physically active workers.

5.1.2.2. The Method of Agreement

There is a single factor that unites many diverse settings. The common factor is thought to be the disease's cause. For example, the prevalence of long-term respiratory conditions like emphyzema and asthma tends to rise wherever air pollution is present. This finding supports the theory that lung illnesses may be exacerbated by air pollution, if it exists.

5.1.2.3. The Method of Concomitant Variation

A disease's frequency varies based on a factor's potency. This correlation implies that the factor is the disease's causal agent. Numerous studies have demonstrated, for instance, the connection between the incidence of lung diseases (e.g., lung cancer, bronchitis, emphyzema, and lung cancer) and the quantity of cigarettes smoked: Smoking increases the risk of developing lung cancer and other lung conditions.

5.1.2.4. The Method of Residues

Using the residues method, one can ascertain which factor or combination of factors has the biggest influence on a dependent variable by deducting potential causal factors. When studying heart disease, statistical techniques akin to the residues method (e.g., multiple regression analysis) have been employed to ascertain the potential correlation between various risk factors and the development of a coronary heart attack or cardiac death. It is possible to quantify how much a person's blood lipid level, diet, stress level, and heredity all contribute to CHD. The most influential factor can then be identified.

5.1.2.5. The Method of Analogy (Additional Criterion from MacMahon and Pugh)

The pattern of the distribution of an illness with an unclear etiology is comparable to that of a known illness, which epidemiologists have studied in greater detail. According to this information, there may be some similarities between the causes of known and unknown diseases. There are numerous instances of the analogy method in the field of infectious diseases. Unknown diseases that are localized to specific regions and spread during the summer may be spread by a vector, such as (e.g., mosquito). Another example is the symptoms of Legionnaires' disease, which resembled those caused by an infectious respiratory disease agent that could be bacterial or viral in origin. Epidemiologists found that Legionnaires' disease is caused by a bacterium that only survives in water (e.g., in cooling towers for air conditioning), and could aerosolize, potentially leading to airborne transmission. MacMahon states that the method of analogy was applied in two cases, sometimes incorrectly: the first involved the hypothesis of an infectious agent for multiple sclerosis (MS), based on the similarity between the geographic distribution of MS and that of polio; the second involved the hypothesis of a relationship between smoking and tuberculosis, based on the analogy of smoking and lung cancer.

5.1.3. Three Approaches to Descriptive Epidemiology

Cross-sectional studies, case series, and case reports (counts) are the three methods used in descriptive epidemiology. While counts can be useful in epidemiologic disease descriptions, they are typically more informative when expressed as a proportion relative to a denominator. The most basic type of descriptive epidemiology could be thought of as collections of case reports, or counts. A case report can serve as a basis for investigating underlying causal mechanisms and introducing preventive interventions. Astute clinical observations of unusual cases can also catalyze further investigations to see if a large number of cases with similar presentations exist.

Here is an example of a case report:

Methylene chloride, a volatile chemical used in paint strippers, produces a highly toxic vapor. Workers who use methylene chloride-based strippers must wear protective equipment such as respirators. The Centers for Disease Control and Prevention reported a death associated with use of a chemical for stripping bathtubs. "In March 2010, the coowner of a Michigan-based bathtub refinishing company, aged 52 years, was refinishing a bathtub in an apartment bathroom that was approximately 5 feet by 8 feet ... He was using an aircraft paint stripper product that contains 60–100% methylene chloride ... The [bathroom] fan was off. The man wore latex gloves and did not wear respiratory protection ... Approximately 90 minutes after the man began working on the tub, he did not answer a call to his cellular telephone. An apartment maintenance man entered the apartment to look for the man and found him behind the closed bathroom door, unresponsive, and slumped over the tub ... [After treatment by emergency responders and transportation to a hospital], the man was declared dead at the hospital.

A series of cases is the second strategy. Expanding a single observation to a series of cases may be desirable because it can be challenging to make definitive conclusions from a single case report. This series usually consists of an overview of the features of a list of patients from one or more primary clinical settings presented in chronological order. Summaries measures can be produced from a collection of observations to aid in the distillation of typical features. As an illustration, consider the five cases of hantavirus pulmonary syndrome (HPS) among five pediatric patients that the CDC reported in 2009. The extremely deadly HPS disease is linked to rodent contact. There were five cases in 2009 from the CDC were:

- **Case 1:** (May 16, 2009)—a boy aged 6 years who lived in Colorado was hospitalized for a severe illness. Within 2 hours of admission to the hospital, the boy died from apparent cardiac failure secondary to shock. Rodent droppings and nesting materials were found under the boy's bed and near his home.
- **Case 2:** (June 7, 2009)—an adolescent boy aged 14 years went to a Washington emergency department

with a 5-day history of shortness of breath, chest pain, cough, and fever. The boy subsequently recovered. Rodent fecal contamination was found in a container of corn that the youth reported hand grinding.

- **Case 3:** (July 12, 2009)—a boy aged 6 years went to a Colorado emergency department with a 5-day history of fever and later recovered. The boy had been bitten on the finger by a mouse.
- **Case 4:** (July 12, 2009)—a girl aged 9 years who lived in Arizona went to a New Mexico hospital with chest pain and shortness of breath. The patient was hospitalized until August 5. Evidence of rodents was found in several houses that the girl had frequented.
- **Case 5:** (November 25, 2009)—an adolescent boy aged 13 years went to a California emergency department with a five-day history of fever and other symptoms. The patient recovered after a period of hospitalization. Mice had been trapped in the youth's kitchen and garage approximately three months before the disease onset.

Cross-sectional studies carried out at different times are used in the third main method of descriptive epidemiology. These are population surveys used to determine the frequency of a condition or exposures. Data from multiple cross-sectional surveys conducted at various times can occasionally be used to look at trends over time in the prevalence of a disease or risk factors.

5.1.4. Advantage and Disadvantage of Descriptive Epidemiology

1. Advantages of Descriptive Epidemiology

i. **Identification of Disease Patterns:** Descriptive epidemiology enables the identification of patterns and trends in disease occurrence within a population. By examining factors such as time, place, and person, epidemiologists can discern spatial clusters, seasonal variations, and demographic disparities in disease distribution. This information is essential for detecting outbreaks, understanding endemic patterns, and targeting public health interventions effectively.

ii. **Early Detection of Outbreaks:** Descriptive epidemiology plays a crucial role in the early detection of outbreaks and emerging infectious diseases. By monitoring changes in disease incidence over time and across geographic regions, public health authorities can swiftly identify unusual spikes or clusters of cases that may indicate a potential outbreak. Timely detection allows for rapid response efforts, including case investigation, contact tracing, and implementation of control measures to contain the spread of disease.

iii. **Assessment of Disease Burden:** Descriptive epidemiology provides valuable insights into the burden of disease within a population. By quantifying disease frequency and distribution, epidemiologists can estimate disease prevalence, incidence rates, and mortality rates, thus assessing the public health impact of specific diseases. This information is essential for prioritizing health resources, planning healthcare services, and advocating for policy interventions to address the most significant health challenges facing communities.

iv. **Identification of Risk Factors:**

Descriptive epidemiology serves as a starting point for identifying potential risk factors associated with disease occurrence. By analyzing demographic characteristics, geographic locations, and temporal trends, researchers can identify populations at higher risk of disease and explore factors contributing to their vulnerability. This knowledge informs further analytical studies, including analytical epidemiology and experimental research, aimed at elucidating causal relationships between risk factors and disease outcomes.

v. **Planning and Evaluation of Public Health Interventions:** Descriptive epidemiology informs the planning, implementation, and evaluation of public health interventions aimed at disease prevention and control. By understanding the distribution and determinants of disease, policymakers can design targeted interventions tailored to specific population needs. Moreover, descriptive data serve as a baseline for evaluating the effectiveness of interventions over time, allowing for continuous monitoring and adjustment of public health strategies to maximize impact.

2. **Disadvantages of Descriptive Epidemiology**

i. **Limited Causal Inference:** Descriptive epidemiology alone does not establish causal relationships between exposures and disease outcomes. While it can identify associations and patterns in disease occurrence, it does not provide evidence of causation. Without further analytical studies, such as cohort or case-control studies, it is challenging to determine whether observed associations are truly causal or the result of confounding factors.

ii. **Lack of Individual-Level Data:** Descriptive epidemiology often relies on aggregated population-level data, which may obscure individual-level variability and heterogeneity in disease risk factors. This limitation can hinder the identification of specific risk factors and their interactions at the individual level. Moreover, aggregated data may mask disparities within subpopulations, such as socioeconomic or racial/ethnic disparities in disease burden, thus impeding targeted interventions to address health inequities.

iii. **Inability to Control for Confounding Factors:** Descriptive epidemiology does not allow for the control of confounding factors, which may bias the observed associations between exposures and disease outcomes. Confounding variables, such as age, sex, or socioeconomic status, can distort the interpretation of descriptive data and lead to erroneous conclusions about the relationship between exposures and disease. Without analytical techniques to adjust for confounding, the validity of descriptive findings may be compromised.

iv. **Limited Temporal Resolution:** Descriptive epidemiology may have limited temporal resolution, particularly when relying on routinely collected surveillance data or aggregated administrative records. These data sources may have delays in reporting or lack real-time updates, limiting the timeliness of disease surveillance and outbreak detection. In rapidly evolving public health emergencies, such as pandemics or bioterrorism events, delays in data availability can impede rapid response efforts and mitigation strategies.

v. **Incomplete Data and Reporting Biases:** Descriptive epidemiology is subject to biases related to data completeness, accuracy, and reporting practices. Surveillance systems may suffer from underreporting of cases, misclassification errors, or inconsistencies in case definitions, leading to inaccurate estimates of disease burden and trends. Moreover, reporting biases may vary by geographic region, healthcare setting, or demographic group, further complicating the interpretation of descriptive data and limiting their generalizability.

5.2. Characteristics of Persons

5.2.1. Age

When describing the incidence of almost any disease or illness, age is arguably the most crucial factor to take into account because rates of diseases specific to a given age typically vary more than rates defined by nearly any other personal characteristic. For this reason, when comparing the disease burden across populations, public health professionals frequently use age-specific rates. The main causes of death showed varying trends in mortality depending on the age group. Data for 2007 reveal the following trends for specific causes:

- Unintentional injuries—the leading cause of death for persons aged 1–44 years
- Homicide and suicide—important causes of death for the 1–44 years age group
- Stroke, influenza, and pneumonia—among the 10 leading causes of death for the 1–44 years age group
- Chronic diseases (e.g., cancer and heart disease)—leading causes of death among persons aged 45 years and older
- Human immunodeficiency virus (HIV)—among the leading causes in the 20–44 age group

Childhood to early adolescence (1–14 years): Imperaturity and congenital birth defects are two of the leading causes of death for infants in this age group. Certain communicable and infectious diseases' incidence (e.g., the measles, mumps, chicken pox, otitis media (ear infections), and meningococcal disease) tend to strike most frequently in childhood.

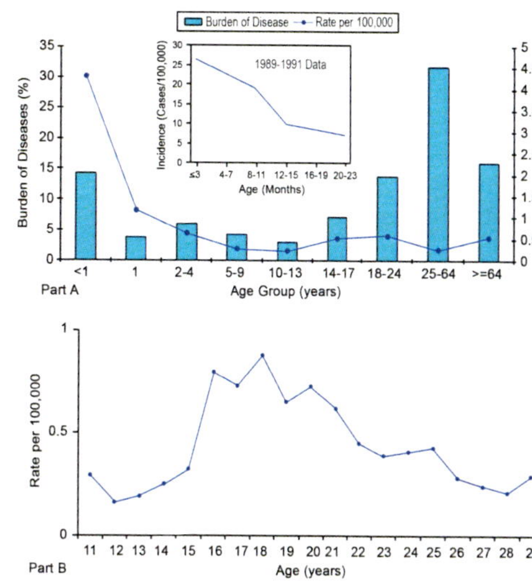

Figure 5.1. *Meningococcal disease.*

Source: Robert H. Friis and Thomas Sellers; Epidemiology for public health practice; ISBN 978-1-4496-5158-9 (pbk.)

Data on the incidence and burden of meningococcal disease (number of cases) per 100,000 people are shown in Figure 5.1 for the years 2000–2009. The disease exhibits a bimodal distribution, with peaks in incidence seen in children under the age of one year and in teenagers (roughly 18 years old, as part B of the figure illustrates). The data from 1989–1991 in the inset of part A shows how the incidence of meningococcal disease decreased from early infancy to roughly age 2. Approximately 16% of cases occurred in infants and 20% occurred in adolescents and young adults over the course of the ten-year period, 2000–2009 (part A).

Unintentional injuries, sometimes referred to as accidents, were the main cause of death for individuals between the ages of 1 and 14 from 1997 to 2007. Heart disease, cancer, and congenital deformities were other significant causes of death. (See part A of Figure 5.2.) Teenage years through young adulthood (15–24 years): Unintentional injuries, homicide, and suicide were the three main causes of death for teenagers and young adults in 2007. Heart disease and cancer ranked fourth and fifth, respectively. (See part B of Figure 5.2.).

Unplanned pregnancies, drug addiction, tobacco use, and binge drinking are additional health issues that impact teenagers. These conditions also affect young adults. Among youths aged 12 to 17, alcohol, marijuana, and tobacco are the most popular drugs. Furthermore, nearly one-twelfth of the youth in this age group abuse prescription medications, including stimulants, opioids, and depressants that affect the central nervous system.

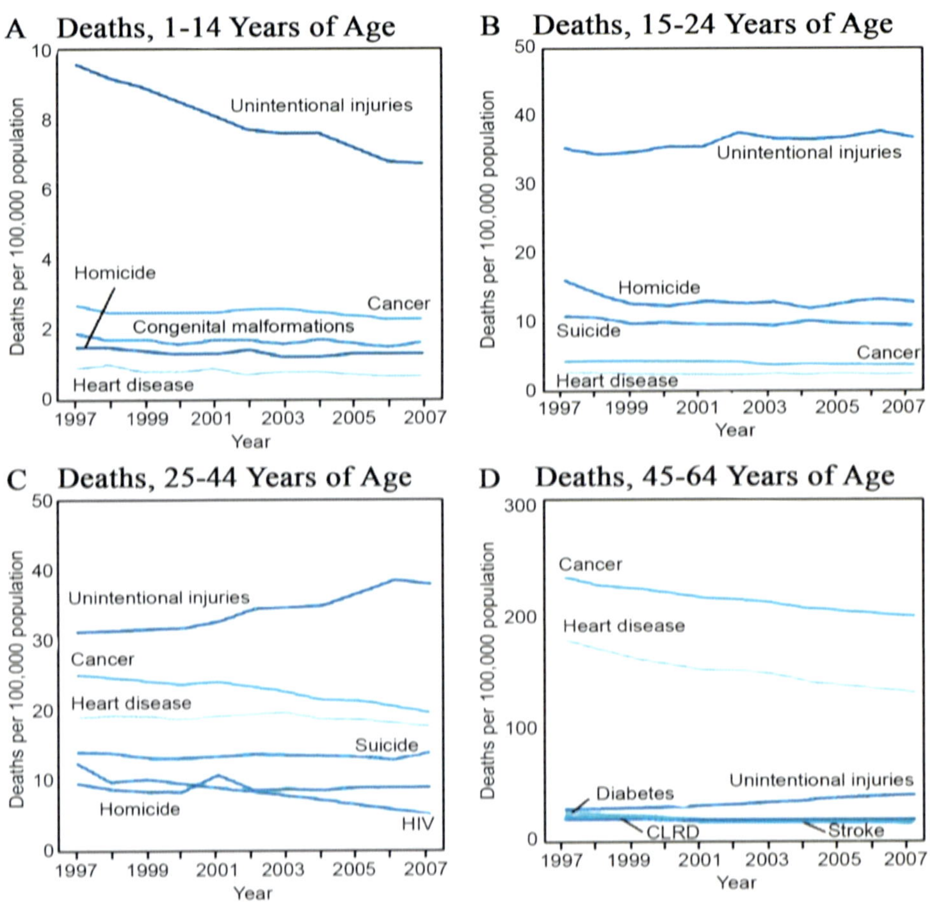

Figure 5.2. *Death rates.*

Source: Robert H. Friis and Thomas Sellers; Epidemiology for public health practice; ISBN 978-1-4496-5158-9 (pbk.)

Additionally, this age group is impacted by poor lifestyle choices. Teenagers love to play with the newest technology, so too much "screen time" can result in obesity, which raises the risk of developing chronic diseases later in life. Young people tend to choose high-fat foods and sugary drinks that are widely available and sold in enormous containers.

Adults (25–44 years old): From 1997 to 2007, unintentional injuries were the main cause of death in this age group. Not only were homicide and HIV disease among the leading causes of death, but also heart disease, cancer, and suicide. The most frequent causes of cancer-related mortality in men were lung, brain, and colon cancers. Cervical, lung, and breast cancers were the most common causes among women. Men had three times the death rate from homicide and suicide as women did. HIV disease, which was the sixth most common cause of death in 2007, has seen a more than 50% decrease in death rates since the 1990s.

Older adults (45–65): After the age of 45, chronic illnesses like cancer and heart disease are the main causes of morbidity and death. These conditions affect younger people as well, but they are the main causes of death for older adults. For instance, the generally linear increase in age-specific incidence rates after age 45 across all racial groups shows that the incidence of cancer rises with age (Figure 5.3).

The elderly (65+): Heart disorders, cancerous neoplasms, cerebrovascular illnesses, chronic lower respiratory diseases (CLRD), and Alzheimer's disease were the top five causes of death in 2007. It should be noted that the apparent decline in cancer incidence (Figure 5.3) around the age group of 80–84 is somewhat misleading due to unstable estimates caused by the very elderly categories' smaller numerators and denominators than those of other age groups. Accidental injuries came in at number eight on the list of the main causes of death.

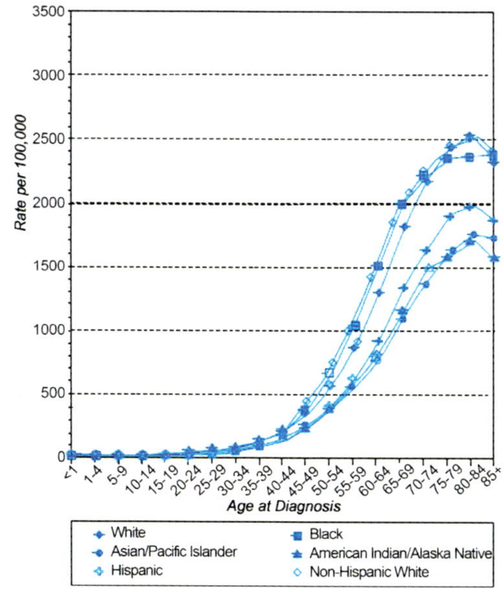

Figure 5.3. *Age-standardized incidence rates of gastric cancer*

Source: Robert H. Friis and Thomas Sellers; Epidemiology for public health practice; ISBN 978-1-4496-5158-9 (pbk.)

As a result of declining physical and mental health, some elderly persons experience impairment of their ability to live independently. In 2010, approximately 4% of seniors aged 65–74 years and 11% aged 75 years and older suffered from limitations in activities of daily living (ADLs). (Refer to Figure 5.4.) The term ADL refers to "needing the help of other persons with personal care needs, such as eating, bathing, dressing, or getting around inside [the] home ... [b]ecause of a physical, mental, or emotional problem." Limitations of instrumental activities of daily living (IADLs) were even more frequent. The definition of IADLs is "need[ing] the help of other persons in handling routine needs, such as everyday household chores, doing necessary business, shopping or getting around for other purposes ... [b]ecause of a physical, mental, or emotional problem."

More than 6% of persons aged 65–74 years and 19% of persons aged 75 years and older had limitations in IADLs.

MacMahon and Pugh suggested four reasons for age associations. These are:

- the validity of diagnoses across the lifespan
- multimodality (e.g., bimodality) of trends
- latency effects
- action of the "human biological clock"

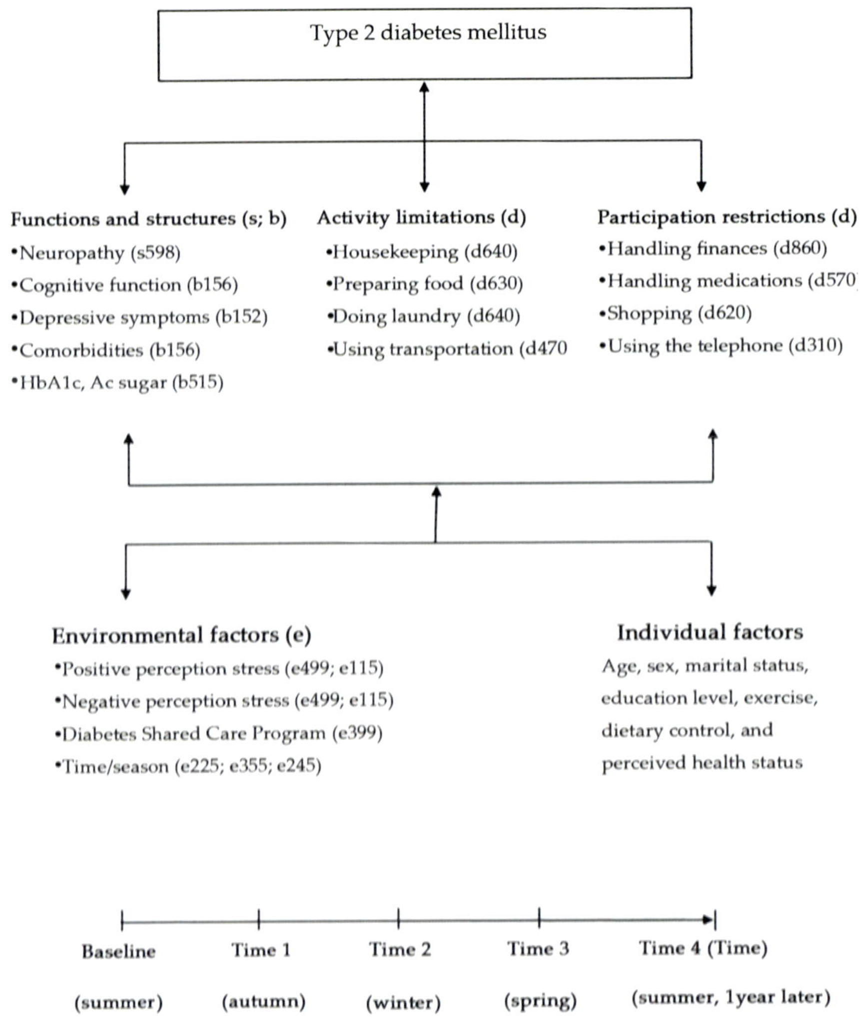

Figure 5.4. *Adults with activity limitations.*

Source: Tai, L.A., Tsai, L.Y. & Chiu, Y.C. Relation of environmental factors with activity limitations and participation restrictions in older adults with diabetes mellitus over time: an international classification of functioning framework perspective. BMC Geriatr 23, 335 (2023). https://doi.org/10.1186/s12877-023-03977-0.

Classification errors may have an impact on the validity of diagnoses throughout the life span. An age-incidence graph may exhibit distortions due to imprecise age-specific incidence rates within older age groups. Errors may arise from the challenge of accurately determining the cause of death in elderly patients, who may have multiple causes of morbidity at the same time.

Certain medical conditions exhibit multimodal age-specific incidence curves, which indicate that the frequency of the diseases varies with age and exhibits multiple peaks and declines. Meningococcal illness and tuberculosis (TB), which peaks between the ages of 0 and 4 and 20 and 29 respectively, are two examples. Hodgkin's disease is a third example, with peaks observed in the mid-20s and early 70s. For these conditions, bimodal (two-peak) distributions might imply two distinct causal mechanisms. For instance, in the case of tuberculosis, the peak in the disease's prevalence during early adulthood may be related to young people's heightened vulnerability to infectious diseases, while the peak during this age group's increased social interaction or changes in the immune system brought on by puberty could be explained.

The lengthy latency period between environmental exposures and the onset of some diseases is another explanation for how age affects mortality. A lengthy latency period can be defined as the years that elapse between first being exposed to a possible carcinogen and the development of cancer later in life. Moreover, older people have had more opportunities than younger people to be exposed to a variety of possible carcinogens. Older people would be more susceptible to the cumulative effects of such exposures than younger people. The term "human biological clock" phenomenon describes an innate mechanism linked to heightened susceptibility to illness. For instance, the immune system may weaken with age, increasing the susceptibility of tissues to illness. The biological clock also manifests itself in the activation of conditions thought to have a genetic origin (e.g., Alzheimer's disease, which typically affects elderly people).

The life cycle and behavioral phenomena are associated with additional causes of age-related changes in rates of morbidity and mortality, which MacMahon and Pugh do not specify. The relative importance of unintentional injuries, homicide, and suicide as causes of death varies significantly depending on the age group; these differences are influenced by personal behavior and risk-taking, particularly in the case of younger people. Diabetes and other chronic diseases are influenced by lifestyle choices, and a large number of these conditions are thought to have important behavioral components. Certain issues related to aging that affect the older end of the age distribution serve as examples of life cycle phenomena. More epidemiologic research on the subjects of falls, the bereavement process, the "retirement syndrome," and other behaviorally related health issues among the elderly will be required as the number of older people rises.

5.2.2. Sex

Numerous epidemiological studies have demonstrated differences between the sexes in a variety of health-related phenomena, such as morbidity and mortality. Data on mortality disparities by sex are discussed in the discussion that follows. Since 1980, the population age-adjusted death rate in the U.S. has decreased, with a few calendar years out of the exception. From birth until the age of 85 and beyond, men typically have greater all-cause age-specific mortality rates than women; in 2005, the ratio of male to female age-adjusted death rates was 1.4 to 1. The 10 primary sites with the highest rates within the categories of race and ethnicity are shown in Figure 5.5, along with the age-adjusted male-female invasive cancer incidence rates. Prostate cancer in men (150.0 per 100,000) and breast cancer in women (119.0 per 100,000) are the cancer diagnoses with the highest incidence rates per 100,000. Lung and bronchus cancer is the second most common type of cancer; the incidence rate is slightly higher in men than in women (86.8 versus 54.3 per 100,000). Lung and bronchus cancer is the primary cause of cancer-related death in both genders.

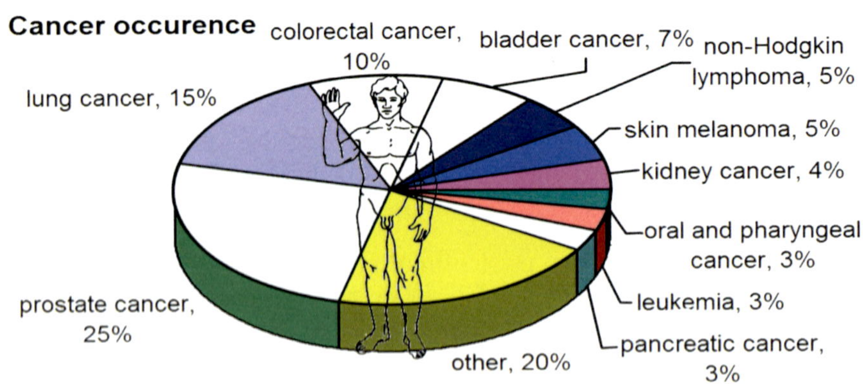

Figure 5.5. *Age-adjusted invasive cancer incidence rates.*

Source: By Mikael Häggström. When using this image in external works, it may be cited as: Häggström, Mikael (2014). "Medical gallery of Mikael Häggström 2014". WikiJournal of Medicine 1 (2). DOI:10.15347/wjm/2014.008. ISSN 2002-4436. Public Domain. or By Mikael Häggström, used with permission. - Own work, using reference: Jemal A, Siegel R, Ward E et al. (2008). " Cancer statistics, 2008&quot. CA Cancer J Clin 58 (2): 71–96. DOI:10.3322/CA.2007.0010. PMID 18287387., Public Domain, https://commons.wikimedia.org/w/index.php?curid=9505746.

5.2.3. Race/Ethnicity

The United States of America is becoming more diverse than it has ever been in terms of race and ethnicity. To a certain degree, race and ethnicity are ill-defined traits that frequently coincide with religion and nativity. The term "natality" describes the place of a person's or a relative's birth. The terms "native-born" and "foreign-born" are frequently used in epidemiology. Scientists have suggested that rather than being a biological construct, race is a social and cultural construct. In Census 2000, the U.S. Bureau of the Census classified race into five major categories: white; black or African American; American Indian and Alaska Native; Asian; and Native Hawaiian and other Pacific Islander. To a degree, race tends to be synonymous with ethnicity because people who come from a particular racial stock also may have a common ethnic and cultural identification. Also, the assignment of some individuals to a particular racial classification on the basis of observed characteristics may be difficult. Often, one must ask the respondent to elect the racial group with which he or she identifies. People may give inconsistent answers to questions about race or ethnicity, or they may respond differently on different occasions based on how they understand the question's intended meaning. Individuals with mixed-race parentage may also have difficulty being classified. An option for respondents to check a multiracial category was introduced in the 2000 census. Modifications to racial category definitions impact the denominators (i.e., the numbers within a specific racial subgroup) of rates used to monitor different health outcomes and the evaluations of unmet needs and social disparities in health that follow. Figure 5.6 demonstrates the racial/ethnic composition of the U.S. population during 2006. At that time, the total population was estimated to be 299,398,485. The largest percentage of the population was white (73.9%). Hispanics and Latinos made up 14.8% of the population (44,252,278). People who self-identify with this ethnic group can be of any race; therefore, Hispanics and Latinos are not shown in the figure.

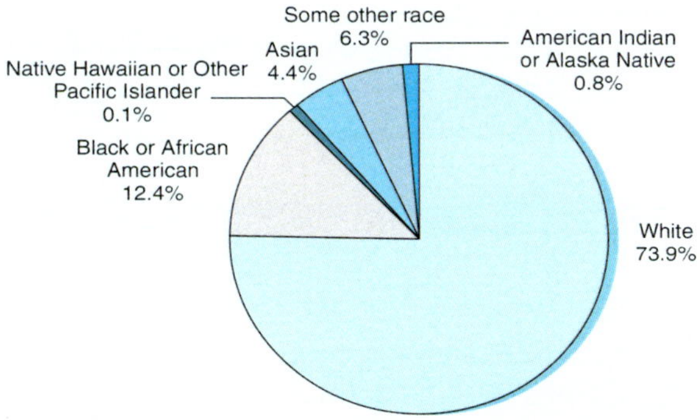

Figure 5.6. *Racial/ethnic distribution of the population of the United States, 2006 estimates. Data for individuals who declare only one race.*

Source: Source: Robert H. Friis and Thomas Sellers; Epidemiology for public health practice; ISBN 978-1-4496-5158-9 (pbk.)

There are many examples of racial/ethnic differences in health characteristics. The following section lists three conditions that show such variations:

- **Asthma:** Individuals who classified themselves as Hispanic had a lower frequency of self-reported asthma than either non-Hispanic whites or non-Hispanic blacks (Figure 5.7).

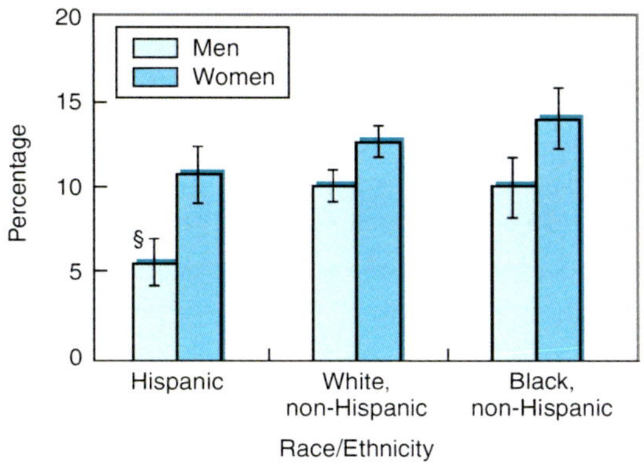

Figure 5.7. *Estimated percentage of adults aged ≥18 years with asthma, by sex and race/ethnicity—National Health Interview Survey, United States, 2006.*

Source: Reprinted from Centers for Disease Control and Prevention, National Center for Health Statistics. QuickStats: Estimated percentage of adults aged ≥18 years with asthma, by sex and race/ethnicity—National Health Interview Survey, United States, 2006. MMWR. 2007;56:1193.

- **No Usual Source of Medical Care:** For persons diagnosed with diabetes, serious heart conditions, and hypertension, non-Hispanic whites and non-Hispanic blacks reported less frequently that they had no usual source of care than Hispanics (Figure 5.8).

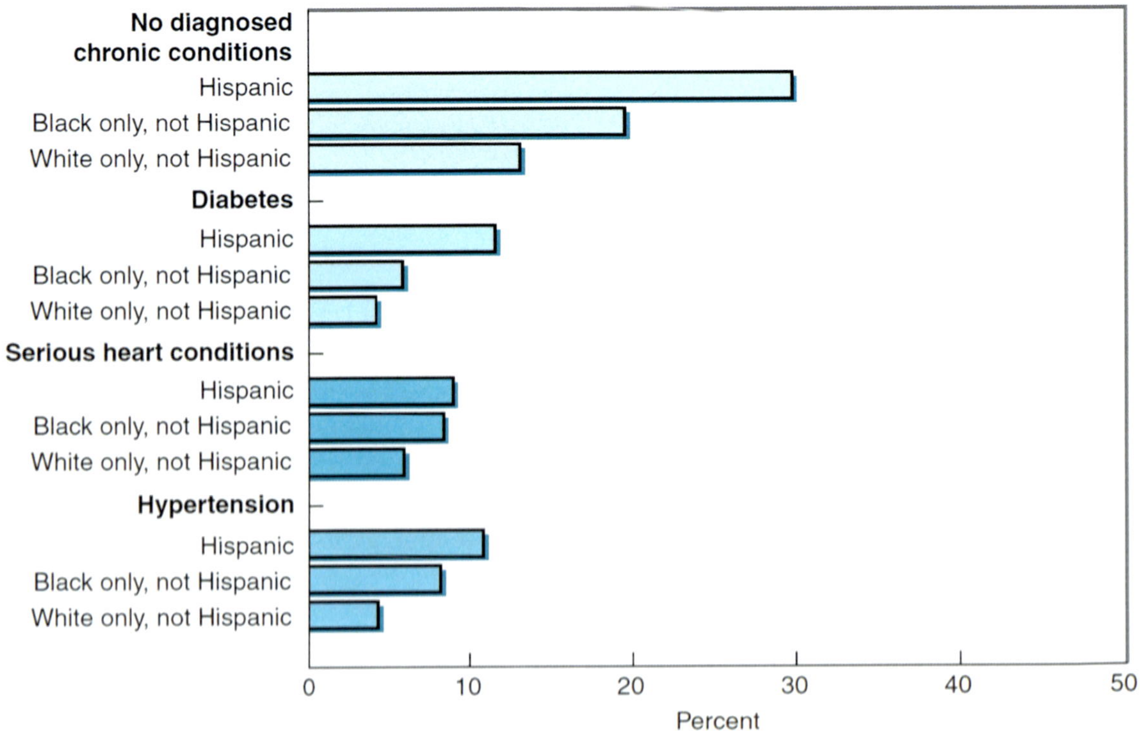

Figure 5.8. *No usual source of care among adults 45–64 years of age, by selected diagnosed chronic conditions and race and Hispanic origin: United States, 2004–2005.*

Source: Reprinted from National Center for Health Statistics. Health, United States, 2007. With Chartbook on Trends in the Health of Americans. Hyattsville, MD: 2007:69.

- **Gonorrhea Incidence:** Black, non-Hispanic individuals had the highest incidence of gonorrhea during 1991 through 2006. However, the incidence of gonorrhea among African Americans declined during this period, although in 2006 it remained above the incidence for other racial and ethnic groups. Non-Hispanic blacks in 2006 had a gonorrhea incidence that was about eighteen times greater than that reported for non-Hispanic whites (Figure 5.9).

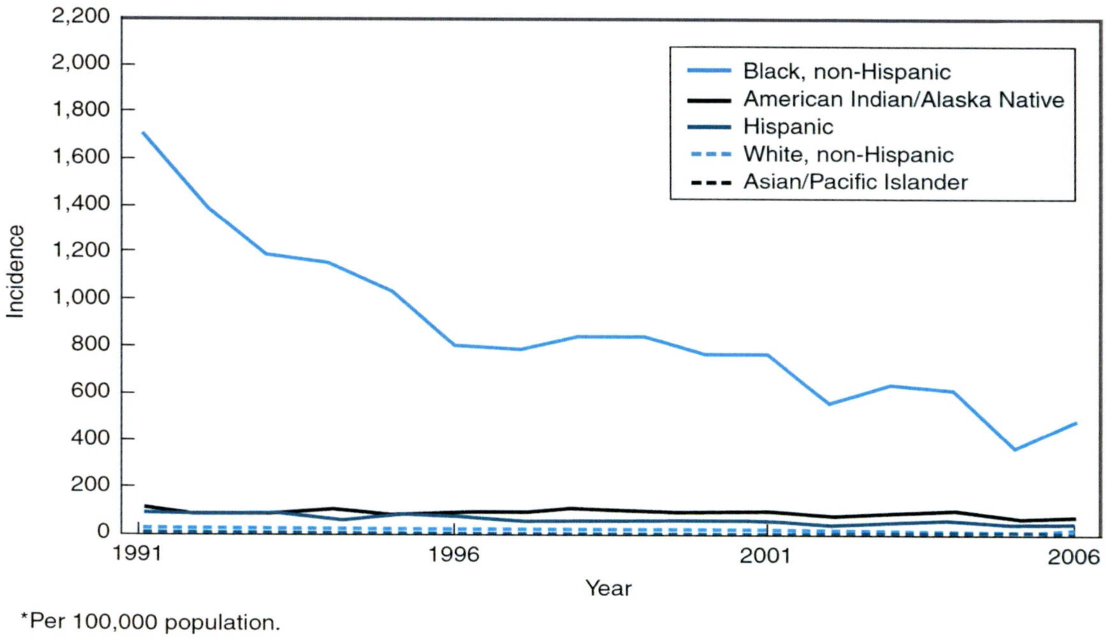

Figure 5.9. *Gonorrhea. Incidence, by race/ethnicity—United States, 1991–2006.*

Source: Reprinted from Centers for Disease Control and Prevention. Summary of Notifiable Diseases—United States, 2006. MMWR. 2008;55:52.

5.2.4. Socioeconomic Status

The term "descriptive term for a person's position in society" refers to socioeconomic status (SES). SES is frequently calculated as a composite measure of three interconnected factors: an individual's income, education, and type of employment. Income level alone is sometimes used as a measure of socioeconomic status (SES); in other situations, two or more of the aforementioned dimensions are combined to create composite variables. People with high SES would be defined by a three-factor measure as those who have the highest levels of income, education, and employment status (e.g., the professions of learning). There is a strong and inverse relationship between the levels of morbidity and mortality and the social class gradient, or the variability in SES from high to low and vice versa. The excess morbidity and mortality experienced by those in the lowest socioeconomic status (SES) categories can be attributed to a variety of factors, including mental health issues, infectious and chronic diseases, and the negative effects of an unhealthy lifestyle.

One of the dimensions of SES—income—may be expressed in several ways in order to assess its impact on health outcomes. For example, poverty is a measure based on before tax income from sources such as earnings, unemployment compensation, interest, and Social Security. Poverty exists when a single person or family has an income that is below a threshold set by the U.S. Bureau of the Census. For a single person younger than 65 years of age, the poverty level in 2006 was annual income below the threshold of $10,488. Poverty status also can be computed for families; the poverty level is a function of the total income of a family in relationship to the poverty threshold. The threshold for poverty in a family is determined by summing the poverty thresholds provided by the U.S. Bureau of the Census for each adult and child living in a family. The poverty threshold for a five-person family that comprises three adults and two children was $24,662 in 2006.

The ratio of income to poverty is the ratio of an individual's or family's income to their poverty threshold. If the five-person family had an annual income of $25,000 in 2006, their income-to-poverty ratio was $25,000/$24,662 or 1.01; this ratio can also be expressed as 101% of poverty. Similarly, all poverty ratios can also be expressed as percentages; to illustrate, 200% of poverty refers to an income that is twice the poverty threshold. The relationship between dental care accessibility and health outcomes is exemplified. Please see Figure 5.10 for an illustration of U. S. data for 2005 regarding individuals who did not visit a dentist in the previous year. The four levels of poverty were used to categorize the respondents. The percentage of people who did not visit the dentist increased stepwise across all age groups as the percentage of the population living in poverty rose. Across all age groups, the group with the highest percentage of people who did not visit the dentist was those who did not make up 100% of the poverty line.

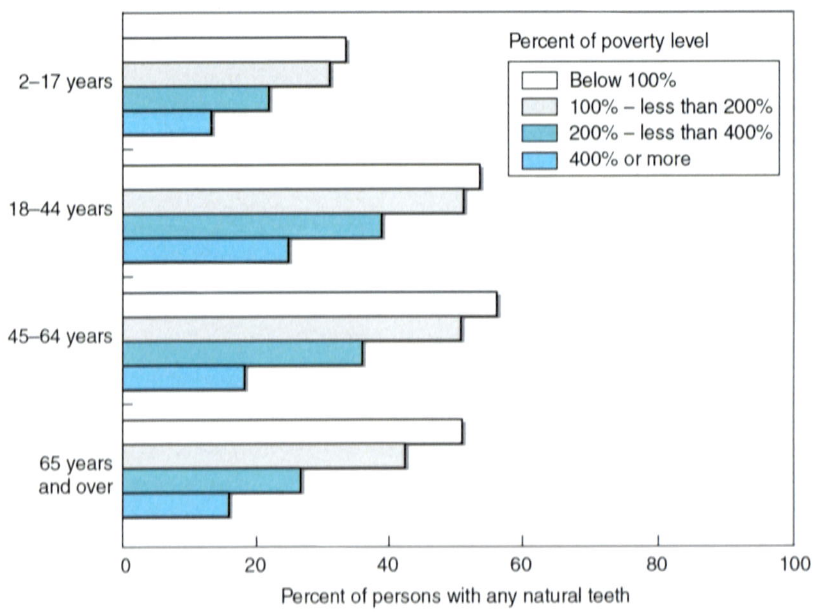

Figure 5.10. *No dental visit in the past year among persons with natural teeth, by age and percent of poverty level: United States, 2005.*

Source: Reprinted from National Center for Health Statistics. Health, United States, 2007. With Chartbook on Trends in the Health of Americans. Hyattsville, MD: 2007:85.

Related to the topic of race (as well as other demographic variables including age, gender, and socioeconomic status) is the term health disparities, which refers to differences in the occurrence of diseases and adverse health conditions in the population. An example is cancer health disparities, defined as "adverse differences in cancer incidence (new cases), cancer prevalence (all existing cases), cancer death (mortality), cancer survivorship, and burden of cancer or related health conditions that exist among specific population groups in the United States." Currently, African Americans have the highest age-adjusted overall cancer incidence and death rates in comparison with four other racial/ethnic groups (Asian/Pacific Islander, Hispanic/ Latino, American Indian/ Alaska Native, and white).

5.3. Characteristics of Place

Place (the geographical regions under comparison) has a significant impact on morbidity and mortality rates. International, national (including regional and urban-rural comparisons within a country), and localized disease occurrences are a few examples of comparisons based on place.

5.3.1. International

The World Health Organization (WHO) is a primary source of data regarding regional differences in disease rates since it funds and carries out continuous surveillance research. International differences in infectious and communicable diseases, starvation, infant mortality, suicide, and other conditions are depicted in WHO statistical studies. As one might anticipate, there is significant national variation in both infectious and chronic diseases. A few of these variations could be related to national eating patterns, access to healthcare, cultural influences, and climate.

Such variations are reflected in great international differences in life expectancy. The United States Central Intelligence Agency reported the ranked life expectancy at birth for 223 countries and indicated that the world life expectancy was 66.1 years (2008 estimate). The three countries with the highest life expectancy in 2008 were Andorra (83.5 years), Macau—technically not a country—(83.3 years), and Japan (82.1 years); the United States ranked number 47 (78.1 years).

The countries ranked as having the three lowest life expectancies were Zambia (38.6 years), Angola (37.9 years), and Swaziland (32.0 years). Life expectancy in many European countries including France, Italy, and Germany exceeded that of the United States. The United States' neighboring country, Canada, ranked seventh in life expectancy worldwide (81.2 years). Polio is one infectious disease that exhibits both decreasing incidence and international variations; at one point, it was a global illness. About 1% of cases of polio result in flaccid paralysis, a type of paralysis.

Polio is a virus infection that, in most cases, is either asymptomatic or causes a nonspecific fever. In the Western Hemisphere, Europe, and numerous other regions of the world, vaccination campaigns have contributed to the eradication of native wild cases of polio.

Figure 5.11 shows how polio spread between 2002 and 2005. In 2002, the Indian subcontinent, Afghanistan, Pakistan, and some regions of Africa were endemic for polio. The wild polio virus was reestablished in a number of African and Middle Eastern nations after polio spread from these endemic areas.

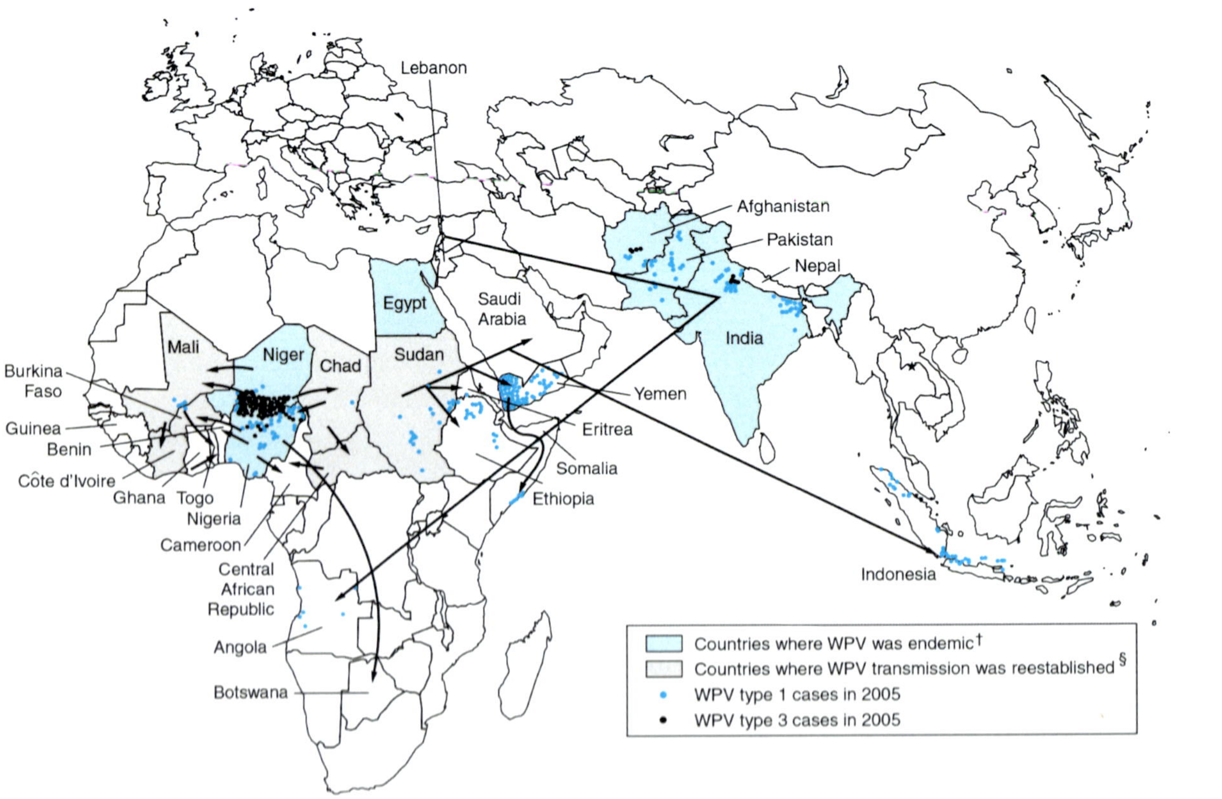

* Routes (not all importation events) indicated by arrows.

† As of February 1, 2006, Niger and Egypt were considered no longer endemic for WPV because neither country had indigenous transmission during the preceding 12 months.

§ Countries were considered to have reestablished transmission if WPV was detected for >1 year after importation. The majority of these countries have not experienced WPV type 1 transmission since July 2005.

Figure 5.11. *Wild poliovirus (WPV) cases in 2005 and WPV importation routes* during 2002–2005—worldwide.*

Source: Reprinted from Centers for Disease Control and Prevention. Resurgence of wild poliovirus type 1 transmission and consequences of importation— 21 countries, 2002–2005. MMWR. 2006;55:147.

5.3.2. National (Within Country)

There are differences in the frequency of diseases within many countries, particularly large ones. The incidence and prevalence of diseases are influenced by regional variations in variables like climate, latitude, and environmental pollution. Comparing disease occurrence by state, county, and geographic region (north, east, south, and west) is common in the United States. The proportion of adults who reported having had a stroke in 2005 is one illustration of variation at the state level. Among the states with the highest percentages were those in the south (e.g., Nevada, as well as Louisiana and Alabama). Please see Figure 5.12.

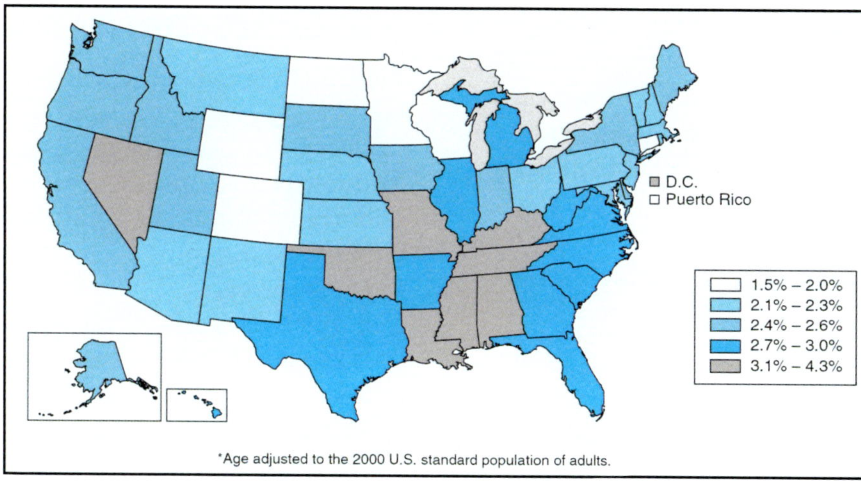

Figure 5.12. *Percentage of respondents aged 18 years who reported a history of stroke, by state/area— Behavioral Risk Factor Surveillance System, United States, 2005.**

Source: Reprinted from Centers for Disease Control and Prevention. Prevalence of stroke—United States, 2005. MMWR. 2007; 56:473.

5.3.3. Urban-Rural Differences

There are differences in morbidity and mortality rates associated with environmental and lifestyle factors between urban and rural areas in the United States. Urban diseases and mortality factors that are associated with urban pollution, dense population, inner-city poverty, and person-to-person contact are more likely to occur. One health problem that affects urban dwellers who may be exposed to lead-based paint from deteriorating older buildings is children's lead poisoning.

For people living in rural areas, agriculture is a significant source of employment. Hazards like poisonous pesticides and unintentional injuries from farm equipment are commonplace for farm workers. The distribution of nonfatal occupational farming injuries by state from 1993 to 1995 is depicted in Figure 5.13, which represents the latest available data. With 14.5 injuries per 100 full-time employees, Mississippi had the highest rate of injury.

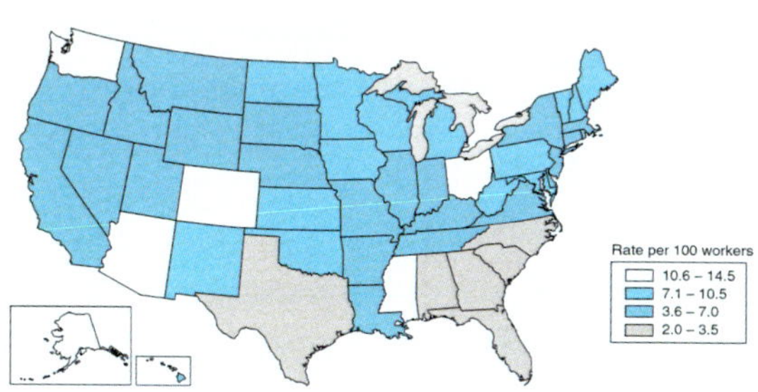

Figure 5.13. *Rates of nonfatal occupational farming injuries by state, 1993–1995.*

Source: Reprinted from Centers for Disease Control and Prevention, National Institute for Occupational Safety and Health. Worker Health Chartbook, 2004. DHHS (NIOSH) Publication No. 2004–146. Cincinnati, OH: National Institute for Occupational Safety and Health; 2004: 203.

Among the workers who could be exposed to health risks related to farming are migrant laborers. Many times, they live in cramped, inadequate housing that exposes them to diseases prevalent in dirty environments. Many of these laborers endure extraordinarily strenuous work environments with little access to restrooms, drinking water, or rest periods.

5.3.4. Localized Patterns of Disease

Disease patterns that are localized are those linked to particular environmental factors that could exist in a given region. Examples include arsenic poisoning connected to elevated levels of naturally occurring arsenic in the water and cancer linked to radon gas found in some geographic areas. Additionally, the local environment may provide a home for disease vectors that would not survive elsewhere.

Dengue fever is an example of a localized pattern of illness. It is a virus spread by a type of mosquito, or vector, that lives along the border between Texas and Mexico close to the Gulf of Mexico. It is believed that localized populations of mosquitoes played a role in the 2005 dengue fever outbreak. The regions impacted are displayed in Figure 5.14.

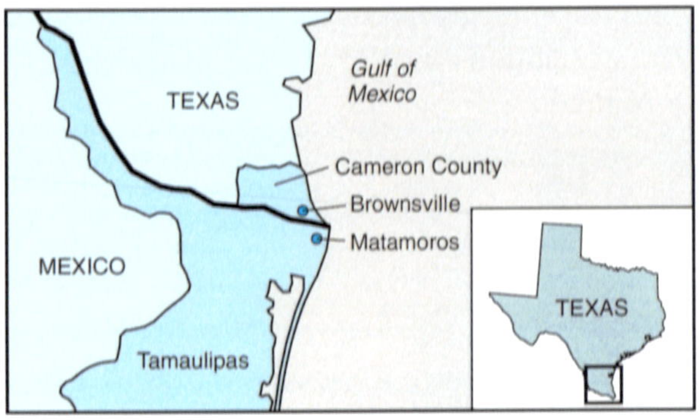

Figure 5.14. *Jurisdictions affected by dengue fever outbreak—Texas-Mexico border, 2005.*

Source: https://samples.jbpub.com/9780763754433/chapter4.pdf.

5.4. Characteristics of Time

Time features include secular time trends, point epidemics, clustering, and cyclic fluctuations. Changes in the disease pattern over time frequently provide crucial insights into the etiology of illness or the identification of new epidemics. Equally significant, if there are seasonal or cyclical fluctuations in the disease rate, the timing of data collection may need to be taken into account when comparing measures of disease frequency between two populations or within a population over time.

5.4.1. Cyclic Fluctuations/Seasonal Trends

The frequency of illnesses and health conditions can fluctuate cyclically over a number of years or even within a single year. These variations frequently mirror seasonal patterns. "[T]he recognition of seasonal patterns in infectious disease occurrence dates back at least as far as the Hippocratic era, but mechanisms underlying seasonality of person-to-person transmitted diseases are not well understood," the author of a thorough review of the seasonality of infectious diseases wrote." One phenomenon that follows a seasonal trend and rises in the early summer is birth rates. Another illustration is the incidence of depressive symptoms, which in a Belgian study peaked in the months of April through May. Seasonal variations are observed in influenza, drownings, unintentional injuries, and heart attack mortality every year. An Australian population's risk of both fatal and nonfatal coronary events increased by 20–40% between winter and spring compared to other seasons, according to an analysis of data from a community registry of heart disease. Seasonal variations can be brought on by endogenous biologic factors, seasonal variations in exposure to infectious or environmental agents, or seasonal changes in the behavior of people who are more susceptible to certain diseases.

The number of deaths from pneumonia-related influenza in the U.S varies annually and exhibits periodic epidemics every few years. Flu cases tend to rise seasonally, starting in the chilly winter months and peaking in February before declining in March and April and finally reaching a minimum in June. Another ailment that seems to fluctuate with the seasons is meningococcal disease, which seems to peak in the winter and diminish in the late summer. Another illness that exhibits seasonality is rotavirus infection, a type of viral gastroenteritis that is more common in young children. For seasonal trends for 2000–2009 (Figure 5.15).

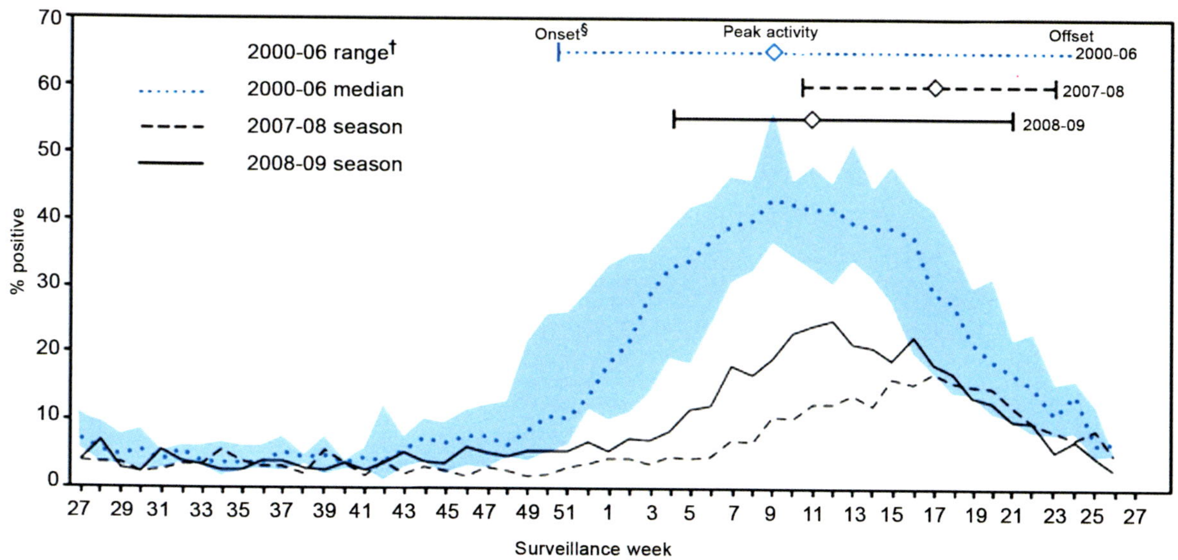

Figure 5.15. *Percentage of rotavirus tests with positive results, by surveillance week–participating laboratories, National Respiratory and Enteric Virus Surveillance System, United States, July 2000–June 2009.*

Source: Reproduced from Centers for Disease Control and Prevention, MMWR. Vol 58, No 41, p 1148, 2009.

* A median of 67 laboratories (range: 62--72) contributed rotavirus testing data to NREVSS during July 2000--June 2009.

† Range created using the maximum or minimum percentage of rotavirus positive tests for each surveillance week during 2000--2006. Maximums and minimums for each week might have occurred during any of the six rotavirus seasons during 2000--2006.

§ The onset of rotavirus season was defined as the first of 2 consecutive weeks during which the percentage of stool specimens testing positive for rotavirus was ≥10%; offset was defined as the last of 2 consecutive weeks during which the percentage of stool specimens testing positive for rotavirus was ≥10%.

Numerous illnesses exhibit periodic ups and downs linked to shifts in the host's lifestyle, variations in the seasonal climate, and the infectious agent's virulence in the case of a communicable disease. Wintertime, when sedentary men are suddenly needed to free their cars from the aftermath of a snowstorm, is when heart disease mortality peaks. While unintentional injuries tend to peak in the summer and Rocky Mountain spotted fever increases in the spring when ticks carrying the rickettsia bacteria become more active, colds become more common when people spend more time indoors and are near one another. There is a noticeable seasonality to the reported cases of malaria in the Americas and some Asian countries, which is linked to the cyclical occurrence of heavy rains. This seasonality can cause occasional epidemics or severe exacerbations of endemicity.

5.4.2. Common Source and Point Epidemics

An outbreak "caused by exposure of a group of persons to a noxious influence that is common to the individuals in the group" is referred to as a common source epidemic. A point epidemic can be defined as the reaction of a confined population to a shared source of infection, pollution, or other etiologic factor to which they were almost simultaneously exposed.

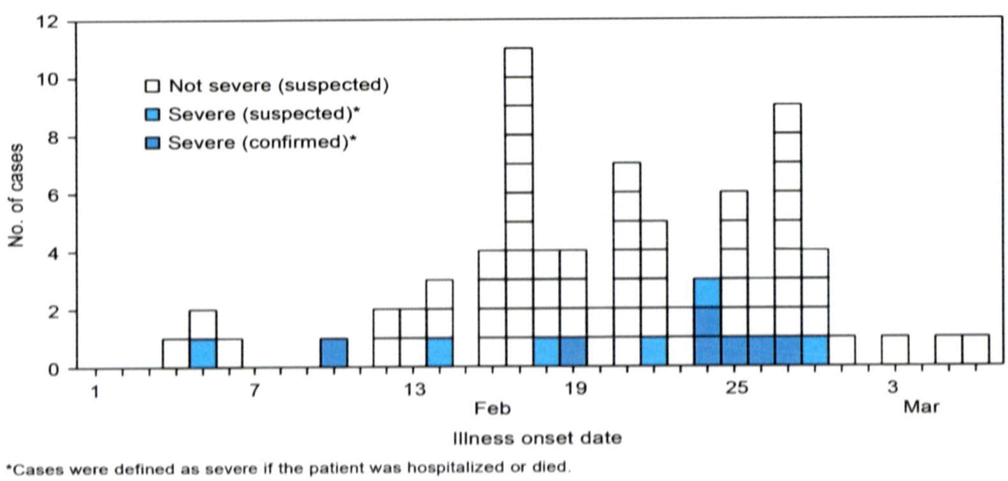

Figure 5.16. *Number of cases of influenza-related illness (n = 76) at a residential facility, by illness onset date and severity–Ohio, 2011.*

Source: Reproduced from Centers for Disease Control and Prevention, MMWR. Vol 58, Nos 51 & 52, p 1730, 2012.

A point epidemic of an infectious disease happens during the disease's incubation period. An epidemic with a common source of exposure that persists beyond the duration of a single incubation period is referred to as a continuous common source epidemic. This kind of outbreak happened in London during the cholera epidemic in 1854. Acute infectious diseases and enteric infections can occasionally follow the pattern of common source or point source epidemics; point source epidemics are those that result from mass illnesses caused by exposure to toxic gases and chemicals. The time clustering of influenza-related illness cases at a residential facility during a CDC-reported outbreak is shown in Figure 5.16. Take note that February 17, 2011, saw the highest number of cases, and that the date of onset varied (e.g., February 10 through February 30). Figure

5.15 illustrates the typical distribution of acute infectious disease outbreaks, foodborne illnesses, and acute reactions to toxic substances. It shows a sharp rise followed by a decline.

5.4.3. Secular Time Trends

As evidenced by variations in the rates of chronic diseases, secular trends are defined as slow shifts in the frequency of a disease over extended periods of time. For instance, the age-adjusted death rate for heart disease decreased by 34%, despite being the leading cause of death in the U.S. from 1970 to 1988; the decrease was 24% for African American men and 37% for White men. These patterns might be the result of unidentified causes as well as the long-term effects of public health initiatives, dietary changes, and improved care. There was a secular increase in lung cancer mortality from the mid-1960s until the 1990s, when the rates leveled off, as more women, particularly teenagers and women of color, began to smoke. Between 1995 and 2004, there were secular declines in breast cancer mortality rates among African Americans and Whites (Figure 5.17).

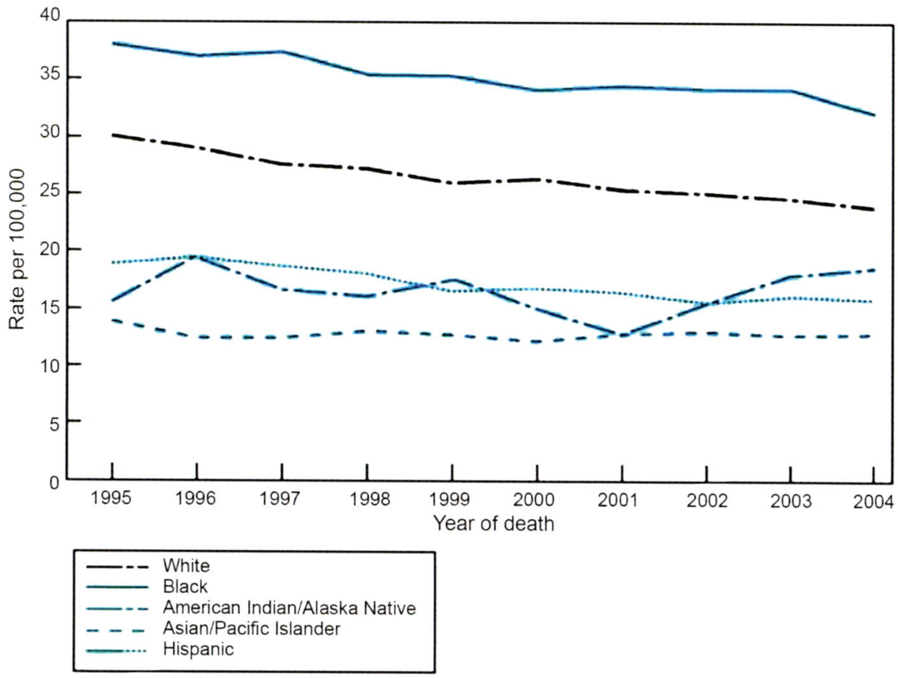

Figure 5.17. *Age-adjusted total U.S. mortality rates for breast cancer, all ages, females for 1995–2004 by "expanded" race age-adjusted to the 2000 U.S. standard population.*

Source: http://repository.stikim.ac.id/file/22-02-25.pdf.

5.4.4. Clustering

An unusual collection of health events grouped together in time or space is referred to as case clustering. The outbreak of Legionnaires' disease in the late 1970s and the cholera epidemic that struck London in 1849 are two instances of infectious disease clustering. Angiosarcoma in workers exposed to vinyl chloride and vaginal adenocarcinoma in daughters whose mothers were prescribed diethylstilbestrol are two instances of noninfectious disease clustering. Clustering studies have also been conducted on asthma, lung diseases related to asbestos exposure, suicides, leukemia, and other cancers. One sort of epidemiologic evidence that may point to a connection between the development of morbidity and mortality and frequent exposure to an etiologic agent is space and time clustering. A common source epidemic, as previously discussed in the chapter, serves as an example. Several issues with cluster analysis include the rarity of health events that exhibit clustering (e.g., specific cancer types), resulting in a limited number of cases, and that some clusters might just happen by coincidence.

5.4.4.1. Temporal Clustering

The emergence of puerperal psychoses and the onset of jaundice in military personnel vaccinated against yellow fever are examples of postvaccination reactions, or adverse reactions to vaccinations, which show temporal clustering. Up to 80% of women experience postpartum depression in the days following childbirth, which can last for several months or longer and range from the "blues" to more severe psychotic episodes.

5.4.4.2. Spatial Clustering

Spatial clustering is the concentration of disease cases in a specific geographic area. It is believed that Hodgkin's disease, a disorder whose etiology is unknown, has an infectious component. An official analysis of the temporal and geographic variability in the incidence of Hodgkin's disease could be used to assess this possibility. According to one study, there was evidence that cases of Hodgkin's disease in Washington State among patients diagnosed after the age of 40 lived closer together than was typical when they were young children and teenagers.

As another illustration, a small community in northern Germany was informed that six children had leukemia. Within a 5-kilometer radius, this occurrence translated to a 460-fold standardized incidence ratio using age-specific population and incidence data. The public may find reports like these to be extremely concerning. It is crucial that they are viewed in context using the proper epidemiologic techniques, even though they may be significant. The definition of the study area's geographic scope is especially important.

Leslie Robison, PhD, and Julie Ross, PhD, colleagues, compare the state of affairs to putting a bull's-eye around arrows that have already been fired. Let's take an example where you have a jar full of 100 marbles and are standing over a large enclosed circle. When the jar is empty, you observe where the marbles fall. Within the circle, there will always be areas that are sparsely scattered marbles and areas that are densely packed. You would notice that the marble pattern would always be random and unlikely to ever appear evenly spaced if you picked up every marble and carried out the procedure repeatedly. Perhaps this description can be compared to disease clusters, like the examples of childhood cancer. In other words, marbles, or cases, may be found within a county, state, or national geographic area, but they can also fall within a smaller, defined area (city). A simple bull's-eye diagram can be used to quickly identify a cluster of cases. One needs to take into account the phenomena's larger geographic context as well as the temporal occurrence of disease in order to properly evaluate such clusters.

A Closer Look

Approaches to Descriptive Epidemiology

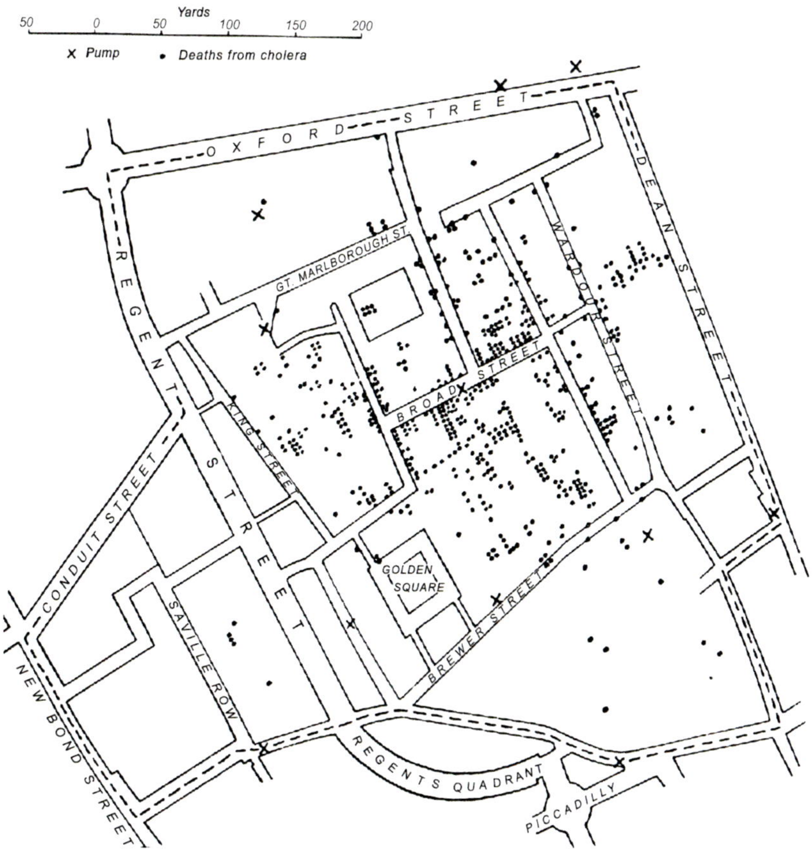

By after John Snow – Unknown sourceTransferred from en.wikipedia to Commons., Public Domain, https://commons.wikimedia.org/w/index.php?curid=403247.

Descriptive epidemiology serves as the foundation for understanding the distribution of diseases within populations, providing valuable insights into patterns, trends, and characteristics of health-related events. Several approaches are employed within descriptive epidemiology to systematically analyze and summarize data, thereby informing public health efforts and guiding further research and interventions.

One common approach to descriptive epidemiology involves examining the distribution of diseases by time. Temporal trends reveal patterns of disease occurrence over time, including seasonal variations, secular trends, and epidemic outbreaks. By analyzing changes in disease incidence or prevalence over different time periods, epidemiologists can identify potential risk factors, assess the impact of interventions, and anticipate future disease trends. This temporal analysis is crucial for detecting emerging health threats, monitoring disease surveillance systems, and guiding the timing of public health interventions.

Another approach to descriptive epidemiology involves assessing the distribution of diseases by place or geography. Geographic variations in disease occurrence provide valuable insights into spatial patterns, clustering, and disparities in health outcomes across different regions or populations. By mapping the geographic distribution of diseases, epidemiologists can identify areas of high disease burden, detect geographic clusters or outbreaks, and explore environmental or social determinants of health. Geographic information systems (GIS) and spatial analysis techniques are commonly used to visualize and analyze spatial data, facilitating the identification of geographic hotspots and guiding targeted interventions to address health inequities.

Furthermore, descriptive epidemiology involves analyzing the distribution of diseases by person or demographic characteristics. This approach focuses on understanding how disease occurrence varies by age, sex, race/ethnicity, socioeconomic status, occupation, and other demographic factors. By examining differences in disease rates and risk factors among various population subgroups, epidemiologists can identify vulnerable populations, assess disparities in health outcomes, and inform strategies for health promotion and disease prevention. This demographic analysis helps prioritize resources and tailor interventions to address the specific needs of diverse populations, ultimately aiming to reduce health inequities and improve overall population health.

Summary

- Descriptive epidemiology serves as the cornerstone of epidemiological investigations, providing a comprehensive overview of the distribution and basic characteristics of diseases or health-related events within populations. This branch of epidemiology focuses on systematically collecting and analyzing data to answer key questions about the "who, what, when, and where" of diseases. By examining patterns in terms of person, place, and time, descriptive epidemiology aims to identify trends, disparities, and potential risk factors associated with specific health outcomes.
- The primary goal of descriptive epidemiology is to characterize the distribution of diseases or health conditions in terms of person, place, and time. Epidemiologists gather and analyze data to identify patterns such as the demographics of affected individuals (e.g., age, gender), geographic distribution (e.g., urban vs. rural), and temporal trends (e.g., seasonal variation, secular trends over years).
- The distribution of a disease of unknown etiology bears a pattern similar to that of a known disease, which epidemiologists have investigated more thoroughly. This information suggests that the known and unknown diseases share certain similar causes.
- Socioeconomic status (SES) is defined as a "descriptive term for a person's position in society, . . ." SES is often formulated as a composite measure of three interrelated dimensions: a person's income level, education level, and type of occupation.
- Descriptive epidemiology provides crucial data for public health decision-making. It helps prioritize health issues based on disease burden and identifies high-risk populations or geographic areas requiring targeted interventions. Surveillance systems use descriptive epidemiology to monitor disease trends, detect outbreaks early, and evaluate the effectiveness of public health interventions.
- Morbidity and mortality vary greatly with respect to place (geographic regions that are being compared). Examples of comparisons according to place are international, national (within-country variations such as regional and urban-rural comparisons), and localized occurrences of disease.
- The World Health Organization (WHO), which sponsors and conducts ongoing surveillance research, is a major source of information about international variations in rates of disease. WHO statistical studies portray international variations in fectious and communicable diseases, malnutrition, infant mortality, suicide, and other conditions.

References

1. Abraido-Lanza, A. F., Dohrenwend, B. P., Ng-Mak, D. S., & Turner, J. B. (1999). The Latino mortality paradox: a test of the "salmon bias" and healthy migrant hypotheses. *American Journal of Public Health, 89*, 1543–1548.
2. Armstrong, B., van Merwyk, A. J., & Coates, H. (1977). Blood pressure in Seventh-Day Adventist vegetarians. *American Journal of Epidemiology, 105*, 444–449.
3. Baldwin, L. M., Grossman, D. C., Casey, S., et al. (2002). Perinatal and infant health among

rural and urban American Indians/Alaska Natives. *American Journal of Public Health, 92*, 1491–1497.

4. Benfante, R. (1992). Studies of cardiovascular disease and cause-specific mortality trends in Japanese-American men living in Hawaii and risk factor comparisons with other Japanese populations in the Pacific region: a review. *Human Biology, 64*, 791–805.
5. Büssing, A., Ostermann, T., & Matthiessen, P. F. (2005). Search for meaningful support and the meaning of illness in German cancer patients. *Anticancer Research, 25*, 1449–1455.
6. Castor, M. L., Smyser, M. S., Taualii, M. M., et al. (2006). A nationwide population-based study identifying health disparities between American Indians/Alaska Natives and the general populations living in select urban counties. *American Journal of Public Health, 96*, 1478–1484.
7. Centers for Disease Control and Prevention. (2002). Recent trends in mortality rates for four major cancers, by sex and race/ethnicity—United States, 1990–1998. *MMWR, 51*, 49–53.
8. Centers for Disease Control and Prevention. (2005). Health disparities experienced by black or African Americans—United States. *MMWR, 54*, 1–3.
9. Centers for Disease Control and Prevention. (2005). Racial/ethnic disparities in prevalence, treatment, and control of hypertension—United States, 1999–2002. *MMWR, 54*, 7–9.
10. Centers for Disease Control and Prevention. (2008). Acute renal failure associated with cosmetic soft-tissue filler injections—North Carolina, 2007. *MMWR, 57*, 453–456.
11. Centers for Disease Control and Prevention. (2008). Primary amebic meningoencephalitis—Arizona, Florida, and Texas, 2007. *MMWR, 57*, 573–577.
12. Centers for Disease Control and Prevention. (2009). Hantavirus pulmonary syndrome in five pediatric patients—four states, 2009. *MMWR, 58*(50), 1409–1410.
13. Centers for Disease Control and Prevention. (2010). Summary of notifiable diseases—United States, 2009. *MMWR, 58*(53), 39.
14. Centers for Disease Control and Prevention. (2012). Fatal exposure to methylene chloride among bathtub refinishers—United States, 2000–2011. *MMWR, 61*(7), 119–120.
15. Centers for Disease Control and Prevention. (2012). Percentage of adults with activity limitations, by age group and type of limitation—National Health Interview Survey, United States, 2010. *MMWR, 61*(14), 249.
16. Delgado, J. L., Johnson, C. L., Roy, I., & Trevino, F. M. (1990). Hispanic Health and Nutrition Examination Survey: methodological considerations. *American Journal of Public Health, 80*(suppl), 6–10.
17. Fine, M. J., Ibrahim, S. A., & Thomas, S. B. (2005). The role of race and genetics in health disparities research. *American Journal of Public Health, 95*, 2125–2128.
18. Flack, J. M., Ferdinand, K. C., & Nasser, S. A. (2003). Epidemiology of hypertension and cardiovascular disease in African Americans. *Journal of Clinical Hypertension, 5*(1 Suppl 1), 5–11.
19. Fraser, G. E., Strahan, T. M., Sabate, J., et al. (1992). Effects of traditional coronary risk factors on rates of incident coronary events in a low-risk population: the Adventist Health Study. *Circulation, 86*, 406–413.
20. Friis, R. H., Forouzesh, M., Chhim, H. S., et al. (2006). Sociocultural determinants of tobacco

use among Cambodian Americans. *Health Education Research, 21*, 355–365.

21. Friis, R., Yngve, A., & Persson, V. (1998). Review of social epidemiologic research on migrants' health: findings, methodological cautions, and theoretical perspectives. *Scandinavian Journal of Social Medicine, 26*, 173–180.
22. Garcia-Palmieri, M. R., Costas Jr., R., Cruz-Vidal, M., et al. (1978). Urban-rural differences in coronary heart disease in a low incidence area: the Puerto Rico Heart Study. *American Journal of Epidemiology, 107*, 206–215.
23. Gold, L. D., & Krumholz, H. M. (2006). Gender differences in treatment of heart failure and acute myocardial infarction: A question of quality or epidemiology? *Cardiology Review, 14*, 180–186.
24. Guralnik, J. M., & Leveille, S. G. (1997). Annotation: race, ethnicity, and health outcomes—unraveling the mediating role of socioeconomic status. *American Journal of Public Health, 87*, 728–729.
25. Hammond, J., Salamonson, Y., Davidson, P., et al. (2007). Why do women underestimate the risk of cardiac disease? A literature review. *Australian Critical Care, 20*, 53–59.
26. Hazuda, H. P., Haffner, S. M., Stern, M. P., & Eifler, C. W. (1988). Effects of acculturation and socioeconomic status on obesity and diabetes in Mexican Americans. *American Journal of Epidemiology, 128*, 1289–1301.
27. Helwig-Larsen, K., & Juel, K. (2000). Sex differences in mortality in Denmark during half a century, 1943–92. *Scandinavian Journal of Public Health, 28*, 214–221.
28. Hirschman, J., Whitman, S., & Ansell, D. (2007). The black: white disparity in breast cancer mortality: the example of Chicago. *Cancer Causes Control, 18*, 323–333.
29. Holman, R. C., Curns, A. T., Singleton, R. J., et al. (2006). Infectious disease hospitalizations among older American Indian and Alaska Native adults. *Public Health Reports, 121*, 674–683.
30. Ikeda, A., Hiroyasu, I., Hideaki, T., et al. (2007). Marital status and mortality among Japanese men and women: the Japan Collaborative Cohort Study. *BMC Public Health, 7*, 73.
31. Knowler, W. C., Bennett, P. H., Hamman, R. F., et al. (1978). Diabetes incidence and prevalence in Pima Indians: a 19-fold greater incidence than in Rochester, Minnesota. *American Journal of Epidemiology, 108*, 497–505.
32. Krieger, N. (2000). Editorial: counting accountably: implications of the new approaches to classifying race/ethnicity in the 2000 census. *American Journal of Public Health, 90*, 1687–1689.
33. Kung, H. C., Hoyert, D. L., Xu, J. Q., & Murphy, S. L. (2008). Deaths: Final data for 2005. *National Vital Statistics Reports, 56*(10). Hyattsville, MD: National Center for Health Statistics.
34. Levin, J. S. (1994). Religion and health: is there an association, is it valid, and is it causal? *Social Science & Medicine, 38*, 1475–1482.
35. Liu, H., & Umberson, D. J. (2008). The times they are a changin': marital status and health differentials from 1972 to 2003. *Journal of Health and Social Behavior, 49*(3), 239–253.
36. Lund, R., Holstein, B. E., & Osler, M. (2004). Marital history from age 15 to 40 years and subsequent 10-year mortality: a longitudinal study of Danish males born in 1953. *International Journal of Epidemiology, 33*, 389–397.

37. Luoma, J. B., & Pearson, J. L. (2002). Suicide and marital status in the United States, 1991–1996: Is widowhood a risk factor? *American Journal of Public Health, 92*, 1518–1522.

38. Markides, K. S., & Eschbach, K. (2005). Aging, migration, and mortality: current status of research on the Hispanic paradox. *Journal of Gerontology B: Psychological Sciences and Social Sciences, 60*(Spec No 2), 68–75.

39. Marmot, M. G., & Syme, S. L. (1976). Acculturation and coronary heart disease in Japanese-Americans. *American Journal of Epidemiology, 104*, 225–247.

40. McKenney, N. R., & Bennett, C. E. (1994). Issues regarding data on race and ethnicity: the Census Bureau experience. *Public Health Reports, 109*, 16–25.

41. Morales, L. S., Kingston, R. S., Valdez, R. O., et al. (2002). Socioeconomic, cultural, and behavioral factors affecting Hispanic health outcomes. *Journal of Healthcare for the Poor and Underserved, 13*, 477–503.

42. National Center for Health Statistics. (2011). *Health, United States, 2010: with Special Feature on Death and Dying*. Hyattsville, MD: National Center for Health Statistics.

43. National Center for Health Statistics. (2012). *Health, United States, 2011: with Special Feature of Socioeconomic Status and Health*. Hyattsville, MD: National Center for Health Statistics.

44. Osborne, C., Ostir, G. V., Du, X., et al. (2005). The influence of marital status on the stage at diagnosis, treatment, and survival of older women with breast cancer. *Breast Cancer Research and Treatment, 93*, 41–47.

45. Schneider, E. (2005). Tuberculosis among American Indians and Alaska Natives in the United States, 1993–2002. *American Journal of Public Health, 95*, 873–880.

46. Schoenborn, C. A. (2004). Marital status and health: United States, 1999–2002. *Advance Data from Vital and Health Statistics, 351*. Centers for Disease Control and Prevention.

47. Singh, G. K., & Miller, B. A. (2004). Health, life expectancy, and mortality patterns among immigrant populations in the United States. *Canadian Journal of Public Health, 95*, 114–121.

48. Syme, S. L. (1974). Behavioral factors associated with the etiology of physical disease: a social epidemiological approach. *American Journal of Public Health, 64*, 1043–1045.

49. Syme, S. L., & Marmot, M. G., Kagan, A., Kato, H., & Rhoads, G. (1975). Epidemiologic studies of coronary heart disease and stroke in Japanese men living in Japan, Hawaii and California: introduction. *American Journal of Epidemiology, 102*, 477–480.

50. U.S. Department of Health and Human Services, Office of Disease Prevention and Health Promotion. *Healthy People 2020*. ODPHP publication no. B0132. Washington, DC: U.S. Department of Health and Human Services.

51. Verbrugge, L. M. (1976). Females and illness: recent trends in sex differences in the United States. *Journal of Health and Social Behavior, 17*, 387–403.

52. Waldron, I., Weiss, C. C., & Hughes, M. E. (1997). Marital status effects on health: are there differences between never married women and divorced and separated women? *Social Science & Medicine, 45*, 1387–1397.

53. Williams, C. L., & Berry, J. W. (1991). Primary prevention of acculturative stress among refugees. *American Psychologist, 46*, 632–641.

54. Williams, D. R. (2003). The health of men: structured inequalities and opportunities. *American Journal of Public Health, 93*, 724–731.

55. Williams, D. R., Mohammed, S. A., Leavell, J., & Collins, C. (2010). Race, socioeconomic status and health: complexities, ongoing challenges and research opportunities. *Annals of the New York Academy of Sciences, 1186*, 69–101.

56. Wong, M. D., Tagawa, T., Hsieh, H. J., et al. (2005). Differences in cause-specific mortality between Latino and white adults. *Medical Care, 43*, 1058–1062.

57. Xu, J., Kochanek, K. D., Murphy, S. L., & Tejada-Vera, B. (2010). Deaths: final data for 2007. *National Vital Statistics Reports, 58*(19). Hyattsville, MD: National Center for Health Statistics.

58. Yano, K., Blackwelder, W. C., Kagan, A., et al. (1979). Childhood cultural experience and the incidence of coronary heart disease in Hawaii Japanese men. American Journal of Epidemiology, 109, 440–450.

Chapter 6

CLINICAL EPIDEMIOLOGY AND ITS RELEVANCE FOR PUBLIC HEALTH

Contents

Introduction

The current medical approach must take into account the use of clinical epidemiology in healthcare settings and with patients. In general, epidemiologic research, with its analytical designs and clinical trials, allows for advancements in management and treatment, as well as the definition of ever-more-sophisticated auxiliary exam quality through test-of-test design and cost-benefit analysis. Conversely, field epidemiology is used in descriptive studies of the health status of the population using analytical methods for Situational Health Analysis (SHA), the investigation of epidemic outbreaks, and the assessment of the response from community interventions. In this way, it makes it possible to manage epidemiology comprehensively, both individually and communally, leading to the eventual development of public health and preventive medicine. Clinical epidemiology is most useful when it comes to managing and treating diseases. It also helps identify risk factors for specific illnesses and is still a key component of evidence-based medicine. For these reasons, clinical epidemiology education is crucial because it will help professionals become more capable of making wise decisions and using the best available options for diagnosis and treatment. It also encourages the training of future researchers because it is assumed that conducting clinical epidemiology will result in new research.

The development of research necessitates the use of tools that will increase research efficiency. These tools include online text writing and editing programs like Google Docs, ZOGO, and OneNote, scientific literature search engines that will enable us to find evidence to support our work in healthcare systems, and sometimes even tools we don't even need to look for, like Google Reader and RSS/XML applications, accessing portals devoted to Evidence Based Medicine, or statistical calculators like Epidat that can streamline our statistical analysis. Social epidemiology is another idea to take into account. It has gained popularity in recent years and supports the study of the social determinants of health status. The integration and multidisciplinary nature of this approach have raised high expectations, but there is some skepticism that links it to the idealism of a political strategy tool. However, the positivist paradigm forms the basis of social epidemiology, just as it does for clinical epidemiology, and statistical methods serve as the foundation for analysis. Furthermore, it's vital to note that a brand-new field of study centered on social determinants has emerged recently, and young researchers face new obstacles as a result of the critical use of multilevel statistical models and cutting-edge technologies. The current trend in medical science is concentrated on producing evidence that influences patient outcomes and has aided in its development. Although it is acknowledged that community interventions through public health deserve to be recognized as significant events that have had an impact on the population's health, this EBM approach is primarily expressed in the care related to drugs and medical devices. Thus, it's important to acknowledge the existence of research aimed at demonstrating the significance of public health's range of initiatives. Evidence-Based Public Health maintains the cause-and-effect relationship while allowing the inclusion of health determinants like culture, environment, and lifestyles in the scientific framework, which is often what determines whether an intervention is implemented successfully or not. A new movement known as "Evidence Based Public Health" unites efforts to provide the best data possible for effective political decision-making. When it is focused on studying the health problems of a population, whether in the community or in a hospital setting, it significantly advances public health, particularly in our developing nations, by helping to solve a wide range of local and regional realities.

Orientation and Directional Terms

Term	Definition	Illustration
Number Needed to Harm Vs Treat	Number Needed to Harm Vs Treat is the number of people that need to be treated in order to help one person benefit from a treatment.	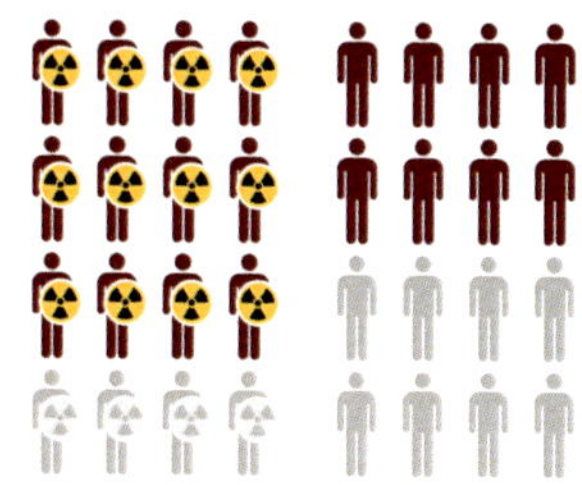
Intermediate Epidemiology	Intermediate Epidemiology exposes students to a variety of key concepts and methods when carrying out epidemiologic studies and teaches students applied skills in analyzing epidemiologic data and interpreting study findings appropriately.	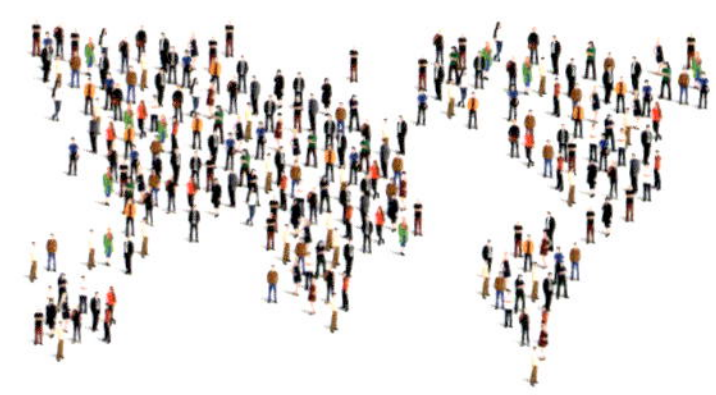
Epidemic Intelligence Service (EIS)	Epidemic Intelligence Service (EIS) was established in 1951 at the Centers for Disease Control and Prevention (CDC), Atlanta, Georgia, as a combined training and service program in the practice of applied epidemiology.	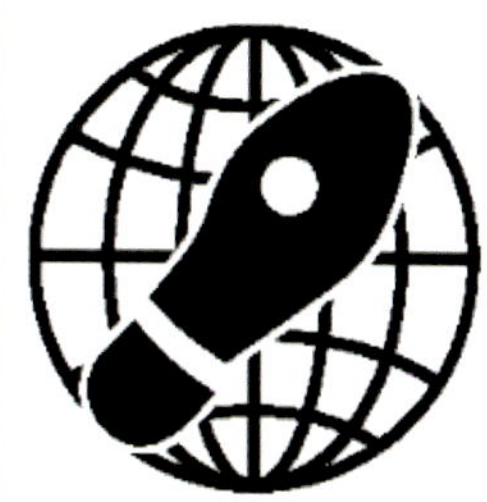
Evidence-Based Medicine (EBM)	Evidence-based medicine (EBM) uses the scientific method to organize and apply current data to improve healthcare decisions.	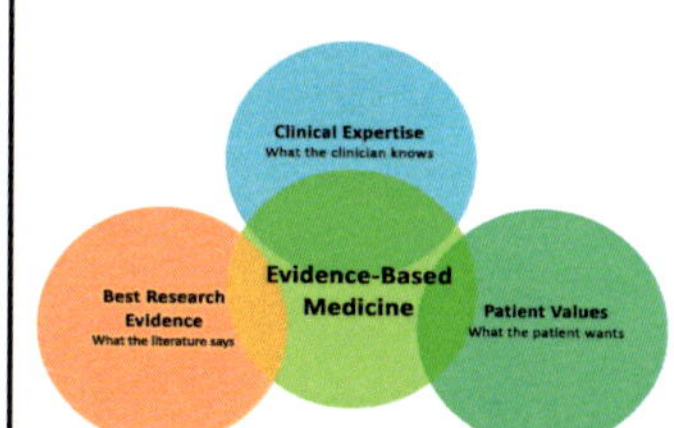
Clinical Trials	Clinical trials are research studies that test a medical, surgical, or behavioral intervention in people. These trials are the primary way that researchers determine if a new form of treatment or prevention, such as a new drug, diet, or medical device (for example, a pacemaker), is safe and effective in people.	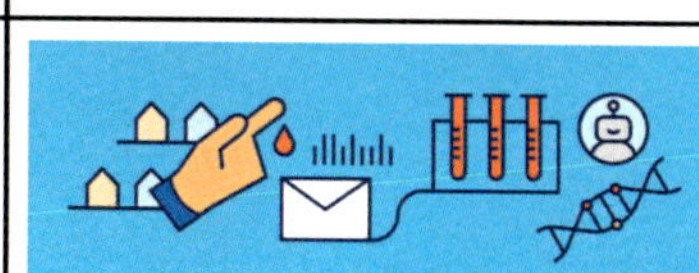

6.1. Differences Between Clinical Epidemiology and Field Epidemiology

6.1.1. Classic or Field Epidemiology

Epidemiology is a long-standing field of study with roots in rational and scientific frameworks that are grounded in actual experience. It is crucial for public health, and in recent years, its influence on clinical medicine has grown. When clinical and field epidemiology are compared, it may be possible to find parallels and differences that will help both approaches achieve their ultimate goal of improving people's health.

The main goals of field epidemiology are to locate the origin or cause of infectious disease outbreaks, stop their spread, and arrange for the prompt medical care of afflicted individuals. Practice is predominant over theory, with information gathering and action taking place "in the field," or in the epidemic territory. The field epidemiologist puts in a lot of overtime during an outbreak to gain control over it. Its execution by professionals from various specialties, including nurses, veterinarians, biologists, technicians, etc., is another distinctive aspect.

The goal of the Training Programs in Epidemiology and Public Health Interventions Network (TEPHINET), which was established in 1997 and is presently spread across 53 nations, is to improve the capacity of field epidemiologists for public health on an international scale. To address the shortage of epidemiology specialists in Peru, the Field Epidemiology Residency Program (PREC) was created to train professionals from various specialties to act in their respective jurisdictions.

This national Program had 4 stages: I Introduction to Epidemiology (2 months), II Basic Epidemiology (4 months), III Intermediate Epidemiology (6 months) and IV Specialized Epidemiology (12 months). The designated participants for each Regional Health Direction started to take the classes in their own offices, taught by specialists from the General Epidemiology Office and professors from a macro regional level University's headquarters with on-line tutoring, as well as field practices. Stages II and III were carried out in the University's headquarters and the selection of the participants to continue on to the next stages were done with a pyramidal system, according to weighted averages and additional exams. The last stage was carried out only in Lima-Peru, though it was still open to other provinces.

It is discussed that in the absence of a theoretical framework, field epidemiology would likely act. This tendency stems from its closest source, the Epidemic Intelligence Service (EIS) of the Centers for Disease Control and Prevention (CDC), a government agency in the United States. As an administrative body with military ties to the intelligence service, the CDC gives them a more appealing image than a functional role, more akin to a covert agent focused on action—protecting a community from a germ invasion, avoiding social alarm, and fostering population insecurity. Every day, field epidemiology uses traditional methods to carry out its intervention in micro spaces that are typically institutional, such as restaurants, schools, nursing homes for the elderly, and hospitals that may experience outbreaks.

Thacker SB and Buffington J., who belong to the CDC, call field epidemiology as the 21st century applied epidemiology, based on the philosophy of 'learn by doing,' supervised by experienced epidemiologists on field research, database analysis, vigilance system evaluation, presenting and publishing scientific research and answering to public questions. On the other hand, it has to be directed toward action regarding the main Public Health problems, the reduction of social inequality, having a greater consideration for psychosocial elements of the illness process, the incorporation of contents and methods from social sciences and working in multidisciplinary teams.

The use of epidemiologic methods for disease prevention and population health promotion is a feature of field or applied epidemiology, also known as general epidemiology. Its goal is to effectively achieve public health objectives by attempting to apply primary prevention.

6.2. Clinical Epidemiology

Clinical epidemiology was first used by Jean Paul in 1938, and he described it as "a new basic science for preventive medicine." Consequently, a crucial component of evidence-based medicine and clinical decision-making is the practical application of clinical epidemiology. Clinical epidemiology is a discipline that applies epidemiologic principles to the clinical setting with a patient-centered approach. Its hallmark is the integration of epidemiologic techniques with social clinical activity goals, namely accurate diagnosis and effective patient treatment. The information is combined with what is discovered through critical reading of scientific literature and thorough bibliographic research. It is currently regarded as Evidence Based Medicine's cornerstone.

Clinical epidemiology primarily relies on its clinical trials, which assess diagnostic techniques, discuss prognoses, participate in treatment development, and attempt to set up a controlled, randomized study in opposition to treating patients with placebos or other recommended medication. To be honest, it was hard to separate this work from what would eventually be referred to as Evidence Based Medicine (EBM), a term coined in 1992 by the same team that had established Clinical Epidemiology (CE) years earlier.

However, both disciplines: field epidemiology and clinical epidemiology share the same methodology and tool, the difference relies on the place where these are applied (Table 6.1).

Since epidemiologic research, with its analytical designs and clinical trials, allows for advancements in treatments and management, the current medical approach must take into account the application of clinical epidemiology in healthcare facilities for the benefit of patients. It also defines the quality of increasingly sophisticated auxiliary exams through test-of-test design and its economic approach (cost-benefit, cost-utility, cost-effectiveness), without neglecting the general population. Field epidemiology is applied in the community, where it is used to conduct descriptive studies of the health status of the populace with analytical approaches to Situational Health Analysis, study epidemic outbreaks and the interventions that follow, and propose global preventive measures and hygiene standards for improved health and disease prevention. In this sense, both collective and individual integral management is being carried out, leading ultimately to public health and preventive medicine. David Sackett drew attention to the need to integrate the evidence with the clinical experience and the value of patients in clinical decision-making, referring to it as Clinical Epidemiology and defining it as: 'the application of epidemiologic principles and methods to the problems challenging clinical medicine. The basic aim of clinical epidemiology is to promote the clinical observation and interpretation methods, which result in valid conclusions.'

Table 6.1. Clinical vs. Field Epidemiology

Aspect	Field Epidemiology	Field Epidemiology
Fundamental objectives	To identify the causes or sources of outbreaks. To carry out the prevention of diseases and promotion of health in the population.	To evaluate methods and the quality of diagnostics and patient treatment.
Place of action	Community, population	Health establishments (hospitals, clinics, etc.)
Intervention or study population	General population of the community	Patients in health establishments.
Professionals in charge	Multidisciplinary: doctors, nurses, technicians, veterinarians, biologist, etc.	Multidisciplinary: with a greater emphasis in doctors for carrying out diagnostic and treatment activities.
Methods	Action without an extended theoretical background, it is practice, applied.	Bibliographic research and critical reading, applying Evidence Based Medicine.
Basic prevention	Primary	Secondary and Tertiary
Study type	Observational	Experimental : clinical trial (mostly)
Situation at work	It is dealt with unexpected problems and has to travel and work in the field, giving immediate answers in a limited time.	Hospitalized patients are evaluated; applying the validity and reliability of diagnostic tests and choosing the best alternative for the patient's treatment.

Source: Daz-Vlez, C., Soto-Cceres, V., E., R., Apolaya Segura, M. A., & Galn-Rodas, E. (2013). Clinical epidemiology and its relevance for public health in developing countries. InTech. doi: 10.5772/54901.

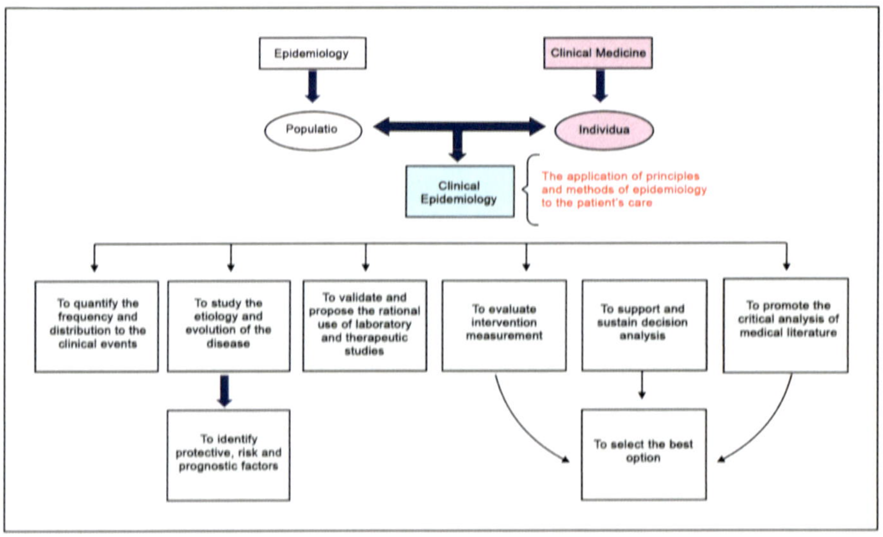

Figure 6.1. *Uses of Clinical Epidemiology.*

Source: Daz-Vlez, C., Soto-Cceres, V., E., R., Apolaya Segura, M. A., & Galn-Rodas, E. (2013). Clinical epidemiology and its relevance for public health in developing countries. InTech. doi: 10.5772/54901.

The creation and identification of reliable tests, as well as their logical extension, are the goals of clinical epidemiology. It is evidence-based medicine, or EBM, that seeks to apply evidence judiciously to each patient's diagnosis and course of care. Clinical epidemiology is the evolution of classic epidemiology, which was originally focused on broad approaches to community group public health, to encompass clinical judgments regarding the treatment of individual patients (Figure 6.1).

6.2.1. Evolution of Clinical Epidemiology

The field of clinical epidemiology has played a pivotal role in five recent advancements, or even revolutions, in the healthcare industry. These advancements include the creation of evidence, critical assessment, effective storage and retrieval, evidence-based medicine, and evidence synthesis (Table 6.2).

Table 6.2. Evolution of Clinical Epidemiology

Evolution	Change	Description
1° Evolution	Evidence generation	Increase of reports, especially clinical trials, followed by prognostic and diagnostic studies.
2° Evolution	Critical evaluation	Critical evaluation of the validity of medical literature.
3° Evolution	Efficient storage and recovery	Implementation of databases and scientific literature search engines.
4° Evolution	Evidence Based Medicine	Number Needed to Harm (NNH)
5° Evolution	Evidence synthesis	Start of the Cochrane Collaboration (http://www.cochrane.org)

Source: Daz-Vlez, C., Soto-Cceres, V., E., R., Apolaya Segura, M. A., & Galn-Rodas, E. (2013). Clinical epidemiology and its relevance for public health in developing countries. InTech. doi: 10.5772/54901.

Applying epidemiologic principles has had an impact beyond merely enhancing the application of clinical judgment and removing the implicit epistemic component from clinical reasoning. Decades of psychological research on decision-making, according to Arthur Elstein, have shown that: clinical judgment from experts was not as expert as we thought it was; knowledge transference was more limited than we expected; and judgment errors are not exclusive to medical students nor do they go away with experience. Instead, they can be made worse by the reliance on "experts opinion," which is a cognitive error that is inherent to clinical reasoning.

In Sackett DL (1992). and Col. chose to replace the term "Evidence Based Medicine" with "Clinical Epidemiology," indicating that all medical interventions, including diagnosis, prognosis, and treatment, must be supported by quantitative, reliable evidence derived from the best available epidemiologic and clinical research. And so, Sacket DL. he stated that "conscious, explicit, and reasonable use of the best current evidence to make decisions regarding the care of individual patients" was one of the first definitions of evidence-based medicine (EBM).

Sackett D.L. highlights the duality that exists between the art of clinical epidemiology's intuitive judgments and the science of epidemiologic reasoning. The individual came to the realization that the accuracy and efficacy of diagnosis and prognosis could be significantly enhanced by applying these epidemiologic principles, along with a little additional biostatistics, to the beliefs, judgments, and intuitions that comprise the medical art. EBM is a practice that combines individual clinical experience with the best external clinical evidence gleaned from systematic research. It was recently defined as "the integration of the best research evidence, of clinical experience and the patients' values" in a paper published in 2000. In the interim, Cuestas E. describes it as "the discipline that handles the study of the events surrounding medical decisions' determinants."

Clinical epidemiology, in its broadest sense, studies patient events, which include the onset of the disease and its outcome, such as recovery, complications, or death. Since sick people are typically found in medical facilities, the study subjects are also medical professionals, and their input is valuable, particularly for disease diagnosis and secondary and third prevention.

There are two types of clinical epidemiology: analytical and descriptive. While the analytical section focuses on the primary predictors of prognosis, diagnosis, and treatment—all of which are crucial ideas in clinical epidemiology and clinical medicine practice—the descriptive section concentrates on the variation in clinical prognosis (Figure 6.2). Furthermore, although clinical epidemiology focuses more on the individual, demographic epidemiology primarily targets the general public (Figure 6.1).

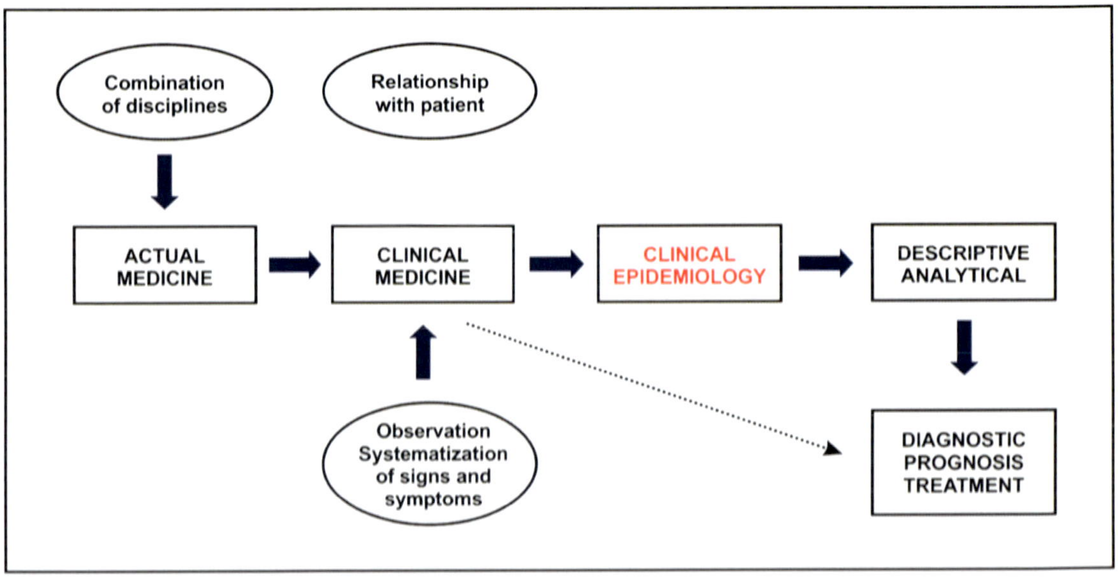

Figure 6.2. *Actual medicine, clinical medicine and clinical epidemiology.*

Source: Daz-Vlez, C., Soto-Cceres, V., E., R., Apolaya Segura, M. A., & Galn-Rodas, E. (2013). Clinical epidemiology and its relevance for public health in developing countries. InTech. doi: 10.5772/54901.

The EBM is motivated by the need to address the overabundance of information in the medical field, patient demands for the best diagnosis and care, and cost control—since it is well known that the global trend in healthcare costs is rising. These factors encourage critical evaluation of laboratory tests to make the most efficient use of the few resources available. Executing a cost-benefit analysis is what that means. Due to the necessity of conducting assessments in the areas of resource utilization, patient security, health economy, and quality of care, clinical epidemiology has grown "extremely important" for the healthcare system in recent years. The concepts of clinical epidemiology form the foundation of all these aspects.

Nowadays, there have been many misunderstandings about EBM, which arise because it has been adopted by functionaries and academicians in Public Health, and by health managers, who for better or for worse, are 'too far from patients,' giving interpretations like 'they remain sitting comfortably in their desks,' 'they manage abusively and without a criterion, telling clinical doctors how to treat the patients in cost-effective ways'...; points of view far from what was originally planned for the integral approach of clinical practice and clinical epidemiology.

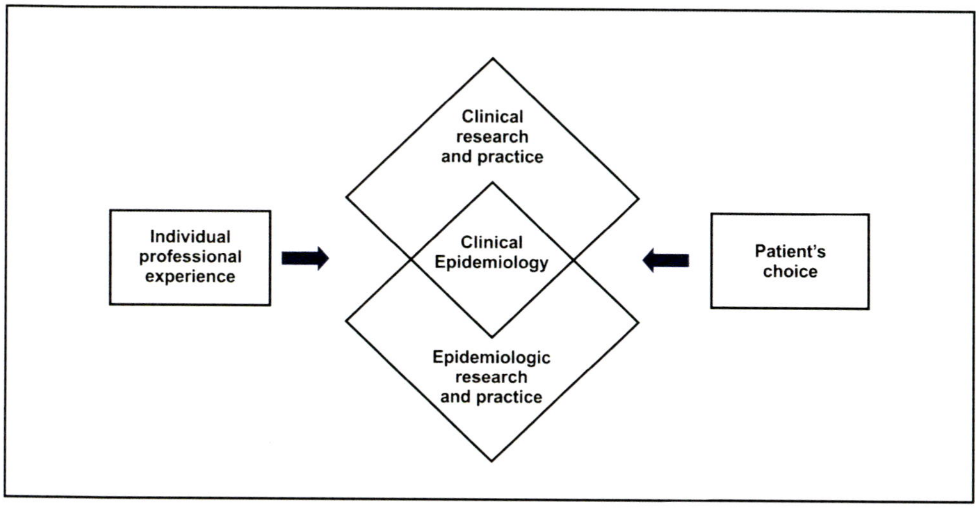

Figure 6.3. *Interactions of the clinical epidemiology.*

Source: Daz-Vlez, C., Soto-Cceres, V., E., R., Apolaya Segura, M. A., & Galn-Rodas, E. (2013). Clinical epidemiology and its relevance for public health in developing countries. InTech. doi: 10.5772/54901.

However, we also need to remember that, contrary to popular belief, the EBM is not a "cookbook" because it calls for the integration of the best available external evidence with the patient's choice, the professional's experience, and individual professional judgment. While clinical evidence can be helpful, it cannot replace the unique clinical experience. This information is required to assess whether the external evidence can be applied to the specific subject in order to determine how to enhance the clinical outcomes for the patient (Figure 6.3). Similarly, it is incorrect to view EBM as a "cost-reducing" medical approach because physicians who employ EBM may actually raise healthcare costs rather than lower them by identifying and implementing the most effective interventions to maximize patient quality of life.

6.2.2. From Epidemiology Teaching and Practice to Research

EBM, clinical medicine, and clinical epidemiology have all received a lot of attention as ways to improve patient care. To do this, physicians must be able to use the findings from clinical trials to present the patient with the available therapeutic options for a shared decision-making process. Subsequently, it becomes crucial to accurately interpret research findings, appropriately communicate this information to patients, and make the best decisions regarding diagnosis and treatment.

Significant advancements in the search, evaluation, and synthesis of scientific literature have been made possible by systematic reviews, meta-analyzes, and clinical practice guidelines. Medical journals frequently use terms like "likelihood ratio" and "number needed to harm." Numerous epidemiologic risk indicators are also employed in medical literature to convey the outcomes of therapeutic intervention efficacy. Relative risk (RR), relative risk reduction (RRR), absolute risk reduction (ARR), hazard ratio (HR), and number needed to harm (NNH) are the most commonly used metrics. All of these indicators show various ways to convey the same outcome.

Research conducted at the start of the decade revealed that physicians in practice had a restricted understanding of the numerical data provided by the study findings. The questions concerning relative risk reduction (87.7%), sensibility (84.6%), and specificity (80%) had the highest proportions of correct answers in Estellat C's study. Calculus and the use of likelihood ratio (16.9% and 9.2%, respectively), as well as the interpretation of the kappa coefficient (19.2%), had the lowest proportions of correct answers. Only 32% of the respondents could apply a diagnostic test's sensitivity or specificity in a clinical setting, even though over 80% of them could calculate these metrics. Similarly, while 30% of respondents accurately defined the likelihood ratio, less than 10% of respondents were able to use it to estimate the probability of a disease at test completion.

In the same study, the subjects who had had previous training in statistics, epidemiology or critical evaluation of medical literature scored significantly higher than those who did not have this training. The average score (the highest score being 7) was 5.9 (IC95% 5.3–6.5) and 4.5 (IC95% 4.0–5.0), respectively ($p<0.01$). Therefore, their capacity to interpret quantitative data from medical scientific literature may be limited, which can deplete the information given to the patient for the decision-making.

The five tasks involved in EBM practice are as follows: (1) developing a clinical question based on the patient's problem; (2) learning how to search the medical literature for the best available evidence; (3) critically evaluating the evidence; (4) applying and integrating the evidence to the patient's healthcare; and (5) evaluating (how to evaluate the process of helping the patient?). As a result, EBM is now taught in undergraduate courses and graduate programs in continuing medical education across the globe.

For instance, the majority of medical schools in France have included a formal clinical epidemiology course in their curricula because the critical evaluation of a medical article is a requirement for passing the national residence exam. Nonetheless, the majority of physicians in teaching hospitals tend to overlook clinical epidemiology and EBM. This is primarily because these subjects demand an understanding of technical statistics and epidemiology terms, which can make them difficult for some doctors to understand or simply uninterested.

As a result, when the risk indicators that were utilized to guide the outcomes of clinical trials were assessed in students and residents, it was discovered that 19.4% of them were unable to identify any of the indicators, and 81.4% of them were unable to compute them. The most commonly recognized indicator was the relative risk reduction (55.2%), which was followed by the hazard ratio (9.5%), absolute risk reduction (26.6%), and "number need to harm" (51.6%). It was determined that medical students and residents are unable to identify and accurately compute the risk indicators utilized in clinical trials.

Similar research was conducted in the faculties of a northern Peruvian city (unpublished data), involving 139 medical students, two groups comprising those who had completed Clinical Epidemiology and another finishing Classic Epidemiology. The most commonly recognized indicator was NNH (number needed to harm), at 58.9%, followed by RRR (relative risk reduction) at 56.8%. Furthermore, 13.7% of the students were unable to identify any indicators, while 30.9% of them acknowledged at least one. When they were asked to calculate the indicators, though, this was different because they discovered that RR (30.9%) and ARR (35.9%) had the most accurate calculations. Similarly, 56.1% of respondents calculated at least one of them incorrectly, and 11.5% of respondents calculated at least one of them adequately. Only slightly over 10% could identify and compute the risk indicators. There was a significant difference (p<0.05) between the ability of the two groups to identify and compute the indicators (Table 6.3).

Table 6.3. Comparison of Mean Scores Obtained

Indicators	Clinical Epidemiology	Classic Epidemiology	p
Recognizes*	3.12 ± 0.89	0.79 ± 1.19	p<0,05
Calculates&	2.94 ± 0.96	1.45 ± 0.79	p<0,05
Total§	6.06 ± 1.43	2.21 ± 1.53	p<0,05

**Maximum score: 4. &Maximum score: 4. §maximum score: 8.*

Source: Daz-Vlez, C., Soto-Cceres, V., E., R., Apolaya Segura, M. A., & Galn-Rodas, E. (2013). Clinical epidemiology and its relevance for public health in developing countries. InTech. doi: 10.5772/54901.

Typically, medical students enter their classes with a strong sense of curiosity and a desire to better the human condition. However, they quickly discover that their coursework is extensive and passive and that their direct involvement in patient care is minimal. Certain courses are challenging for learners, and the outcomes frequently impact patient care right away. This clearly extends beyond the fact that students apply the theory to made-up scenarios. The situation would be better if students used the EBM to select clinical problems for patients, enabling them to find and assess relevant articles that will support the patient's treatment. Their critical thinking abilities and practical approach to real teamwork may be enhanced by these exercises.

Dunn K. and Col. in the last decade they were already channeling the teaching of EBM, looking to create competencies in students such as (1) elaboration of researchable clinical questions, (2) access to the best and most recent literature, (3) evaluation and scoring of the literature for its validity and pertinence, and (4) cost-performance-benefit analysis and the interpretation of meta-analysis. Rucker L also mentions the 'EBM recipe' as a useful tool to bring EBM closer to healthcare, which consisted in posing clinical questions relevant during rounds at hospitals, which would later be solved by the students with the help of teachers. A similar progress occurs at the Canadian Institute of Health Research, implementing a 'teaching recipe,' which allows the resident to take note of the doubts from a concrete clinical case, and answer them following a methodology based on the PICO model (problem/patient, intervention, comparison and result) and finally designate a date and a person in charge to deliver the answer. The development of scientific research marked the beginning of the evolution of clinical epidemiology, which then spread to critical reading, the creation of databases and their search engines, EBM, and information synthesis (Table 6.2). This indicates that research has surrounded it from the start and throughout its entire evolution. But what really sticks out is that in a study conducted in 2005 with 1484 medical students from 13 Peruvian faculties, we discovered a relationship between being a member of a research group and having good knowledge, with 53.7% of students having good knowledge and 71.9% having an adequate attitude toward research. In a later study by Cabrera-Enríquez JA et al., this decreased by 7% and 34. 2%, respectively. Additionally, 68% did not take any extracurricular courses, and of those who did, only 3.28% and 6. 24%, respectively, could perform critical reading and statistics. This study found a significant correlation between knowledge level and attitude toward research ($p<0.05$), and only 51% had participated in or were currently participating in a study.

Even though the Latin American environment is not the best for training researchers, undergraduates can still support research by participating in student societies. In university institutions, research lines are not always sufficiently developed. Furthermore, hospital research receives greater funding, particularly from the pharmaceutical industries, while primary healthcare research is underdeveloped and not even explicitly stated. When we consider the fact that there are few local publications (due to previously mentioned factors) and that 75% of them cover subjects that are not of regional or national importance, along with the knowledge of the social, ethnic, and cultural diversity among communities, what further evidence do we have to dispel our clinical doubts?

In this regard, a strong research mindset coupled with an integrated approach to the field offers undergraduates and recent graduates alike an alternative to developing a strong research mindset and intelligence in terms of scientific work capacity. In addition, as university instructors, we have been advocating for certain activities, such as undergraduate students graduating by publication as a substitute for raising university scientific output.

There are instances of EBM and research education everywhere in the world. Among other fundamental competencies, the University of California, San Francisco's Accreditation Council for Graduate Medical Education covers EBM and practice-based learning. To address this, the "PRIME curriculum" program (EBM/clinical research program) was created. It employs journal clubs, didactic lectures, progress evaluation sessions, and active tutoring to enable residents to complete a clinical research project while they are in residence.

The development of topics like statistical power calculation, qualitative research methods, survey research, decision analysis and treatment threshold, cost-effectiveness analysis, ethical use of patients in research, community research and research process evaluation with international support, use of administrative data, and spreadsheet management are all motivated by the didactic lectures, which make up the first component of the "PRIME curriculum" program. Small journal clubs (evaluating diagnostic tests, case-control studies, cohort studies, controlled randomized clinical trials, meta-analyzes, decision-making, cost-effectiveness analyzes, clinical practice guidelines, etc.) meet once a week in the evenings as part of the second component.), which are created by students and last for fifteen minutes. The tutor then moderates a debate afterward. The third element is the quarterly presentation of interactive seminars on resident projects, which are intended to refine the project author's concepts. Thus far, these experiences have proven to be fruitful, possibly because participating residents explicitly anticipate that the findings of their research will be published, which in turn encourages teachers to volunteer their time as mentors. Nonetheless, we think that the structured curricula, the mentors' willingness to help, and most importantly, the residents' enthusiasm all play a major role in the exit.

Upon successful completion of the program, the student will have gained knowledge of the fundamental forms of research design, such as quasi-experimental studies, randomized clinical trials, cohort and case-control studies, and concepts of health measurement and evaluation in epidemiologic studies. They will also be able to critically assess medical literature and use and interpret a variety of statistical programs for data analysis.

However, there are limits to the EBM that, according to Cuestas E., might be: (a) the frequently conflictive results of randomized and controlled trials (RCT); (b) the inexistence of evidence in an enormity of topics; (c) the questionable quality of many RCT and meta-analysis; and (d) many time the RCT are not easy to conduct due to practical reasons, or impossible to do because of ethical reasons. Besides, it is necessary to integrate the best scientific evidence available with the preferences of the patient, with limits such as economic, social, ethnic, moral, cultural and health organization of the system.

The Internal Medicine Residence and Postgraduate Curriculum Working Group in the United States proposes that since medical students do not always acquire these skills in the classroom or during medical or teaching rounds, the EBM concepts ought to be a fundamental component of the undergraduate and residency curriculum.

6.2.3. Clinical Epidemiology Competences

- Understanding of how bias and chance can affect the accuracy of observations in individual patients.
- Evaluation of the validity of original articles over diagnosis, prognosis, treatment and prevention.
- Knowing the strengths and weaknesses of randomized clinical trials, case-control studies, cohort studies (prospective and retrospective) and meta-analysis.
- Using practical strategies to judge the validity of clinical evidence synthesis (i.e., reviews).
- Comprehension of the meaning, uses and limits of the statistic power, the values of 'p' and the confidence interval, relative risk, attributable risk and NNH (number needed to harm).
- Knowing how to measure the patients' preferences.
- Comprehension and usage of the sensibility analysis and the cost-effectiveness analysis.

6.2.4. Competences for Quantitative Clinical Reasoning

- Comprehension of the way to calculate the pre-test disease probability and how to use the Bayes theorem to calculate the post-test probability.
- Defining and using sensibility, specificity and likelihood ratio of the diagnostic information.

- Knowing and being capable of detecting possible bias in calculations of sensibility and specificity.
- Comprehension of the value of decision trees and decision-making.

The range of options for health professionals to receive clinical epidemiology education and training has gradually increased. The International Clinical Epidemiology Network, which is made up of research and clinical epidemiology training centers as well as clinical epidemiology units worldwide, has a regional member in South America called LatinCLEN (Latinamerican Clinical Epidemiology Network), which works to promote the field's growth. (Table 6.4).

After considering all of the above, it is clear that both field epidemiology and clinical epidemiology use the same methodology and tools; the only differences are in the settings in which they are applied. The current medical approach must take into account the application of clinical epidemiology in healthcare facilities, patients, and epidemiology researchers. Clinical trials and their analytical designs enable advancements in treatment and management, as well as the definition of increasingly complex auxiliary exams through testing and economic approaches (cost-benefit, cost-utility, and cost-effectiveness).

Table 6.4. Clinical Epidemiology world Network

Network	Country members	Website
LatinCLEN	South American countries	www.latinclen.org
INCLEN-África	African countries	www.inclenafrica.org
CanUSACLEN	Canada and the USA	www.canusaclen.org
ChinaCLEN	China	www.chinaclen.org.cn
INCLEN – Euro-Med	Europe countries	www.recif.univ-lyon1.fr
IndiaCLEN	India	www.indiaclen.org
INCLEN – Southeast Asia	Asian countries	www.cim.edu.ph

Source: Daz-Vlez, C., Soto-Cceres, V., E., R., Apolaya Segura, M. A., & Galn-Rodas, E. (2013). Clinical epidemiology and its relevance for public health in developing countries. InTech. doi: 10.5772/54901.

The general public cannot be overlooked because it is in the community that field epidemiology is used, along with the analytical method of Situational Health Analysis, descriptive study of the health situation, analysis of epidemic outbreaks and the corresponding interventions, and planning of global preventive measures and hygiene for improved life quality and disease prevention. Finally, the value of clinical epidemiology in clinical research is acknowledged in ways that classic epidemiology has not been able to, but it is based on the expertise of medical professionals and is always evolving, so it remains valid. In this way, an essential management of epidemiology will be conducted, both individually and societally, leading to preventive medicine and public health.

6.2.5. Informatics Tools for Health Research

During health professionals' daily practice, the need to keep informed about the new scientific evidence comes up as a responsibility towards patients and, of course, to oneself. It is not strange to see yourself in front of a patient with a specific pathology to which certain treatments haven't had an effect, and ask yourself: what is new to treating this condition? Or, on the other hand, in front of a research, lecture or speech about any topic, trying to have the most updated information about the topic. Considering its etymologic origin, the word 'investigation' comes from the Latin word *invenio, invenire*, which means 'to find.' By association and as a logical consequence, to find you must first search. And for that, we must know how to and where to search. This searching implies knowing the principal sources of information to which, as professionals, we must access. However, the task does not end there, for, once we find the information, we must do a critical reading of it and select the most relevant, which in the context of a research study must be adequately cited. Informatics tools, mostly available online, make research easier. They include information sources, user-friendly interfaces for quick access and navigation, bibliographic reference managers, and statistical software that lets us perform calculations that would be extremely difficult if done the traditional way.

6.2.6. Information Sources

Search resources to which we normally turn are general search engines (Google, Yahoo, Altavista, Metacrawler, etc.) Google (http://www.google.com) has the biggest demand, but the health information available in this engine may come from a non-reliable source, so it is important to distinguish which are the most adequate websites to find the health- related information, which implies evaluating the quality of these websites, an activity that sometimes is quite tedious for the researcher.

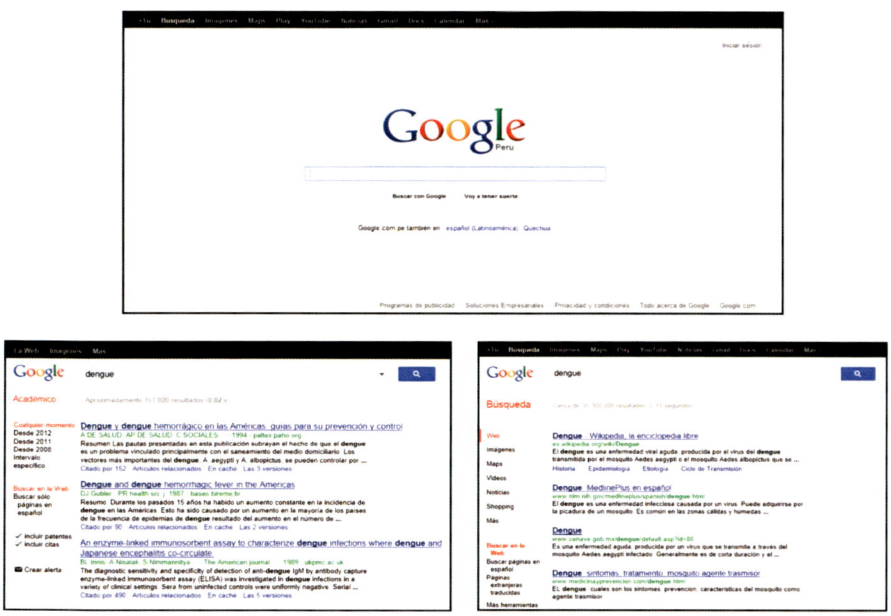

Figure 6.4. *Google-google scholar.*

Source: Daz-Vlez, C., Soto-Cceres, V., E., R., Apolaya Segura, M. A., & Galn-Rodas, E. (2013). Clinical epidemiology and its relevance for public health in developing countries. InTech. doi: 10.5772/54901.

Given the wealth of information it retrieves the conventional search engine Google, and considering the existence of dubious sources, Google implemented Google Scholar (Google Scholar) oriented search scientific references (http://scholar.google.es), which are listed in order of relevance, and provide information about the source, year of publication, authors, times the number that have been cited and other versions of the publication, and also, you can access related articles (mentioning or are cited by the text), the content in HTML, PDF, DOC or other formats, it is recommended to do the advanced search preference (Figure 6.4).

One of the best online medical bibliographic databases is MEDLINE, which has been produced by the National Library of Medicine (NLM) in the United States since 1966. The most comprehensive article bibliographic resource available to us in the biomedical sciences is MEDLINE. The three indexes that comprise the database are the International Nursing Index, the Index Medicus, and the Index to Dental Literature. For researchers worldwide, it is the most consulted database at the moment. A 34.1% reference was provided by a study conducted on professional biomedical researchers who speak Spanish.

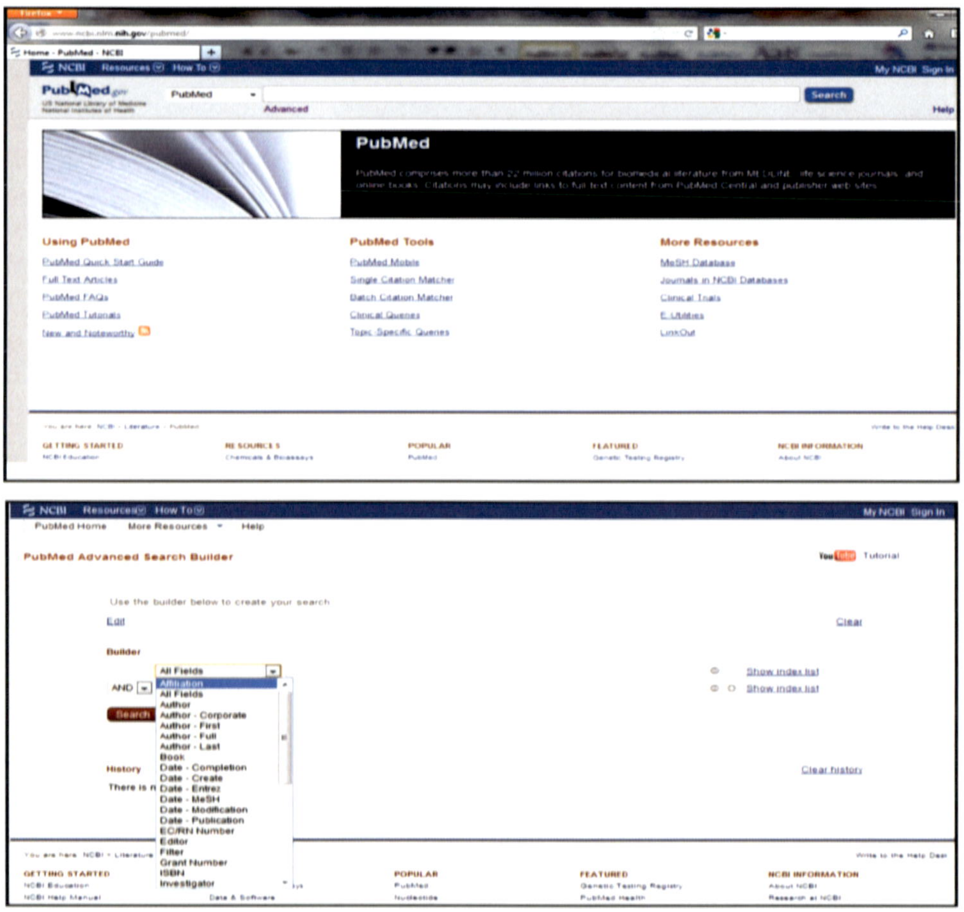

Figure 6.5. *Pubmed specialized search engine of the National Library of Medicine (MEDLINE).*

Source: Daz-Vlez, C., Soto-Cceres, V., E., R., Apolaya Segura, M. A., & Galn-Rodas, E. (2013). Clinical epidemiology and its relevance for public health in developing countries. InTech. doi: 10.5772/54901.

MEDLINE includes general topics, such as microbiology, health prevention, nutrition, pharmacology and environmental health. However, the covered categories by the database include anatomy, organisms, diseases, drugs, techniques, equipment, psychiatry, biological sciences, physical sciences, social sciences and education, technology, food, industry, humanities, and communication sciences. All of these are related to health. The search is done via PUBMED: http://www.pubmed.gov (Figure 6.5). Here, the searches are in English based on Boolean operators: AND, intersection, automatic term mapping; OR, conjunction and isolation; NOT, excludes the final term; uses a MeSH (Medical Subject Headings) controlled vocabulary and the subheadings described by the Index Medicus, where most of the abstracts have the link to the editorial where the full-text article can be found.

Another large database, not as extensive as MEDLINE, is 'Literatura Latinoamericana y del Caribe en Ciencias de la Salud' (Latinamerican and the Caribbean Literature on Health Sciences – LILACS). It can be accessed through the Virtual Health Library (Regional Medicine Library – BIREME): http://www.bireme.br, the same that includes other sources of information in biomedical sciences. One of them is the catalog of the library hosting the Panamerican Health Organization (PAHO) and the World Health Organization (WHO). Here you can access full-text articles that are included in the Scientific Electronic Library Online (SciELO): http://www.scielo.org, which includes Argentina, Brazil, Chile, Colombia, Costa Rica, Cuba, Spain, Mexico, Portugal, Venezuela, Public Health, Social Sciences and developing initiatives like Bolivia, Paraguay, Peru, South Africa and Uruguay (Figure 6.6).

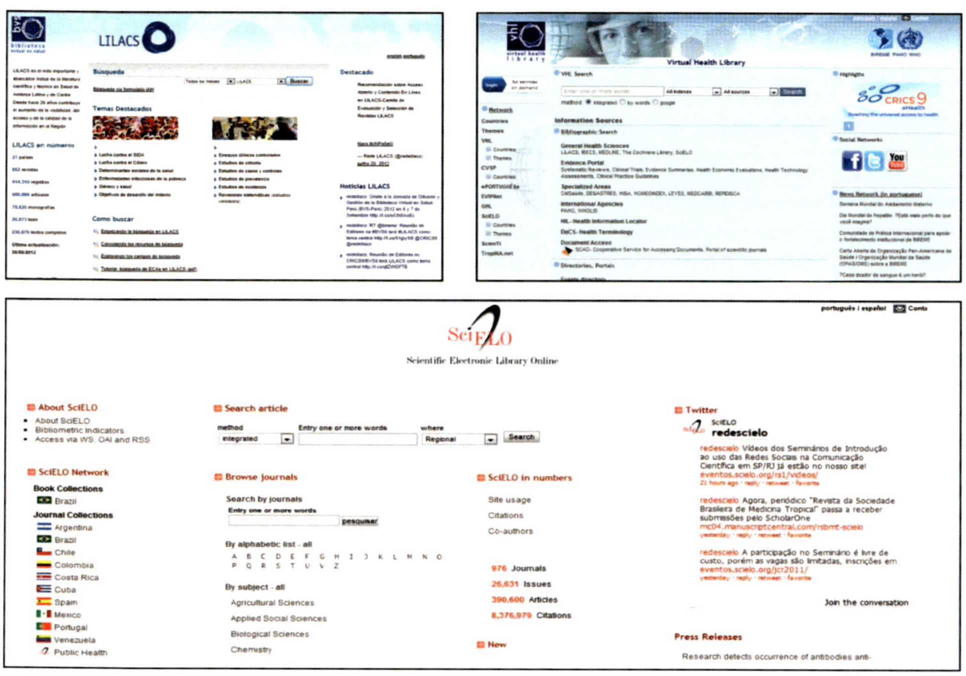

Figure 6.6. *Latin American and the Caribbean literature on health sciences (LILACS), virtual health library and scientific electronic library online (SCIELO).*

Source: Daz-Vlez, C., Soto-Cceres, V., E., R., Apolaya Segura, M. A., & Galn-Rodas, E. (2013). Clinical epidemiology and its relevance for public health in developing countries. InTech. doi: 10.5772/54901.

An important resource is the Cochrane Library: (http://www.bibliotecacochrane.org/) (Figure 6.7), whose aim is to prepare, keep and spread systematic reviews regarding the effects of healthcare, mostly based on controlled clinical trials, and are highly structured and systematized, for they include the evidence according specific quality criteria.

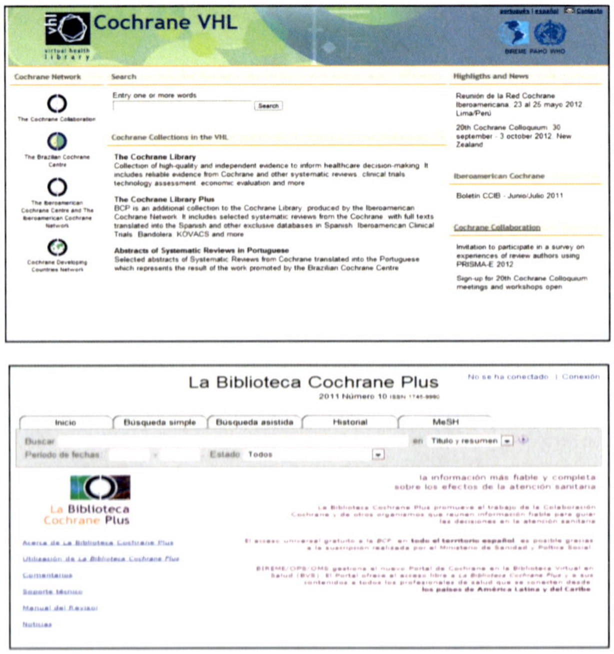

Figure 6.7. *Cochrane library.*

Daz-Vlez, C., Soto-Cceres, V., E., R., Apolaya Segura, M. A., & Galn-Rodas, E. (2013). Clinical epidemiology and its relevance for public health in developing countries. InTech. doi: 10.5772/54901.

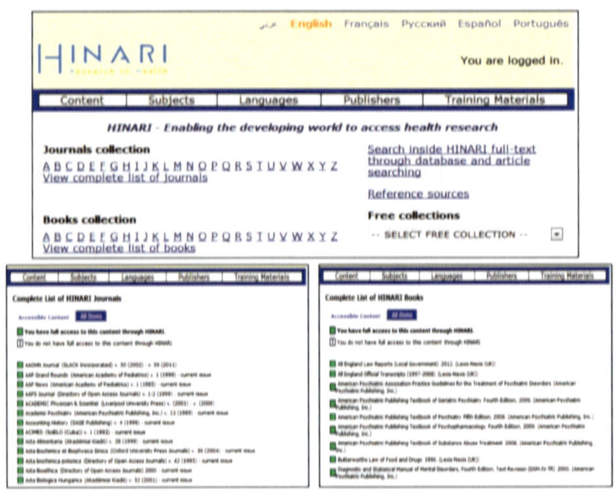

Figure 6.8. *Health internetwork access to research initiative (HINARI).*

Source: Daz-Vlez, C., Soto-Cceres, V., E., R., Apolaya Segura, M. A., & Galn-Rodas, E. (2013). Clinical epidemiology and its relevance for public health in developing countries. InTech. doi: 10.5772/54901.

Health Inter Network Access to Research Initiative (HINARI) in: http://extranet.who.int/hinari/en/journals.php (Figure 6.8) is a program established by the WHO, in partnership with publisher, and gives an easier access to one of the most extensive biomedical and health literature collections. It contains more than 8 500 information resources, in 30 different languages, which are available for health institutions in more than 100 countries.

Global representative health organizations, such as the PAHO, offer in their website important links, as well as free access to their publications (http://new.paho.org/) (Figure 6.9). The WHO allows us to access important articles on disease control, vigilance systems and public health. The information is in three languages, including Spanish (http://www.who.int/en/) (Figure 6.9).

The Center for Disease Control and Prevention (CDC), whose objective is to promote health and quality of life, gives updated information on the control of disease, lesions and disabilities (http://www.cdc.gov/) (Figure 6.9).

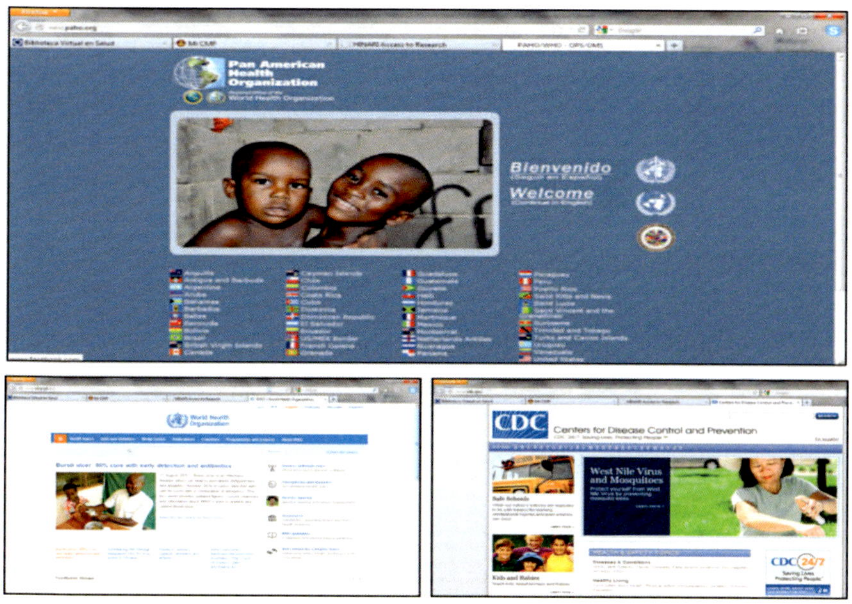

Figure 6.9. *Pan-American Health Organization, World Health Organization, The Center for Disease Control and Prevention (CDC).*

Source: Daz-Vlez, C., Soto-Cceres, V., E., R., Apolaya Segura, M. A., & Galn-Rodas, E. (2013). Clinical epidemiology and its relevance for public health in developing countries. InTech. doi: 10.5772/54901.

To access a consensus, the National Guideline Clearinghouse (http://www.guideline.gov/) (Figure 6.10) contains evidence-based clinical guidelines of the main medical societies in the USA and Canada, National Institute of Clinical Studies, National Institute of Health and Medical Research Council (NHMRC) which collects the CLG developed in Australia (http://www.clinicalguidelines.gov.au/) (Figure 6.10), National Institute for Health and Clinical Excellence (NICE), an independent agency of the NHS in England and Wales (http://www.nice.org.uk) (Figure 6.10) or the Scottish Intercollegiate Guidelines Network (SIGN) which develops these products for the NHS (UK) in Scotland (http://www.sign.ac.uk/) (Figure 6.10).

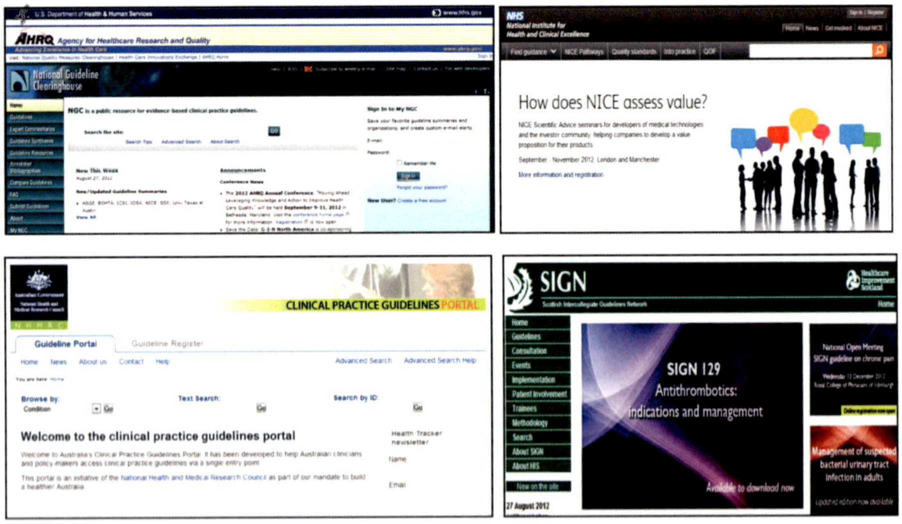

Figure 6.10. *The Nacional guideline clearinghouse (AHRQ), national institute of clinical studies (NHMRC), national institute for health and clinical excellence (NHS) and el Scottish intercollegiate guidelines network (SIGN).*

Source: Daz-Vlez, C., Soto-Cceres, V., E., R., Apolaya Segura, M. A., & Galn-Rodas, E. (2013). Clinical epidemiology and its relevance for public health in developing countries. InTech. doi: 10.5772/54901.

Social media platforms like Twitter are examples of other informatic applications for health information access that support research, share scientific knowledge and funding opportunities, and are highly beneficial for researchers, students, and medical professionals.

6.2.7. Bibliographic Reference Managers

A bibliographic reference (BR) is a basic set of information that makes it possible to identify a publication or a section of it. The number of BR types equals the number of information sources. Journal articles, electronic articles, books, book chapters, theses, standards, technical documents, videos, etc., are a few examples.

Each BR, in turn, consists of a variety of fields, some required and others optional, whose arrangements vary based on the BR format. In actuality, though, each journal selects its own style for BR and citations; the most popular formats are Vancouver style, American Psychological Association (APA), Modern Language Association (MLA), National Library of Medicine (NLM), and others.

The Vancouver Group, subsequently known as the International Committee of Medical Journal Editors (ICMJE), asked the National Library of Medicine to establish guidelines for writing bibliographic references in 1978. The NIH then published the NLM Recommended Formats for Bibliographic References in 1991, which were based on the American National Standard for Bibliographic References. The goal was to standardize the wide variety of available formats. Numerous software programs, the most well-known of which is the Endnote, have been made available for the management of BR in response to the need for a more effective and flexible approach to managing the BR. The primary purpose of this commercial reference and photo software is to organize, store, and search bibliographic references in a personal reference library. Additionally, it enables the organization of images, including equations, tables, graphics, and pictures, giving each one a caption and set of keywords. Other free access resources exist, though, such as the enhanced and free version of the Firefox-Mozilla Add-on Zotero (The University of Washington). With the help of this software, we will be able to create our BR library, automatically save our Pubmed search results, and directly cite every individual using Microsoft Word, Outlook, and other programs (Figure 6.11).

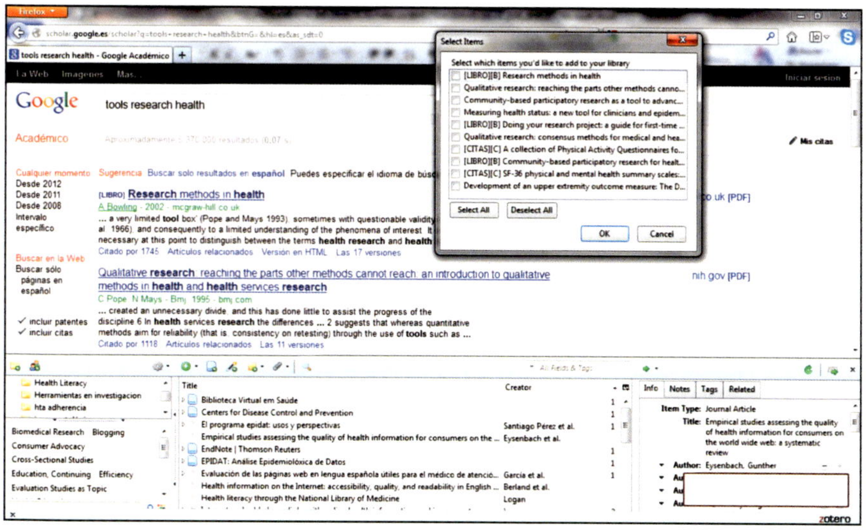

Figure 6.11. *Applications of zotero.*

Source: Daz-Vlez, C., Soto-Cceres, V., E., R., Apolaya Segura, M. A., & Galn-Rodas, E. (2013). Clinical epidemiology and its relevance for public health in developing countries. InTech. doi: 10.5772/54901.

6.2.8. Statistic Applications

A statistical package is a program or collection of programs that enable the application of an infinite number of statistical operations in sync, without exiting the program, to the same data file. The EPIDAT is a free program that the public developed to help epidemiologists and other health professionals manage tabular data. It allows us to perform descriptive analyzes, data filtering and imputation, sampling, parameters inference, contingency tables, matching and consistency, diagnostic tests, rates adjustment, demographics, logistic regression, survival analysis, probability distributions, Bayesian analysis, meta-analysis, public health monitoring, health inequality measurement, and economic evaluation methods, among other statistical applications that are particularly relevant to the investigation.

One of the most widely used and well-known statistical packages is SPSS, a graphical environment system for statistical analysis and data management that does most of the work with the help of straightforward dialog boxes and descriptive menus. It consists of a straightforward interface, a data editor, and features like multidimensional pivot tables, high-resolution graphics, database access, data processing, electronic distribution, and online help (Figure 6.12).

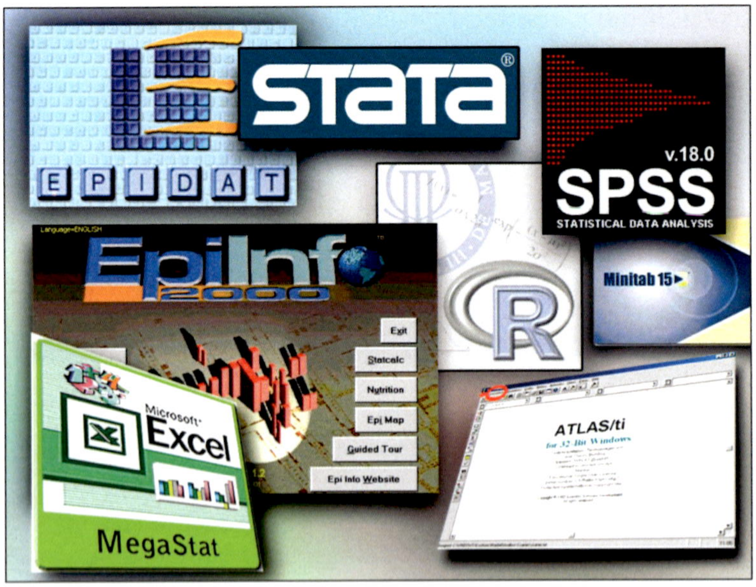

Figure 6.12. *Software statistics.*

Source: Daz-Vlez, C., Soto-Cceres, V., E., R., Apolaya Segura, M. A., & Galn-Rodas, E. (2013). Clinical epidemiology and its relevance for public health in developing countries. InTech. doi: 10.5772/54901.

6.3. Evidence-Based Medicine in Hospital Practice and in Public Health

The current trend in science is to concentrate on producing evidence that influences patient outcomes and advances the field. The application of Evidence-Based Medicine (EBM) is primarily observed in the pharmaceutical and medical device industries. Nonetheless, it is acknowledged that community interventions should be acknowledged as transcendent components that have influenced the population's health. Thus, it is imperative to acknowledge the presence of research that supports and demonstrates the effects of the range of initiatives of Public Health.

Evidence-Based Public Health (EBPH) upholds the logic of cause and effect while permitting the inclusion of health determinants, such as lifestyles, cultures, and environments, within a scientific framework. This is because these factors frequently determine whether an intervention is successful or unsuccessful. In this sense, EBPH represents a novel trend that has been combining forces to provide the best data for the most effective political decision-making.

6.3.1. Evidence-Based Medicine in the Clinical Environment

Doctors and students gain from the application of EBM in the hospital setting because it helps gather data that is chosen for its quality, informatics value, and user-relevantness (see, for instance, McMaster Premium Service Literature [PLUS] and ACP Journal Club Plus). Its ability to focus opinions on methodological quality and potential relevance for its application is one of its current advantages. To give professionals access to the highest caliber and relevance of technical literature, McMaster University created the "McMaster Online Rating of Evidence" (MORE) program.

This is accomplished by a classification made by experts from various latitudes across the globe. In addition, these services give concise and pertinent results and provide the ability to visualize feedback or criticism without requiring management of the data. This information indicates that "the EBM and nuclear fission can be very powerful when they are appropriately used and dangerous if they are not," according to the analogy. This is because the EBM distinguishes between describing the quality of the underlying evidence, the magnitude of the effects, and the applicability of any results in the context, without taking the values and preferences of the patients into account.

Consequently, it is undeniable that EBM has facilitated advancements in the field of medicine. The population's health would improve with the EBM, but its application in the health system has been uneven. The ability to easily incorporate the advancements of EBM is limited by the disparities in health systems around the world in terms of population healthcare, or frequently to a certain degree by political or economic constraints. However, it is noteworthy to mention that research in primary healthcare has indicated a correlation between a high level of EBM knowledge and improved healthcare quality. However, there isn't much data to support the impact of EBM on doctor performance and education when used as a formative performance evaluation method in the workplace. Regarding the application of EBM, it can be noted that public hospitals have a positive mindset. Furthermore, it is acknowledged that physicians who employ the EBM have a more open-minded approach to modifying information and counseling through networks of mutual assistance. Physicians are also aware of the disconnect between the applications of evidence-based medicine and clinical practice, as it is challenging to make decisions without considering clinical experience, peer opinions, or certain non-EBM scientific studies. As more time is spent providing care, decision-making based on clinical experience is more confidently made. Few physicians, nevertheless, advise that clinical experience be the only factor considered. According to the majority of physicians, local evidence gathered from local practice should direct EBM practice since it will enable them to support their decisions in clinical practice. As a result, the ability to automatically manage the evidence would benefit patients with chronic illnesses, for example, and would enable them to pay attention to unhealthy community factors that could be incorporated into the EBM to expand its paradigm. In light of this, it is important to consider the experiences of Canadian family physicians, who gave birth to the EBM. They report a positive attitude toward EBM, acknowledging its ability to improve patient care and the practical application of research findings in the treatment of everyday patients. In clinical practice, however, a demanding patient may impact the decision-making process and necessitate the use of a detection test (OR: 5.15; IC 95%: 2.9–9.2). The patient's preferences should be respected even though there was no therapeutic relationship maintained, and the clinical setting appears to more accurately reflect the clinical reality of EBM and primary care physicians.

6.3.2. Evidence-Based Medicine Compared to Evidence-Based Public Health

The Evidence-Based Medicine (EBM) approach assesses published clinical research and is increasingly being used as a reference for knowledge and in the evaluation of clinical practices. Its methodology primarily relies on the use of evidence, such as systematic reviews and meta-analyzes, to provide answers to specific clinical questions that are supported by statistical evidence. The use of EBM in clinical practice offers many advantages, but it also presents a number of challenges because it is difficult to apply universally without taking into account the socioeconomic, academic, and cultural context of each region. Because of this, using EBM correctly presents a challenge for modern medicine. However, this approach enables the health provider (or other professional) to use EBM to support his clinical practice, such as in a hospital setting. While it is not required, using it helps medical teams that are dedicated to enhancing hospital care.

The EBM approach works in tandem to focus efforts on maintaining evidence that supports health politics and community interventions, despite the known limitations of the EBH's use of evidence for using observational studies that have been consistently underestimated by EBM as a reference. This means that when applied to public health interventions, the EBM approach is not appropriately adjusted because it uses clinical trials as the gold standard, whose use in public health is of difficult extrapolation for when it is applied to the population. Technical evaluation models are currently being developed to act as a filter for evidence and work together to select studies with higher methodological stringency that can be used in public health.

Numerous aspects of the evaluation models used to assess the efficacy of public health interventions remain consistent. On the other hand, there is still no universal agreement on it. Among the tactics that should be mentioned is TREND (Transparent Reporting of Evaluations with Non-randomized Designs), which assesses the quality of publications that provide information on public health interventions. The capacity to enhance the systematization of data pertaining to public health interventions can be supplemented by the use of the MOOSE (Meta-analysis Of Observational Studies in Epidemiology) for reading observational studies meta-analysis or the STROBE (strengthening the Reporting of observational studies in Epidemiology) for cohorts and case-control studies. In general, it can be said that the EBM and EBPH have a common origin, which is the use of epidemiology as a decisive tool for the selection, evaluation and recommendation of evidence for its use, whether in hospital clinical practice of the social environment, which is Public Health.

In addition to budgetary constraints, it can be argued that there are other barriers to the integration of research in politics. Though if politicians were trained in this method, the EBM could be useful in helping them recognize and assess high-quality data. In this manner, scientists and health policy designers can work together to create the best possible decisions for the nation and its citizens. For upcoming health politics, this can serve as a generation and intervention experience exchange network.

6.3.3. The Cause-Effect Logic in the Public Health Interventions

As such, epidemiology supports the health sciences in their understanding of the various causal mechanisms through which the cause-effect relationship contributes to the evidence that defines health issues. In this sense, public health is one of the specialties that makes use of it as a crucial tool to present trustworthy data that will aid in comprehending the various health issues that different populations face. However, it is evident from the way the causal map is currently organized that a large number of the public health causal factors depend on social determinants. However, the issue with public health is complex and multifaceted. The analysis demonstrates that the challenge facing epidemiology is identifying a critical causal path that works in concert to comprehend how altering an event sequence (factors) can be induced to produce the anticipated result in a population's health problems; this event sequence is the critical causal path.

According to what it is stated, a group of steps that aid to develop this critical causal path will be explained, which will be used as an axis for the diverse approaches of the public health's interventions.

Step 1: Identify the public health issue: Primary or secondary data for the problem evaluation approach in public health can be obtained from various sources. Primary sources are the hardest to locate because obtaining scientific studies that compile the health problems facing divers requires time and resources. Utilizing secondary sources to problematize a population's health status is generally more practical given the technical and political context. The Health Situation Analysis (HAS) methodology, which enables the evaluation of three crucial factors, is one of the primary management tools utilized in accordance with geographic space. These factors include social determinants (socio-economic, cultural, lifestyle, commerce, environmental, etc.) the social response (health systems, health institutions, human resources in health, equipment, etc.) and morbidity and mortality (child mortality rate, maternal death rate, major diseases and death causes, etc.) which, when examined holistically, can reveal the primary health issues in a particular region and how they interact with national interventions. Finally, the health issue that needs to be considered in its true context must be emphasized.

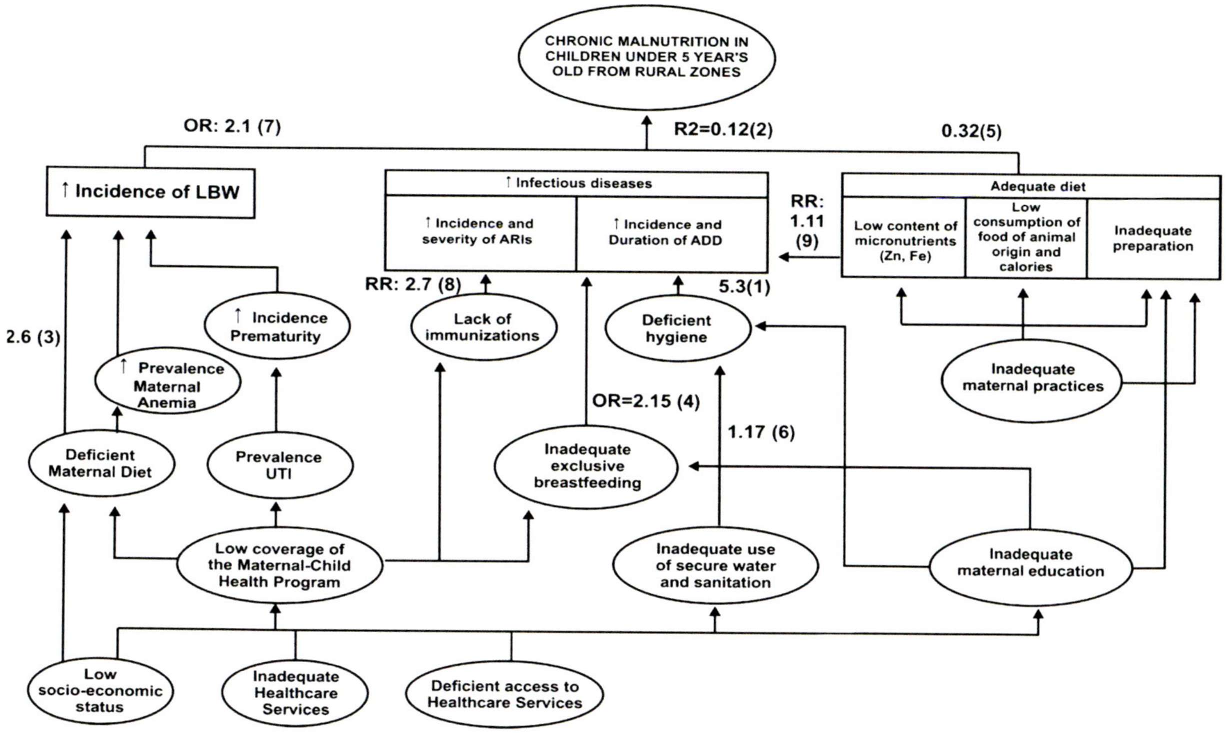

Figure 6.13. *Causal map of chronic malnutrition in children under 5 years old from rural zones.*

Source: Daz-Vlez, C., Soto-Cceres, V., E., R., Apolaya Segura, M. A., & Galn-Rodas, E. (2013). Clinical epidemiology and its relevance for public health in developing countries. InTech. doi: 10.5772/54901.

Step 2: Causal mapping with an evidence-based approach involves systematically evaluating evidence to explain a health problem and its causes and effects. When displayed in a causal map, this approach illustrates the cause-effect relationships supported by scientific evidence. This aids health decision-makers in understanding the complex web of factors contributing to the health problem, maintaining a multifactorial perspective. To create a causal map, researchers should gather the best available scientific evidence through a thorough literature search using digital tools and reputable scientific sources, while also ensuring the selected articles adhere to the methodological rigor expected in Evidence-Based Public Health (EBPH). As an example, it can be shown in Figure 6.13, the causal map of the health problema: "Chronic malnutrition in children under 5 years old from rural zones."

The causal map's arrows can be used to define the cause-and-effect logic. The numbers next to the arrows indicate the scientific evidence supporting the causal relation, which can be gathered into an evidence table like in Table 6.5. By analyzing how variables interact in relation to a health issue, health policy decision-makers can identify the root causes on a causal map. These causes may be linked to social determinants, like low socio-economic status, which may not be easily addressable in the short to medium term. However, there are variables that can be altered, and changing these may trigger a chain reaction of effects. This can lead to the development of a critical causal pathway.

Step 3: Establish key causal relationships: When searching for evidence in Public Health to create interventions that address health issues, it is important to understand how direct and indirect variables are connected to these problems. This understanding helps provide guidance on what needs to be modified. Critical causal pathways visually display the interaction between these variables, allowing decision makers to evaluate various paths for health interventions. For example, in the causal map shown in Figure 6.14, a pathway is outlined to assess the potential impact of fortified food programs on reducing chronic malnutrition in children under 5 years old.

Table 6.5. Evidence of the Causal Map of Chronic Malnutrition in Children Under 5 Years Old from Rural Zones

Evidence	Place	Type of Study	Interventions/ Results	Evidence level	Quality of vidence	Value
1. N Etilera. S Velipasaoglub. M. Aktekinc. Risk factors for overall and persistent diarrhoea in infancy in Antalya. Turkey: a cohort study. Public Health (2004) 118, 62-69. (13)	Turley	Cohort	Evaluation of lack of hygiene and increase of ADD.	II-2	3	RR:5.3
2. Peter G. Lunn. The impact of infection and nutrition on gut function and growth in childhood. Medical Research Council, Ke Peter Lunn1@tesco.net CAB International PNS Proceedings of the Nutrition Society (P185@ N4S N 9u9tr-ilti1o6nC Slion cicieatly nutrition in childhood P. G. Lunn147 2000)@ Nutrition Society 2000 59. (14)	Gambia	Review	Papers done in Gambia on the association between digestive infections and chronic malnutrition are evaluated.	II-3	4	R^2:0.12

3. Matete K. Virtanen S.M. Chilhood malnutriition and its predictor in rural Malawi. Paediatric & Pennatal Epidemdogy. volume 17. Number 4. October 2003, pp. 384-390. (15)	Malawi	Case-Control	Evaluates the association between deficient maternal diet and the increase in LBW.	II-2	3	RR:2.6
4. Alex K Anderson, Grace Danuo. Sara Young. Donna Chapman. A Randomized Tnal Assessing the Efficacy of Peer counseling on Exclusive Breastfeeding in a predominantly Latina Low income Community. Arch Pediatric Adolesc Med 2005: 159. 836-841. (16)	Latin communities	Randomized Clinical Trial	Association between breastfooding and ADD	II-1	1	RR:2.15
5. Bhandari N. Mazumder S. Bahl R. Marton J. Black R and Bhan M. An Educational Intervention to Promote Appropriate Complementary Feeding Practices and Physical Growth in Infants and Young Children in Rural Haryana. India.J. Nutr. 134:2342-2348. September 2004 (17)	India	Cluster Clinical Trial	Evaluation of the educational intervention in feeding practices and malnutrition.	II-2	1	Difference in growth 0.32 cm and 0.5cm
6. Merchant AT. Jones .C. Kiure A. Kupka R. Fitzmaunce G. Herrera MG. Favai WW. Water and sanitation associated with improved child growth European purnal of clinical nutrition 2003 Dec57 12 1562-8 (18)	India	Observational	Association between inadequate water-drainage services and inadequate practices.	II-3	3	OR:2.1
7. Institute National de EstadIsbca e Informatics PRISMA -Direction de Invesbgacson. Detenninantes de la desnutncien aguda y crtinica on nabs menores de 3 anos. Un sub-analisis de La ENDES 1992 y 1996. (19)	Peru	Observational	Association between low birth weight and malnutrition	II-3	3	OR:2.1
8. Deb SK. Acute respiratory disease survey in Tripura in case of children below five years of age J Indian Med Assoc. 1998 Apr;96(4)-111-6. (20)	India	Cohort	Association between immunizations and ARIs.	11-2	3	RR: 2.7
9. Tarun Gem. H P S Sachdev Effect of iron supplementation on incidence of infectious illness in children systematic review. BMJ vol 325 16 Nov 2002 (21)		Systematic Review	Effect of iron on infections in ADD	I-1	1	RR 1.11

Source: Daz-Vlez, C., Soto-Cceres, V., E., R., Apolaya Segura, M. A., & Galn-Rodas, E. (2013). Clinical epidemiology and its relevance for public health in developing countries. InTech. doi: 10.5772/54901.

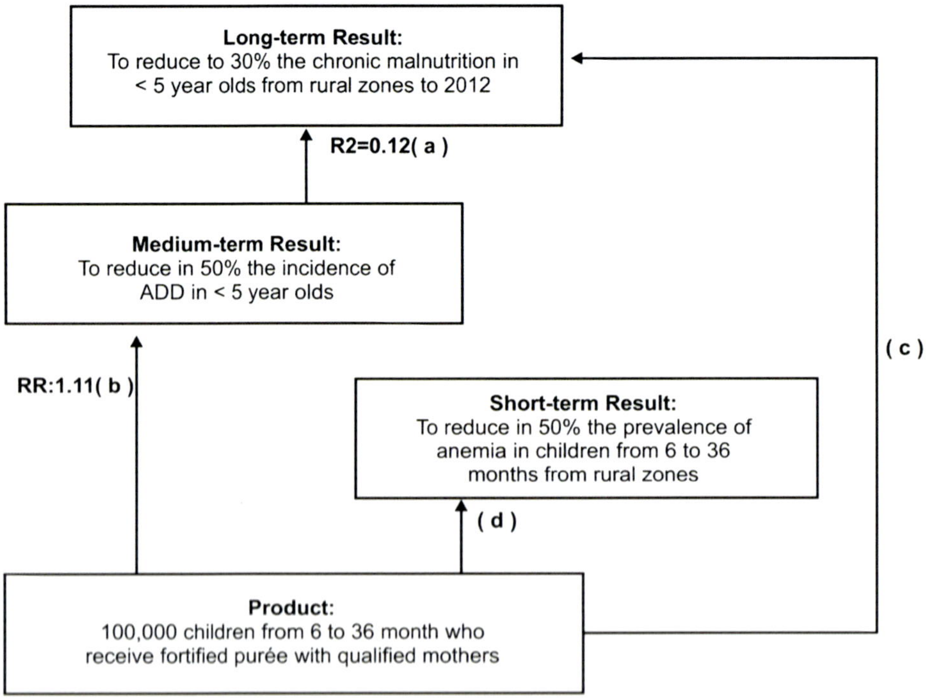

Figure 6.14. *Critical causal chain of the fortified food program to reduce the chronic malnutrition in children under 5 years old from rural zones.*

Source: Daz-Vlez, C., Soto-Cceres, V., E., R., Apolaya Segura, M. A., & Galn-Rodas, E. (2013). Clinical epidemiology and its relevance for public health in developing countries. InTech. doi: 10.5772/54901.

Table 6.6. Evidence That Sustains the Causality Relationship

Author	Design	Outcome	Population	Effect	Degree of recommendation	Evidence level
Peter G (a)	Analytical	Chronic malnutrition	Children	Diarrhea increases chronic malnutrition (R2 : 0.12)	B	III
Tarun Gera (b)	Review	Diarrhea	Children	Iron supplement RR: 1.11	A	Ia
Apolaya M (c)	Review	Chronic malnutrition	6 to 36 months	Non conclusive	A	Ia
Assunção MCF (d)	Review	Anemia	Infants	Non conclusive	A	Ia

Source: Daz-Vlez, C., Soto-Cceres, V., E., R., Apolaya Segura, M. A., & Galn-Rodas, E. (2013). Clinical epidemiology and its relevance for public health in developing countries. InTech. doi: 10.5772/54901.

It's also critical to place the health intervention proposals in the context of the economic aspects of each and the methodologies as economic evaluations created by each nation. This forces us to reconsider the need to acknowledge that socio-political factors have a significant impact on the health issues or interventions that are likely to be implemented. Nevertheless, as technical authorities, it is our goal to demonstrate, in the most objective, efficient, and effective manner possible, how to handle these factors in this task with the assistance of scientific data via the MBE or SPBE (Table 6.6).

A Closer Look

Clinical Epidemiology

Clinical epidemiology is a field that applies epidemiological methods to study the distribution and determinants of health and disease within clinical settings, with a focus on improving patient outcomes and healthcare delivery. It integrates principles of epidemiology with clinical research methodologies to generate evidence that informs clinical decision-making, healthcare policies, and the delivery of patient care.

One key aspect of clinical epidemiology is the study of disease etiology and risk factors within clinical populations. By investigating the factors that contribute to the development and progression of diseases among patients, clinical epidemiologists aim to identify modifiable risk factors, genetic predispositions, and other determinants of health outcomes. This knowledge helps clinicians and healthcare providers understand the underlying mechanisms of disease and develop targeted interventions to prevent, diagnose, and treat illnesses effectively.

Clinical epidemiology also plays a crucial role in evaluating the effectiveness and safety of healthcare interventions and treatments. Through randomized controlled trials, observational studies, and systematic reviews, clinical epidemiologists assess the efficacy, safety, and comparative effectiveness of medical therapies, surgical procedures, diagnostic tests, and preventive interventions. This evidence-based approach guides clinical decision-making by providing clinicians with reliable information on the benefits, harms, and uncertainties associated with different treatment options, ultimately aiming to optimize patient care and outcomes.

Moreover, clinical epidemiology contributes to the practice of evidence-based medicine by synthesizing research evidence with clinical expertise and patient values. By critically appraising scientific literature and synthesizing findings from multiple studies, clinical epidemiologists provide clinicians with up-to-date, reliable evidence to inform diagnostic and therapeutic decisions at the individual patient level. This integration of research evidence with clinical judgment and patient preferences ensures that healthcare interventions are tailored to the unique needs and circumstances of each patient, optimizing the quality, safety, and effectiveness of care.

In addition, clinical epidemiology plays a vital role in healthcare quality improvement and healthcare delivery research. By applying epidemiological methods to analyze healthcare processes, outcomes, and healthcare-associated infections, clinical epidemiologists identify opportunities for quality improvement, patient safety initiatives, and healthcare system optimization. This continuous monitoring and evaluation of healthcare practices contribute to the delivery of high-quality, evidence-based care and promote patient-centered outcomes within clinical settings.

Summary

- Clinical epidemiology has its application peak in the solution of treatment and management of diseases, contributing the identification of risk factors to certain illnesses and being to date the fundamental part of Evidence Based Medicine, and for that it becomes important the teaching of clinical epidemiology, for it will aid in the education of professionals with judicious capacity and rational use of the best alternatives in diagnostic and treatment, as well as helping to stimulate the training of researchers, because it's implied that the execution of the clinical epidemiology will lead to the development of research.
- Field epidemiology's primary function is to identify the cause or source of infectious diseases' outbreaks, containing its dissemination and organizing the infected patients' treatment as soon as possible.
- Field epidemiology executes its intervention on a daily basis in micro spaces, generally institutional: schools, restaurants, elderly residencies, hospitals whose services can present outbreaks, and uses conventional methods.
- Clinical epidemiology is based mainly on its clinical trials, examining the diagnostic methods, discussing the prognosis, taking part in the evolution of treatments, trying to organize a controlled and randomized study opposite to sick people getting placebos or another indicated drug.
- Clinical Medicine, Clinical Epidemiology and EBM have been widely promoted as an improvement in patient's healthcare. For that, doctors must be capable of showing the patient the therapeutic options for a shared decision making, using the results obtained in clinical studies. Then it becomes important to correctly interpret the results of a study, to transmit appropriately this information to the patients, and to take the best diagnostic and therapeutic decisions.
- A bibliographic reference (BR) is a minimal group of data that allows the identification of a publication or a part of the same. There are as many types of BR as information sources. Among them, journal articles, electronic articles, books, chapters of books, thesis, norms, technical documents, videos, etc.
- The Evidence Based Public Health (EBPH) maintains a cause-effect logic, and allows to add the health determinants, like lifestyles, culture and environment, in a scientific context, because many times it's them who characterize the good or bad performance of a certain intervention. This way, EBPH is a new tendency that has been joining efforts to give the best information for the most efficient politics decision making.

References

1. Altman, D. G., & Bland, J. M. (1994). Statistics Notes: Diagnostic tests 2: predictive values. *BMJ, 309*, 102.
2. Berger, J. S., Roncaglioni, M. C., Avanzini, F., Pangrazzi, I., Tognoni, G., & Brown, D. L. (2006). Aspirin for the primary prevention of cardiovascular events in women and men: a sex-specific meta-analysis of randomized controlled trials. *JAMA, 295*, 306–313.

3. Garg, A. X., Adhikari, N. K., McDonald, H., Rosas-Arellano, M. P., Devereaux, P. J., Beyene, J., et al. (2005). Effects of computerized clinical decision support systems on practitioner performance and patient outcomes: a systematic review. *JAMA, 293*, 1223–1238.
4. Grimshaw, J., Eccles, M., & Tetroe, J. (2004). Implementing clinical guidelines: current evidence and future implications. *Journal of Continuing Education in the Health Professions, 24*, S31–S37.
5. Jackson, R. T. (1996). Guidelines for managing raised blood pressure: Evidence based or evidence burdened? *BMJ, 313*, 64–65.
6. Jackson, R., Barham, P., Bills, J., Birch, T., McLennan, L., MacMahon, S., et al. (1993). The management of raised blood pressure in New Zealand. *BMJ, 307*, 107–110.
7. Jamrozik, K., Vessey, M., Fowler, G., Wald, N., Parker, G., & Van Vunakis, H. (1984). Controlled trial of three different antismoking interventions in general practice. *BMJ, 288*, 1499–1503.
8. Lloyd-Jones, D. M., Leip, E. P., D'Agostino, R., Beiser, H., Wilson, P. W., Wolf, P. A., & Levy, M. I. (2006). Prediction of lifetime risk for cardiovascular disease by risk factor burden at 50 years of age. *Circulation, 113*, 791–799.
9. Manuel, D. G., Lim, J., Tanuseputro, P., Anderson, G. M., Alter, D. A., Laupacis, A., et al. (2006). Revisiting Rose: strategies for reducing coronary heart disease. *BMJ, 332*, 659–662.
10. Mendis, S., Abegunde, D., Yusuf, S., Ebrahim, S., Shaper, G., Ghannem, H., et al. (2005). WHO study on Prevention of Recurrences of Myocardial Infarction and Stroke (WHO-PREMISE) (Phase I) Study Group. *Bulletin of the World Health Organization, 83*, 820–828.
11. Murray, C. J., Lauer, J. A., Hutubessy, R. C., Niessen, L., Tomijima, N., Rodgers, A., et al. (2003). Effectiveness and costs of interventions to lower systolic blood pressure and cholesterol: a global and regional analysis on reduction of cardiovascular disease risk. *Lancet, 361*, 717–725.
12. Stewart, A. W., Beaglehole, R., Jackson, R., & Bingley, W. (1999). Trends in 3-year survival following acute myocardial infarction 1983–92. *European Heart Journal, 20*, 803–807.
13. Wald, N. J., & Law, M. R. (2003). A strategy to reduce cardiovascular disease by more than 80%. *BMJ, 326*, 1419–1424.
14. Whitehead, M., Dahlgren, G., & Evans, T. (2001). Equity and health sector reforms: can low-income countries escape the medical poverty trap? *Lancet, 358*, 833–836.

Chapter 7

SOCIAL EPIDEMIOLOGY: PAST, PRESENT, AND FUTURE

Contents

Introduction

A subfield of epidemiology that focuses on comprehending how social organization affects the distribution of health and disease has seen a rise in usage over the past 30 years: social epidemiology. A variety of systems and structures, such as social and economic ties, laws and regulations, and customs, are included in social organization. It encompasses a wide range of elements, including social hierarchy and the degree of inequality, the economy, the way resources are distributed and labor is organized, the relationships between different racial and ethnic groups, cultural aspects, and social norms. Social epidemiology is distinguished from other subfields of epidemiology by its emphasis on the wide range of social conditions that influence numerous health-related outcomes, as opposed to other subfields that are defined by the health outcome.

Even though it could be argued that all epidemiology requires taking the social world into account, the term "social epidemiology" allowed explicit emphasis on the social production of disease as a potent explanatory paradigm and as crucial to determining the policies required to improve population health in an environment where epidemiologic research has been heavily influenced by a biomedical and individualistic approach. This field of study is particularly difficult due to the complexity of the social and biological worlds and how they interact to impact health, but it is also a great place to develop new ideas and critical thinking skills for epidemiology and population health research in general.

Orientation and Directional Terms

Term	Definition	Illustration
Ethnicity	Ethnicity or ethnic group is a group of people who identify with each other on the basis of perceived shared attributes that distinguish them from other groups. Those attributes can include a common nation of origin, or common sets of ancestry, traditions, language, history, society, religion, or social treatment.	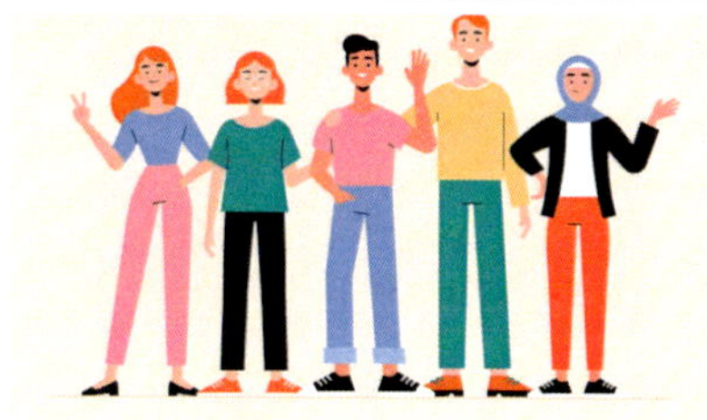
Social Determinants of Health	The social determinants of health are the economic and social conditions that influence individual and group differences in health status.	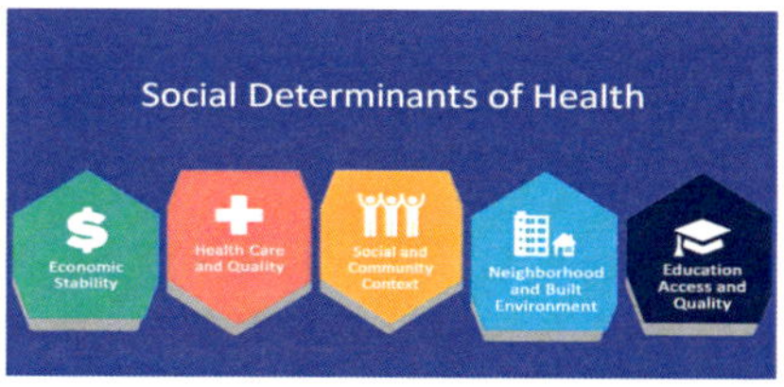
Health Outcomes	Health outcomes are defined as those events occurring as a result of an intervention. These may be measured clinically (physical examination, laboratory testing, imaging), self-reported, or observed (such as gait or movement fluctuations seen by a healthcare provider or caregiver).	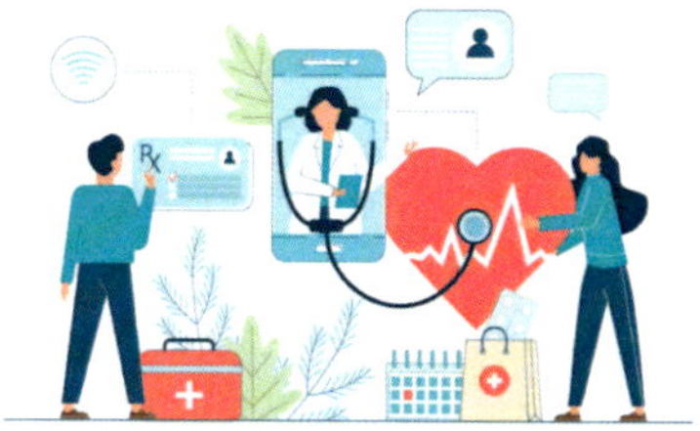
Social Networks	Social networks are websites and apps that allow users and organizations to connect, communicate, share information and form relationships.	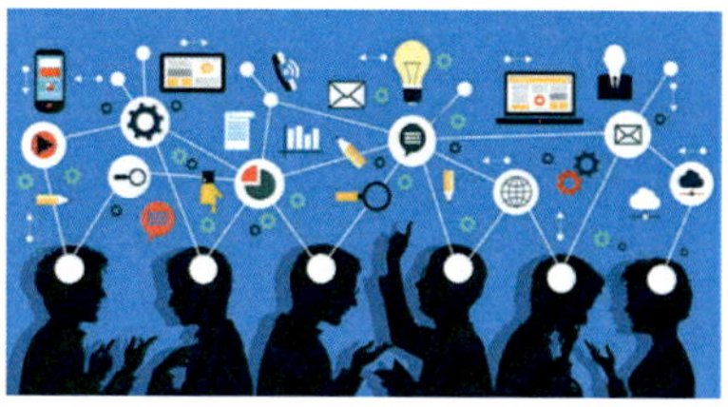
Psychosocial Factors	Psychosocial factors are characteristics or facets that influence an individual psychologically and/or socially. Such factors can describe individuals in relation to their social environment and how these affect physical and mental health.	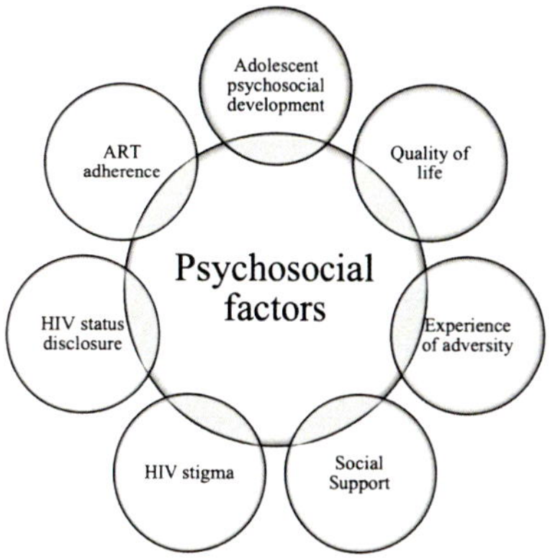

7.1. Major Substantive Areas of Focus

Over the past 30 years, social epidemiology has focused on a wide range of substantive topics. Building the evidence base for the claim that societal conditions have a major influence in the development of illness has occupied a large amount of the research effort. In order to better understand causality in biological processes—which frequently cannot be fully understood without reference to the social context in which they operate—a related body of work has concentrated on pinpointing the precise mechanisms through which this social causation operates. Examining the effects on health of interventions or policies that target social determinants in particular has gained traction in recent years.

7.1.1. The Social Patterning of Health: Describing and Inferring Social Causation Writ Large

The explanation of the social patterns of health has been essential in proving the significant effects of social organization on health. Population health is significantly shaped by social processes related to economic systems and inequality, systemic racism, and residential segregation, as suggested by the straightforward measurement of health disparities by social class, race and ethnicity, or place of residence. In order to support the notion that there are substantial health disparities by class, race, and neighborhood that require attention, regardless of the underlying processes causing these differences, a great deal of work in social epidemiology has concentrated on characterizing and quantifying this social patterning. Social position has been conceptualized in a variety of ways in research on social stratification and health. Even though terms like social class, socioeconomic position, and socioeconomic status are occasionally used synonymously, their connotations are derived from the fundamental theory of social stratification. Research has quantified the size of social differences, explored the nature of the relationship between social position and health, and investigated heterogeneity in social patterning over time and place. These measures, which serve as proxy measures of social status, socioeconomic position, or class, include income, education, and occupation. Separating the relative significance of particular dimensions, like wealth, income, or education, has been the focus of other research. Studies on the relationship between health and social stratification have also looked at health across the life course, showing how social position can have independent or interacting effects at different times in life.

The recording of racial and ethnic disparities in health has received significant attention as well. The terms "race" and "ethnicity" refer to socially constructed population groups that are associated with physical characteristics, shared cultural and linguistic traits, perceived ancestry or geographic origin, and that reflect unequal access to resources and power in society. Beyond scientifically dubious attributions of racial/ethnic differences to biological or genetic variations, social epidemiologic research has brought attention to the contributions of social organization to racial differences. Numerous studies have shown how racial disparities exist in social, economic, and environmental contexts (e.g., factors that could impact health include neighborhoods, work conditions, wealth, income, and education. Systemic racism and structural inequality are historical and social processes that have historically and socially driven racial and ethnic differences. It has also been established that a person's personal experience with racism or discrimination influences their health. According to social epidemiologists, racial disparities in health result from a system that allocates resources, opportunities, and exposures based on race. An associated field of social epidemiologic research has concentrated on how immigration and acculturation affect health. This research has demonstrated the significant and varied health effects that can result from the process of assimilating into a new nation's customs and way of life, also known as acculturation or assimilation. The effects of migration history and acculturation on health are closely related to the health effects of racism and inequality because immigrants are frequently members of marginalized groups in their new nation.

There has been much discussion over whether formal causal inference techniques are necessary to reach generalizations about the social determinants of health. Causal inference methods designed to quantify the short-term causal impact of changes in very specifically defined factors, with all other factors held constant, are often not easily applicable to the broad causal questions of interest in social epidemiology, because the social processes leading to differences in health by social position, race, or immigration history involve the functioning of systems with multiple interacting pathways and long causal chains. Nonetheless, it would be challenging to make the case that, in the setting of unfair and racist systems, social causation cannot be deduced from the copious evidence of marked disparities in health (across a wide range of health outcomes) linked to social stratification and race. Even in the lack of exact counterfactual comparisons, the argument that social organization influences the distribution of health and disease depends heavily on these descriptive analyzes. Later in this review, we will revisit the subject of causal inquiry in social epidemiology.

7.1.2. Beyond Individuals: From Multilevel Determinants to Systems Approaches

The inclusion of factors at various organizational levels in conceptual models and empirical analyzes has been a significant focus in social epidemiology. The idea that epidemiology should consider factors other than individual-level health outcomes has been formalized as a result of the focus on multiple levels. Additionally, there has been a great deal of discussion in epidemiology regarding the implications of this multilevel approach for study design and analytical techniques. The kinds of interventions and policies that may be determined to be pertinent to health may be significantly impacted by the expansion of epidemiologic research to explicitly include variables defined at levels above individuals. Among many other levels of organization, social epidemiology has shown interest in neighborhoods, workplaces, schools, and states. This multilevel approach has been pioneered by three substantive areas, which are the health impacts of income inequality, social capital, and neighborhood features.

Since it can be addressed through policy and is widespread throughout the world, income inequality has drawn a lot of attention. A long history of ecologic analyzes has shown without a doubt that nations with higher levels of income inequality typically have poorer health outcomes, even after controlling for gross domestic product or summary measures of income. These correlations may be partially explained by the two facts that are generally true in more unequal societies: the number of people living in poverty (or at lower income levels) is higher, and income is strongly (though not always linearly) correlated with health across the income spectrum. Whether people who live in more unequal societies have worse health regardless of their own level of income is a topic of extensive discussion that arose in the early 2000s. Some predicted that the psychosocial effects of relative deprivation would act as the main mediator of these associations. Some suggested that variations in the social investments and policies linked to income inequality were probably the cause of any contextual effect of income inequality. Multilevel studies that sought to separate the contextual effects of income inequality from individual-level social position proliferated as a result of discussions about whether income inequality itself (above and beyond any effects of individual-level income) affected health. Discussions about the proper scale for measuring income inequality (e.g., states, neighborhoods), the potential time lags involved, the degree to which confounders were suitably controlled for in the studies, and the mechanisms relating the degree of income inequality in the population to health. The relationship between income inequality and health serves as an excellent example of the difficulties in determining the health effects of a population-level attribute that is relevant to policy, is correlated with a wide range of other population attributes, may act through a complex web of interrelated mechanisms (including the effects of individual-level income), and may operate over an extended period of time.

A lot of focus was also placed on the idea of social capital. The definition of social capital is "the resources available to members of social groups, such as the exchange of favors, the maintenance of group norms, the presence of trust, and the exercise of sanctions." Social connections as defined by the formal analysis of social networks and social cohesiveness (solidarity and trust, norms, and the capacity for collective action) are all included in social capital. The definition of social capital and appropriate metrics for measuring it have been the subject of much debate. Higher levels of social capital have been linked in studies to improved health, which suggests that social capital may be a source of resilience. However, studies have also shown that social capital has a negative impact on health through the social spread of unhealthy behaviors and negative effects in some people, possibly as a result of exclusion.

The multilevel approach has included the study of neighborhood effects on health as a third and primary area of focus. This field has included a wide range of neighborhood-level constructs, from physical environment characteristics (e.g., walkability and resource accessibility) to social variables (e.g., social cohesion, collective efficacy, and measures of neighborhood violence, deprivation, and segregation). Due to the significance of neighborhood health effects for so-called place-based interventions, they have drawn particular attention. The definition of the neighborhood (or, more precisely, the spatial context relevant to the process being studied), the measurement of neighborhood attributes, the appropriate time frame for expected effects, and challenges with causal inference—particularly those pertaining to appropriately accounting for individual-level confounders—have all been significant obstacles in this field of study. Through sophisticated longitudinal studies that include direct measurement of a wide range of neighborhood attributes and the application of improved analytical techniques to support causal inferences, the field has progressed from initially crude approaches that sought to isolate a contextual effect of neighborhood disadvantage. Additionally, research in this field has extended to the use of systems modeling, randomized trials, and policy evaluation.

Over time, consideration of factors at multiple levels of organization has become the norm rather than the exception in population health research, stimulated by the focus on this approach in social epidemiology. The use of multilevel approaches has expanded to encompass a broad range of questions, including the health impacts of gender equality and residential segregation, among others. But social epidemiologists have also recognized the need not only to include factors at multiple levels of organization but also to capture the dynamics of the systems that underlie the social patterning of health. Social epidemiology has been at the forefront of efforts to bring systems thinking and the tools of complex systems approaches to population health. The systems approach is quite different from traditional approaches to causal inference in that it explicitly accounts for feedbacks, dependencies generated via social networks or other processes, nonlinearities, and conditional effects. Systems approaches include a large set of approaches and tools ranging from qualitative and participatory methods to social network analyzes to sophisticated mathematical modeling using agent-based models or systems dynamics models. A number of applications of systems approaches to social epidemiology questions have emerged, illustrating the potential but also the challenges involved. Multilevel and systems thinking are two important ways in which social epidemiology has broadened conceptualization as well as empirical analyzes in population health more generally.

7.1.3. Processes and Mechanisms: Tracing the Specific Pathways Through Which Social Organization Impacts Biology

The identification of particular mechanisms by which social factors influence health has been a focus of attention in the field of social epidemiology. An understanding of mechanisms can provide significant scientific insight into the broader causes of disease. Furthermore, it strengthens causal inferences in social epidemiology by elucidating the particular mechanisms through which the postulated social causation functions.

A large body of work has examined the extent to which behavioral factors mediate social differences in health, the underlying hypothesis being that environmental and resource constraints and social influences shape the distribution of behavioral risk factors that then impact health. Debate ensued about what might explain social differences that persisted after behavioral factors were accounted for. Psychosocial factors were hypothesized to contribute to associations that remained after adjustment for behavioral risk factors. The set of psychosocial factors hypothesized as mediators of social differences include some that are more psychological in nature (e.g., depression, anxiety, anger, status perceptions) and others that are more social (social support) and encompass a broad set of domains, including stressors, emotional responses, and resources. Perceived discrimination has also been proposed as an important stressor in racist societies and posited to contribute to race and ethnic differences in health.

It has also been suggested that work environment variables, such as employment status, psychological aspects, and chemical and physical risks, play a role in the disparities in health between social groups. Complex models of psychosocial aspects of the workplace, such as demands, control over the work process, effort-reward imbalance, and social support, were developed and empirically investigated in connection to health outcomes. The impact of work organization on health was persuasively demonstrated by this study. Disparities in the availability and caliber of healthcare services have also been proposed as contributing to social disparities in health, despite the fact that social epidemiologists examine these issues less frequently.

An increasing amount of research has also looked at the connections between particular biological processes and social factors.

Prior research concentrated on biomedical measurements and conditions like blood pressure, weight, and diabetes; however, interest later shifted to biological domains related to inflammation and markers of inflammation. In order to understand how repeated exposure to stressors causes wear and tear on the body, interest in stress biomarkers and measures of cumulative biological dysregulation, such as allostatic load, has also grown. Scholars have argued in favor of including social factors in gene-by-environment interaction studies and have looked into the relationship between social factors and gene expression and epigenetic markers. In additional research, scientists investigated the connections between societal factors and biological aging indicators like telomere length.

The quantification of how different types of factors (or sets of factors) contribute to or mediate social differences (e.g., percentage of effects mediated through different factors) has been challenging, owing to the rudimentary nature of many of the mediation analyzes used, often simple comparisons of associations before and after adjustment, many times using cross-sectional data. Even when longitudinal data are available and when more sophisticated approaches are used, the quantification of mediation is rendered very complex because of the presence of confounders, the multiple mediators likely involved, and the possible interactions between mediators and between mediators and social antecedents. Perhaps the main contribution of mediation studies has been the demonstration of how pervasive the social patterning is of many behavioral, psychosocial, and biological factors linked to health. The fact that all these factors are consistently and strongly socially patterned has buttressed the argument that the social world is a major determinant of health. This patterning demonstrates the notion of embodiment, i.e., the process by which the social world has specific and measurable impacts on biological structure and function.

7.1.4. Policies and Interventions: Intervening on Individuals, Community, and Society

The description of the social patterning of health and etiologic and mechanistic research have received far more attention in social epidemiology than policy and intervention research, as has been mentioned elsewhere. Nonetheless, research on the health impacts of particular policies or interventions is crucial to support causal inference in social epidemiology more broadly as well as to develop the evidence base for particular actions. This area of research is challenging in terms of study design, data availability, and analytical methods because of the wide range of interventions and policies that can be investigated, the hypothesized health impacts, and the time frames over which they can be expected to occur.

In social epidemiology, the policies or interventions that have the biggest effects on the social determinants of health are of particular interest. Interventions can vary in scope from extremely focused and specific (e.g., housing rehabilitation projects or campaigns to improve neighborhood access to fresh produce) to far more extensive and upstream (e.g., lowering income disparity via redistribution and taxation). Even though they might not directly address the social determinants of health, other policies and interventions can help lessen social injustices by focusing on specific behavioral or medical issues or altering them to better suit particular social groups. By obstructing the mechanisms that social causes use to function, these kinds of interventions can lessen inequality. Selected instances of policies and interventions are shown in Figure 7.1, which is categorized based on the intervention's level and the point on the social causation continuum where it primarily functions.

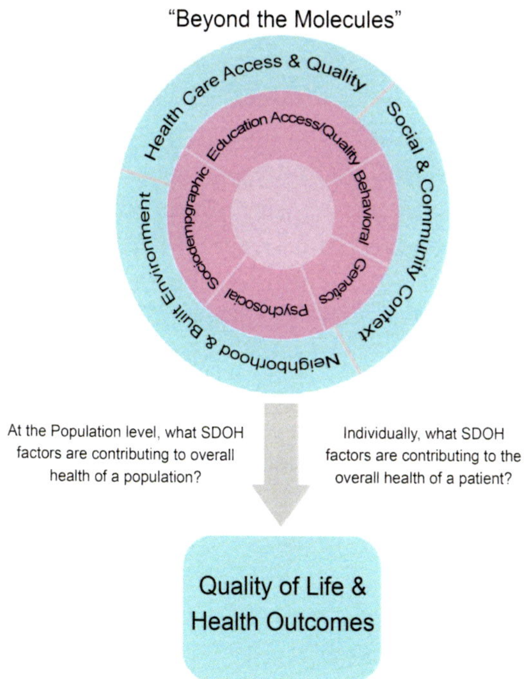

Figure 7.1. *Schematic typology of policies and interventions that address social determinants of health.*

Source: Davidson J, Vashisht R, Butte AJ. From genes to geography, from cells to community, from biomolecules to behaviors: The importance of social determinants of Health. Biomolecules. 2022; 12(10):1449. https://doi.org/10.3390/biom12101449.

Experiments have been used in a growing body of work in social epidemiology to determine the effects of policies or interventions. For instance, the Moving to Opportunity trial is frequently mentioned. It was initially intended to evaluate the effects of a housing voucher program on economic outcomes, but it was later expanded to look at the health effects of moving to a non-poor neighborhood. The Oportunidades trial is a randomized study that examined a conditional cash transfer program that was put into place in Mexico. While both of these studies have provided insight into the effectiveness of the particular interventions tested, they have not addressed more comprehensive policy strategies aimed at addressing health disparities related to neighborhood or income. These tactics might involve spending money in impoverished or segregated areas or using taxes to lower rates of poverty and income inequality. Randomized trials are a far more challenging, if not impossible, way to study these kinds of policies.

Because of the challenges in performing true experiments, many researchers have called for greater use of "natural experiments." A number of efforts have been made to use natural experiments to gain insight into the health consequences of policies that target social determinants of health. Many focus on interventions on neighborhood or community features. Examples include the opening of new food stores, a new public transportation system, vacant lot greening, neighborhood revitalization initiatives, and interventions to improve social capital. Other studies have attempted to estimate the effects of policies that address broader elements of social and economic policy by capitalizing on heterogeneity across geographies or over time in specific policies. For example, Dahl & van der Wel leveraged heterogeneity in social spending across 18 European countries to examine whether more social spending is associated with better health. Ludwig & Miller capitalized on the way in which the Head Start program was implemented in US counties over time to assess the program's impact on child health. Montez et al. used heterogeneity in state policies to estimate effects on differential life expectancy trends by state. Systematic reviews across study designs have also been used to synthesize the impact of policies or interventions focused on the social determinants of health.

It is crucial to remember that laws meant to promote population health may have unforeseen negative effects on health and may also have the unintended effect of exacerbating health disparities due to the way the policies interact with the social structures and systems already in place. An important but understudied area of social epidemiology research is the evaluation of all health or public health policies for their impact on health equity (be it racial, socioeconomic, geographic, or based on other characteristics).

7.2. Challenges and Opportunities

The study of social epidemiology has been incredibly dynamic, spurring discussion about the nature of epidemiology in general and its implications for society. It has also served as an engine for innovation.

7.2.1. Grounding Research in Theoretically Based and Systemic Conceptual Models of the Fundamental Social Drivers of Health

Conceptual models are essential to any field because they help researchers identify analytical implications, clarify theory and assumptions, and frame research questions. The theories that underpin conceptual models clarify the structures, processes, and dynamics that are thought to be responsible for the observed empirical regularities. The questions we pose, the information we gather and examine, and the conclusions we reach all depend on this theory, which must be empirically verified or refuted. Social epidemiology must remember the fundamental role that concepts and theories play in producing reliable and socially useful explanations as it strives to become more methodologically rigorous and empirically grounded.

A myriad of different conceptual models for the social determinants of health have been proposed. One key challenge has been to expand these models so that they reflect levels of organization, time, dynamics (including feedbacks and dependencies), and pathways but still remain parsimonious enough to be useful (i.e., generate insight into fundamental drivers or guide specific empirical analyzes). In some ways, the proliferation of many all-encompassing models has detracted from the generation of significant scientific consensus about what the fundamental factors, dynamics, and processes linking social organization to health are. Given the complexity of the links between social organization and health, it may be more useful to develop more focused models that aim to explain specific phenomena rather than models that attempt to very simply capture a very broad set of social influences on health. These more focused models may allow a better understanding of dynamic relations, something that many existing conceptual models tend to ignore. One example of a focused approach has been the fundamental social cause model proposed by Link et al. Their model proposes a fundamental dynamic and generates testable predictions. Examples of other areas where the development of focused approaches with attention to dynamics would be useful (and are emerging) include the impact of systemic racism on health and the role of environmental factors in generating health inequities.

7.2.2. Implementing a Scientifically Rigorous Yet Realistic Approach to Drawing Conclusions About Social Causes

Causal inference from observational studies has received more attention in social epidemiology in recent years. Further formalization of the assumptions necessary to draw causal inferences from observational studies, the appropriate application of cutting-edge statistical techniques, a greater emphasis on the study of the health impacts of policies or interventions using experiments or natural experiments, and a greater use of tools such as directed acyclic graphs to provide insight into the identifiability of causal effects and the assumptions and analytical approaches required have all been recommended.

Determining which causal questions can be addressed within the framework of the potential outcomes approach to causality has been at the center of a significant methodological discussion that is especially relevant to social epidemiology. There has been discussion about which variables should be the focus of causal inquiry in social epidemiology as a result of the growing interest in formalizing causal inference based on the potential outcomes approach. Some academics have argued that exposures that can be specifically defined as "realistic" or "practicable" interventions should be the focus of causal inference. There are numerous advantages to identifying the relevant causal factor as an intervention. The best analytical strategy, the assumptions involved, and the amount of data required are all better understood by clearly defining the causal question. An additional advantage is that the response to the causal query also directly tackles the potential effects of a theoretical intervention that might be implemented in the real world.

However, because this etiologic understanding is essential to determining potential avenues for actions to improve health, we in social epidemiology are also interested in understanding social causation broadly. There are systems and structures involved in the social production of health. Therefore, a thorough understanding of social causation necessitates an understanding of how the systems function, which cannot be achieved by limiting the study of social causation to determining the results of workable interventions. According to Schwartz et al., social epidemiology's causal inquiry's exclusive focus on "well-defined interventions" favors "interventions that are less social, less upstream, and less system changing."

Therefore, embracing both the developments in quantitative causal inference and the emphasis on policies and interventions without sacrificing a larger focus on comprehending the social structure and systems that give rise to health will be a challenge for social epidemiology in the years to come. Social epidemiologists focus on a variety of "causes" because the field of social epidemiology studies how social organization affects health. These include specific factors, definable interventions, and definable interventions under extremely specific conditions. Broadly defined structural and very distal determinants may operate in a variety of ways and interact with one another. In social epidemiology, causal inquiry and intervention research are far more complex than they are in the medical or even traditional epidemiologic domains because of this wide continuum of causes. Even though the ultimate goal of causal understanding in social epidemiology is to pinpoint actions, studying the effects of particular workable actions taken today alone will not provide us with the comprehensive understanding we require. Our ultimate objective is to gain a deeper understanding of reality, which includes describing phenomena and relationships in addition to narrowly defining causes, in order to identify a variety of potential courses of action. In order to achieve this goal, theoretically sound and empirically supported social explanations for the patterns we observe must be developed, and these explanations must make use of a variety of different types of evidence that, when taken as a whole, improve our comprehension of the most significant factors and their interactions.

7.2.3. Using Complementary Methods to Generate Valid Explanations and Identify Effective Actions

Integrating a wide range of evidence types will be necessary to achieve the comprehensive understanding of social patterning and social causation that forms the basis of social epidemiologic inquiry and is essential to taking effective health-improving actions. These evidence types include true experimental studies, rigorous quantitative causal inference from observational studies, systems modeling, and real-world assessments of interventions and policies under various conditions (including what is known as implementation science), which includes evaluating the equity implications of policies. Experiments and policy evaluation are crucial tools for improving our fundamental understanding of the mechanisms underlying health and health disparities as well as for identifying effective interventions. Other methodological techniques that are frequently overlooked when discussing epidemiologic methods are qualitative comparative analyzes, descriptive methods, and surveillance.

Surveillance has long been used in epidemiology to both identify health issues that require urgent attention and to shed light on possible causes. From historical examples like Goldberger's work on the etiology of pellagra to more recent research outlining and speculating on the causes of the opioid crisis in the U.S, thorough descriptive analyzes have yielded important information that is pertinent to both understanding and policy. Social epidemiology has unique opportunities to improve its descriptions of the social patterning of health and its evolution over time, thanks to the increasing availability and accessibility of georeferenced and linked data on health and social circumstances.

There has been little application of qualitative methods in social epidemiology, despite numerous calls to increase their use in public health. By incorporating a more thorough and nuanced understanding of the phenomena and processes that affect health across levels of organization, with an emphasis on heterogeneity and context, qualitative methods can advance scientific understanding in social epidemiology. In addition to generating hypotheses and enhancing and interpreting the findings of quantitative research, qualitative approaches can directly advance causal understanding by shedding light on processes that quantitative research may miss. For instance, understanding conditional effects and, more precisely, causation resulting from several interacting factors, is particularly well suited to qualitative comparative analysis. Another opportunity for the future is to increase the use of qualitative approaches, and in particular, to create models of how to use mixed methods approaches to advance our understanding of social epidemiology.

7.2.4. Leveraging the Power of Harmonization, Replication, and Big Data

A major challenge in replicating and summarizing findings in social epidemiology has been the differences across studies in the definition and measurement of key social constructs. The large heterogeneity in definitional and measurement aspects is understandable, given the complexity of the factors that are being measured. Moreover, there are many reasons why epidemiologic findings may not fully replicate, including methodological issues (differences in confounder control, for example) as well as substantive reasons, including true heterogeneity in causal effects across samples as a result of different distributions of effect modifiers. Nevertheless, a greater focus on harmonization, replication, and evidence synthesis is a major need in the field. Systematic exploration of the robustness of results using quantitative bias analyzes as well as greater attention to systematically exploring heterogeneity will also help facilitate evidence synthesis.

The rapid growth in the availability of large and often linked data sets ranging from administrative to genomic data and including high-dimensional social data of various types also creates opportunities for research in social epidemiology. Examples of this type of data include geographically referenced electronic health records, cell phone data on mobility, and policy or other contextual data.

The use of these data sets can enhance the description of social patterning and thus yield new insights into how the social world affects health. It may also improve observational studies of social etiology by facilitating the identification of instrumental variables. Longitudinal big data may also create opportunities for the analysis of natural experiments.

The availability of big data has also spurred interest in data discovery approaches such as environment-wide association studies and machine learning approaches focused on pattern recognition and prediction as a complement to the hypothesis-testing approaches more common in social epidemiology.

Although applications of machine learning and data discovery approaches in social epidemiology are rapidly emerging, they are, for the most part, exploratory, and the utility of these approaches in generating new insights remains to be determined. In addition, important questions have emerged regarding how algorithm-driven approaches can perpetuate biases and stereotypes. Finding the balance between theory-based and hypothesis-driven approaches and emerging data-driven approaches spurred by increased data availability and computational power will be an important challenge and opportunity for social epidemiology in the future.

7.2.5. Extending Interdisciplinarity: Beyond Epidemiology, Sociology, and Psychology

One of the defining features of social epidemiology has been its engagement with other disciplines, especially sociology, psychology, and human development. These interdisciplinary collaborations have facilitated the incorporation of new theories, measures, and analytical approaches. A growing interest in the social determinants of health within the clinical and biomedical world has spurred collaborations with medicine and nursing, including the incorporation of measures of social determinants into electronic health records and the use of this information in clinical research. These are important areas for continued work to ensure that the use of social, race, or ethnic indicators does not contribute to stereotyping or perpetuate bias and racism. Growing interest in the health consequences of a range of public policies has also led to engagement with the fields of public policy, transportation, and urban planning. Creating the systems and infrastructures that allow partnerships to be established early to facilitate the rigorous evaluation of the health and health equity impacts of a range of policy actions is also an area of opportunity for social epidemiology.

Another area for greater interdisciplinary collaboration involving social epidemiology is the area of climate and health and environmental factors more generally. Although there have been many examples of work in social epidemiology that has connected social determinants to environmental factors (including the long-standing and growing field of environmental justice), the engagement of environmental and climate scientists has been relatively limited. Today these collaborations need to expand to the area of climate change and health. Significant opportunities include rigorous examinations of how environmental factors operating over the life course contribute to health inequities, the interactions between climate change and health inequities, and the impact of policies to address climate change on health inequities.

Understanding population patterns and social causation can benefit greatly from insights from law and the humanities, including history, ethics and related fields. One prime example is the call to expand the use of concepts, frameworks, and approaches drawn from critical race theory in order to improve the validity and social utility of research in social epidemiology by explicitly acknowledging the multifaceted ways in which systemic racism impacts health as well as the practice of health research itself. These calls challenge researchers to continuously reexamine their assumptions and their approaches, including how the lived experiences of communities are reflected in and inform the work. Another example is the call to move beyond stratification by race and gender to recognize how the intersectionality framework rooted in Black feminist scholarship can aid in understanding the drivers of health inequities. Reflecting on what critical race theory and intersectionality mean for questions, measures, study designs, conclusions, and actions in social epidemiology is a critical need and opportunity to advance scientific insights and actions.

Most importantly, the questions posed in social epidemiology, the data collected, the types of analyzes done, and how results are interpreted are all shaped in part by social and historical contexts and by the experiences and backgrounds of the researchers themselves. For these reasons, ensuring that researchers in social epidemiology reflect diverse backgrounds and lived experiences (in addition to different disciplines) is fundamental to the scientific rigor of the field and the social utility of the work it produces.

7.2.6. Advancing Emerging Critical Approaches to Understanding the Health Impacts of Systemic Racism and Its Policy Implications

Work in sociology and social epidemiology has highlighted the multifaceted ways in which structural racism, cultural racism, and individual-level discrimination affect the health of marginalized racial groups and contribute to health inequities. As noted by Williams et al., "Racism has created a set of dynamic, interdependent, components or subsystems that reinforce each other, creating and sustaining reciprocal causality of racial inequities across various sectors of society". Racism impacts health through a set of interrelated structures and systems and is a fundamental cause [in the sense of Lieberson] of health inequities across race and ethnic groups in a way that is pervasive and operates through multiple evolving mechanisms across generations and over the life course. Despite the recognition of racism as a fundamental cause of ill-health, much work in health research continues to treat race as a purely individual-level descriptor and does not capture or address how racist structures, systems, and policies affect the health of racialized populations. A number of scholars have discussed and questioned how race and racism are studied, discussed, and interpreted in health research, including social epidemiology. Specifically, social epidemiologists and other scholars and practitioners have called for explicit recognition of the health impacts of systemic racism in its many manifestations and have noted that explicit recognition of racism has implications for theories, concepts, and questions; measures and study designs;

and public health practice and policy. Most importantly, public health researchers and practitioners need to question and reflect on how they may perpetuate racism through existing theories, research questions, data collection, measures, and even analytical approaches. Embracing emerging critical work on the links between racism and health; expanding the research agenda on racism and health to explicitly encompass systemic, structural, and policy factors; and considering the implications of this work for research, conclusions, and actions in social epidemiology are critical to both scientific rigor and effective public health and social action.

7.2.7. Going Global

Social epidemiology in the United States and in Europe has been, for the most part, focused on higher-income countries, and standard textbooks of social epidemiology (as well as the vast majority of published papers) tend to be focused on the United States and Europe. The utility of cross-country comparisons of health inequities and policies used to address health inequities has been noted, but rigorous studies of cross-country differences remain relatively rare and these comparisons have not been mined to their full potential. Although many insights about the links between social organization and health may be common across the world, there are likely to be specificities and context-specific factors that affect the social patterning of health. In addition, local descriptions and locally generated knowledge can be powerful motivators of local action. Public health researchers and epidemiologists in lower-income countries have generated important insights and debates about the social determinants of health. Low- and middle-income countries can also provide opportunities for evaluation of the impact of novel policies and interventions. Documenting the magnitude, the determinants, and the impact of policies on health inequities globally remains a critical need.

7.2.8. A Broad Approach to Generating Socially Useful Research

In an insightful article written more than 30 years ago, Carol Weiss reviewed the various ways in which social research relates to policy. It may very well be that social epidemiology affects policy most effectively through the enlightenment model. This assumption is especially appropriate given the nature of the questions addressed by social epidemiology, where the narrowly targeted interventions or policy options that can be evaluated through individual studies likely have only minimal impact because they do not address the complex systemic forces that drive social differences in health. Under the enlightenment model, scientific findings regarding how the world works percolate through many different channels and, over time, provide decision-makers with ways to make sense out of a complex world. Science also identifies new problems and suggests possible solutions (even if it does not specifically evaluate a given policy or intervention) and can in these ways influence the policy agenda in the long run. Most importantly, the enlightenment model also reflects how social epidemiology findings can influence public perceptions more broadly, challenge hegemonic explanations, and motivate social change by modifying how problems are perceived and which actions are considered desirable and even feasible. In this way, social epidemiology findings can expand the policy space. Fostering a greater awareness of the multiple ways in which social epidemiology findings can affect public perceptions and actions (including the empirical research that can shed light on these influences) is also an opportunity for the future (Table 7.1).

Table 7.1. 10 Potential Information and Communication Technologies (ICTs) to "Socialize" Social Epidemiology

	ICT Name	**Features**
1	Magpi	Survey instrument design, data collection & analysis; real-time assessment; SMS, photo, and audio capabilities; geolocation and mapping capability; smartphone deployment; built-in data analysis & visualization tools; collaborative use options; online/offline use
2	Fulcrum	Survey instrument design, data collection & analysis; real-time assessment; photo capability; geolocation and mapping capability; smartphone deployment; built-in data analysis & visualization tools; collaborative use options; online/offline use
3	Kobo ToolBox	Survey instrument design, data collection & analysis; real-time assessment; geolocation and mapping capability; smartphone deployment; built-in data analysis & visualization tools; online/offline use; open source
4	EthnoCorder	Survey instrument design, data collection & analysis; real-time assessment; Text, photo, video, and audio capabilities; geolocation and mapping capability; smartphone deployment; built-in data analysis & visualization tools; collaborative use options
5	MyInsights (MyPanel)	Qualitative and mixed-methods research platform for survey design, data collection and analysis; real-time assessment; Text, photo, video, and audio capabilities; geolocation capability; smartphone deployment; built-in data analysis & visualization tools; collaborative use options
6	QuickTapSurvey	Survey instrument design, data collection & analysis; real-time assessment; text and photo capabilities; geolocation capability; smartphone deployment; built-in data visualization tools; collaborative use options; online/offline use
7	FieldNotes	GPS location-based note taking and data collection & platform; real-time assessment; Text, photo, video, and audio capabilities; geolocation capability; smartphone deployment
8	LiveTrekker	GPS location-based tool for documenting geographic travel and spatial movement patterns; real-time assessment; Text, photo, video, and audio capabilities; geolocation and mapping capability; smartphone deployment; built-in data visualization tools; social media sharing tools

9	Capture365 Journal	Multimedia-enabled journaling platform; Text, photo, video, and audio capabilities; geolocation and weather tracking capability; smartphone deployment; built-in data visualization and social media sharing tools
10	MapYourWorld	Suite of mapping-focused tools geared towards youth participatory research; geolocation and mapping capabilities; built-in data visualization tools; built-in social media sharing tools

Table highlighting a selection of ICTs with the potential to facilitate "socializing" social epidemiology research practice by enabling deeply participatory and collaborative data collection, analysis, and sharing processes.

Source: Petteway R, Mujahid M, Allen A, Morello-Frosch R. Towards a people's social epidemiology: envisioning a more inclusive and equitable future for social epi research and practice in the 21st century. International Journal of Environmental Research and Public Health. 2019; 16(20):3983. https://doi.org/10.3390/ijerph16203983.

A Closer Look

Evaluation of Social Epidemiology

The evaluation of social epidemiology involves assessing the impact of social factors on health outcomes within populations, with a focus on understanding how social determinants influence patterns of disease distribution and health disparities. Social epidemiology examines the complex interplay between social structures, economic inequalities, cultural norms, and health behaviors to identify pathways through which social factors shape health outcomes.

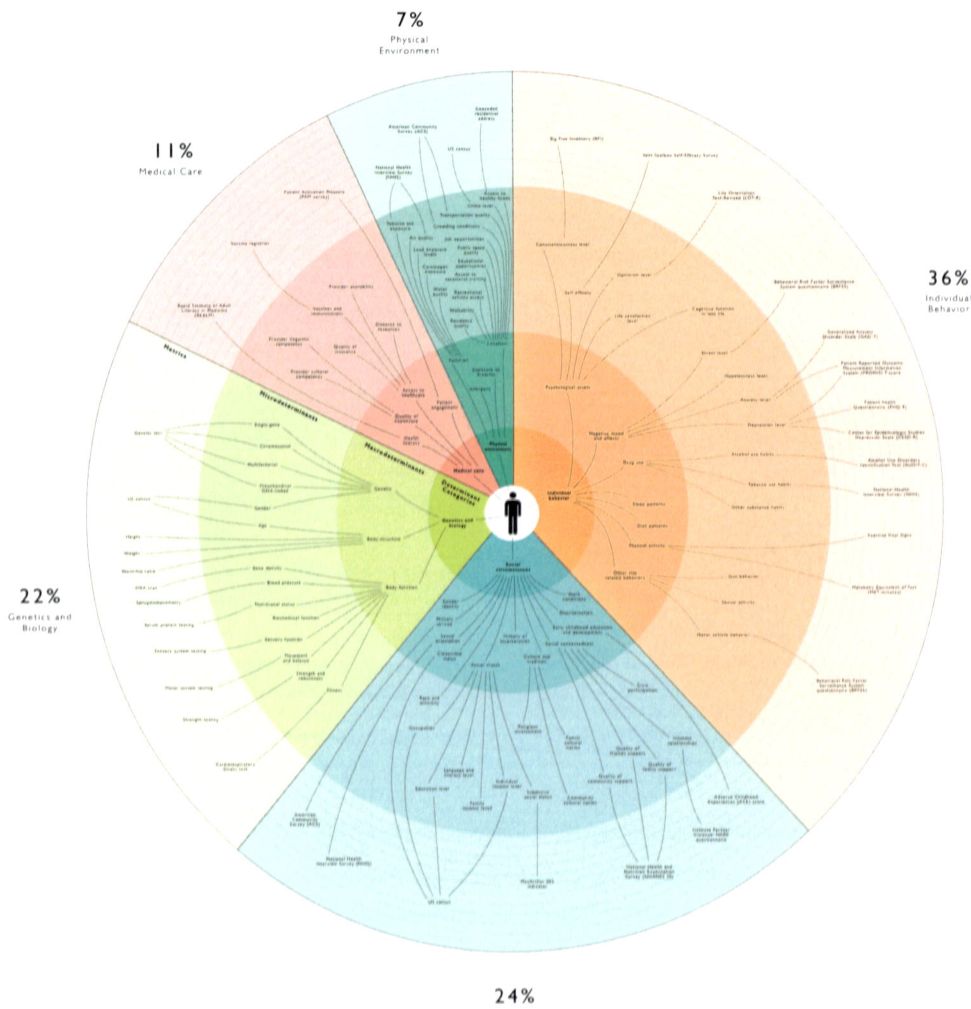

One key aspect of evaluating social epidemiology involves examining social determinants of health and their impact on population health outcomes. Social determinants such as income, education, employment, housing, social support networks, and access to healthcare services play a critical role in shaping health outcomes and influencing health inequities. By evaluating the distribution of social determinants and their association with health outcomes, social epidemiologists provide evidence to inform policies and interventions aimed at addressing underlying social disparities and promoting health equity.

Moreover, the evaluation of social epidemiology involves assessing the impact of social policies and interventions on population health outcomes. Social policies related to education, income support, housing, and healthcare access can have profound effects on population health by addressing social determinants and reducing health inequities. By evaluating the implementation and effectiveness of social policies, social epidemiologists provide insights into the mechanisms through which social interventions influence health outcomes and inform strategies for improving the health and well-being of populations.

Additionally, social epidemiology evaluates the role of social networks, social capital, and social cohesion in shaping health behaviors and health outcomes within communities. Social networks influence health behaviors such as smoking, physical activity, and dietary choices through social norms, peer influence, and social support mechanisms. By examining the structure and function of social networks, social epidemiologists identify opportunities for leveraging social relationships to promote positive health behaviors and prevent disease.

Furthermore, social epidemiology assesses the intersectionality of social determinants and their combined effects on health outcomes among marginalized and disadvantaged populations. Intersectionality considers how multiple social identities such as race, ethnicity, gender, sexual orientation, and socioeconomic status intersect to shape health disparities and experiences of discrimination and disadvantage. By evaluating the intersecting influences of social determinants, social epidemiologists highlight the unique challenges faced by different population groups and advocate for policies and interventions that address the underlying structural inequalities driving health inequities.

Summary

- Social epidemiology examines how social factors influence health outcomes across populations. It explores the complex interplay between social determinants and health, recognizing that health disparities are not solely biological but deeply rooted in social structures, policies, and inequalities.
- Historically, social epidemiology emerged from critiques of traditional biomedical approaches that focused primarily on individual-level risk factors. Instead, social epidemiologists argue for a broader perspective that considers socioeconomic status, education, occupation, housing, neighborhood characteristics, social support networks, and access to healthcare as crucial determinants of health. By investigating these factors, social epidemiology aims to uncover the underlying mechanisms that link social environments to health outcomes, revealing patterns of inequality and identifying opportunities for intervention.
- The construct of social capital also received significant attention. Social capital has been defined as "the resources—for example, the exchange of favors, the maintenance of group norms, the presence of trust, and the exercise of sanctions—available to members of social groups".
- The work environment, including job status, psychosocial factors, and physical and chemical hazards at work, has also been posited to contribute to social differences in health. Sophisticated models of work-related psychosocial dimensions, including demands at work, control over the work process, effort–reward imbalance, and social support at work, were conceptualized and empirically examined in relation to health outcomes.
- In the present context, social epidemiology continues to evolve, increasingly integrating multidisciplinary approaches from sociology, anthropology, economics, and public health. This interdisciplinary approach allows researchers to examine how social structures, policies, cultural norms, and globalization impact health at both individual and population levels. It emphasizes the importance of context in shaping health disparities and highlights the role of social justice in promoting health equity.
- Conceptual models are fundamental to any field because they make explicit theory and assumptions, facilitate the framing of research questions, and allow researchers to identify analytical implications.
- Work in sociology and social epidemiology has highlighted the multifaceted ways in which structural racism, cultural racism, and individual-level discrimination affect the health of marginalized racial groups and contribute to health inequities.

References

1. Abraido-Lanza, A. F., Echeverria, S. E., & Florez, K. R. (2016). Latino immigrants, acculturation, and health: promising new directions in research. *Annual Review of Public Health, 37*, 219–236.
2. Adler, N. E., & Stewart, J. (2010). Health disparities across the lifespan: meaning, methods, and mechanisms. *Annals of the New York Academy of Sciences, 1186*, 5–23.

3. Alang, S., McAlpine, D., McCreedy, E., & Hardeman, R. (2017). Police brutality and Black health: setting the agenda for public health scholars. *American Journal of Public Health, 107*, 662–665.

4. Auchincloss, A. H., & Diez Roux, A. V. (2008). A new tool for epidemiology: the usefulness of dynamic-agent models in understanding place effects on health. *American Journal of Epidemiology, 168*, 1–8.

5. Auchincloss, A. H., Riolo, R. L., Brown, D. G., Cook, J., & Diez Roux, A. V. (2011). An agent-based model of income inequalities in diet in the context of residential segregation. *American Journal of Preventive Medicine, 40*, 303–311.

6. Bailey, Z. D., Feldman, J. M., & Bassett, M. T. (2021). How structural racism works—racist policies as a root cause of U.S. racial health inequities. *New England Journal of Medicine, 384*, 768–773.

7. Bailey, Z. D., Krieger, N., Agénor, M., Graves, J., Linos, N., & Bassett, M. T. (2017). Structural racism and health inequities in the USA: evidence and interventions. *The Lancet, 389*, 1453–1463.

8. Bambra, C., Smith, K. E., Garthwaite, K., Joyce, K. E., & Hunter, D. J. (2011). A labor of Sisyphus? Public policy and health inequalities research from the Black and Acheson Reports to the Marmot Review. *Journal of Epidemiology & Community Health, 65*, 399–406.

9. Bannister-Tyrrell, M., & Meiqari, L. (2020). Qualitative research in epidemiology: theoretical and methodological perspectives. *Annals of Epidemiology, 49*, 27–35.

10. Blane, D. (2006). The life course, the social gradient, and health. In M. Marmot & R. G. Wilkinson (Eds.), *Social Determinants of Health* (2nd ed., pp. 54–77). Oxford, UK: Oxford University Press.

11. Borrell, L. N., Elhawary, J. R., Fuentes-Afflick, E., Witonsky, J., Bhakta, N., et al. (2021). Race and genetic ancestry in medicine—a time for reckoning with racism. *New England Journal of Medicine, 384*, 474–480.

12. Bowleg, L. (2012). The problem with the phrase women and minorities: intersectionality—an important theoretical framework for public health. *American Journal of Public Health, 102*, 1267–1273.

Chapter

EPIDEMIOLOGICAL BURDEN OF TUBERCULOSIS IN DEVELOPING COUNTRIES

8

Contents

Introduction

One infectious disease called tuberculosis (TB) is brought on by various *Mycobacterium* species. One of the leading causes of death worldwide is tuberculosis, along with malaria, human immunodeficiency virus infection (HIV)/acquired immunodeficiency syndrome (AIDS), and other AIDS-related illnesses. *Mycobacterium tuberculosis*, commonly referred to as Koch's bacilli (Figure 8.1), is the primary cause of disease in humans and can affect any organ or tissue in the body. In certain cases, *M. bovis*. However, the primary body area impacted by this mostly tropical pathogen is the lungs, which have specific symptoms like a cough with expectoration lasting longer than 15 days. Before receiving a microbiological diagnosis, those in these situations are referred to as respiratory symptomatic.

In addition to these indications, hemoptisis, fever, sweating at night, general malaise, thoracic pain, anorexia, and weight loss can also be symptoms of the disease. Due to its high transmissibility, this disease is still a serious public health concern, despite being a potentially treatable and preventable condition.

Furthermore, mycobacterial diseases are becoming a global public health concern in the context of HIV and other immunosuppressive illnesses.

Human health is still at risk from tuberculosis, which is still a major public health issue worldwide, but especially in developing nations.

These days, this coinfection, along with the burden of HIV infection, accounts for the majority of tuberculosis morbidity and mortality in many areas (e.g., Africa) and complicates both its reduction and control in numerous ways. In 2010, there were 8.8 million (range, 8.5–9.2 million) incident cases of TB, 1.1 million (range, 0.9–1.2 million) deaths from TB among HIV-negative people, and an additional 0.35 million (range, 0.32–0.39 million) deaths from HIV-associated TB, according to the World Health Organization's (WHO) Global Tuberculosis Control Report 2011—the most significant and official document regarding the epidemiology and other aspects of tuberculosis worldwide.

The World Health Organization (2011) has released some significant new global findings, including the following: a) the absolute number of TB cases has been declining since 2006 (rather than rising slowly as indicated in previous global reports); b) TB incidence rates have been declining since 2002 (two years earlier than previously suggested); c) estimates of the number of TB-related deaths annually have been revised downward; and d) nearly 10 million children were left orphaned in 2009 as a result of parental deaths brought on by TB (Figure 8.1).

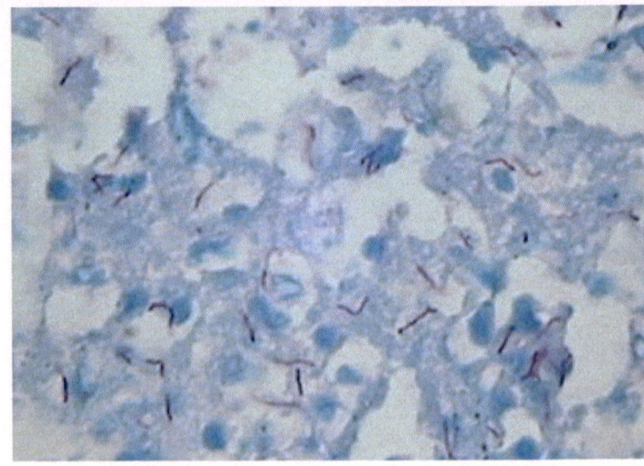

Figure 8.1. *Acid fast-bacilli in a Ziehl-Neelsen stain from a sample of a patient with pulmonary TB (400 X).*

Source: Diana M. Castañeda-Hernández and Alfonso J. Rodriguez-Morales. (2013). Epidemiological burden of tuberculosis in developing countries. InTech. doi: 10.5772/53363.

In addition to clinical factors, the epidemiology of tuberculosis can be impacted by a variety of local and national demographic, geographic, and social factors as well as the nation's current state of development as indicated by indicators like the Human Development Index (HDI). There, it was discovered that there are negative correlations between HDI and tuberculosis-related morbidity and mortality, with lower TB-related morbidity and mortality found with higher HDI levels. The burden of diseases like tuberculosis (TB) can impede the achievement of the Millennium Development Goals, as has been noted with other diseases with high prevalence in developing nations. Then, methods for lessening its effects and enhancing population health—which is frequently neglected—should be put into practice.

The paucity of tuberculosis research that is typically conducted in developing nations is another factor that influences this. For instance,

Colombia produces relatively little scientific research on tuberculosis (TB) when compared to developed nations (USA, 4. 08 articles/100,000 hab.) but also with other countries in Latin America, like Chile (19 cases/100,000 hab), which have an even lower TB incidence.) but with a 2.19 times greater productivity (1.09 articles/100,000 hab). Increased research funding, starting with undergraduate studies, improved public-private sector collaboration, increased academic collaboration, and increased international cooperation would all help to close these gaps, boost scientific publication, and enable domestic application of the knowledge gained to enhance TB epidemiology and other disease-related aspects.

Beyond its epidemiology, of which pulmonary disease accounts for the majority (Figure 8.2), other major forms of disease also constitute a major global burden. Extrapulmonary tuberculosis is the term for infection that affects organs other than the lungs.

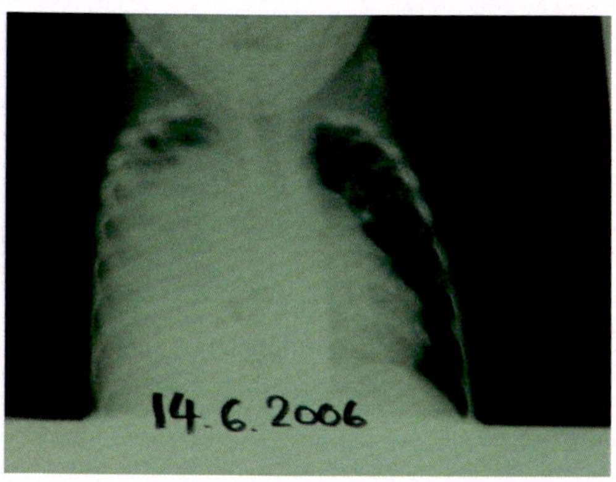

Figure 8.2. *Pulmonary TB in a very young child from Tanzania, Africa.*

Source: Diana M. Castañeda-Hernández and Alfonso J. Rodriguez-Morales. (2013). Epidemiological burden of tuberculosis in developing countries. InTech. doi: 10.5772/53363.

The pleura is where this disease most frequently manifests, followed by the lymphatic nodes. Depending on the organ involved, extrapulmonary tuberculosis can present with a variety of symptoms. The disease's prognosis and progression period can also differ based on the organ that is impacted.

The spectrum of diseases varies and can start as a latent infection or reactivation that gradually progresses into a focal or widespread spread that involves multiple organs. This makes it challenging for clinicians and other healthcare professionals to diagnose, and they frequently fail to do so in a timely manner.

Meningitis (TB meningitis) is one of the most severe forms of extrapulmonary tuberculosis (TB) and is caused by bacilli spreading hematogenously into the subarachnoid space. This is a primary tuberculosis complication that can arise years later from either exogenous reinfection or endogenous reactivation of a latent tuberculosis. Presently, developing nations typically rely solely on the PPD to diagnose latent tuberculosis. Lately, though, there have been new options for diagnosing these cases: latent tuberculosis infection (LTBI) can now be detected with IFNγ release assays (IGRAs). In fact, this is suggested for the benefit of public health in developing nations.

Given the variety of factors that contribute to the occurrence and persistence of tuberculosis in human societies, it is a complex disease. The *Bacillus* (viability, transmissibility, and virulence) and the host (immune status, genetic susceptibility, duration and intensity of exposure) are the first factors to consider, followed by the bacillus-host interaction (place of affection, severity of illness).

Second, clinical factors include the prevalence of undiagnosed or untreated pulmonary tuberculosis, overcrowding, malnutrition, immunosuppression from any source (diabetes, cancer, HIV infection, immunosuppressive drug use, chronic renal failure, silicosis, alcoholism, and drug addiction), and more. In developing nations, tuberculosis (TB) can also be highly prevalent in a number of epidemiological contexts compared to the general population. These contexts include jails, homeless shelters, and indigenous communities.

Protective factors at the community public health interventional level include the BCG (Bacille Calmette Guerin) vaccine, which is used in developing nations. It offers protection prior to exposure and prevents the development of severe infection forms, particularly in infants and early children, providing up to 80% protection against the development of disease forms like meningeal and miliary TB.

In addition to the clinical implications, changes in the susceptibility of the causative agent to drugs used in therapy have created more challenges in managing TB. The problem with TB now largely stems from the fact that a third of the global population is infected with Mycobacterium tuberculosis. Even in the 21st century, TB remains a leading cause of death from infectious diseases. This is due in part to the increasing resistance of the bacterium to anti-TB drugs. Cases of drug-resistant TB, classified by the World Health Organization (WHO) as primary, initial, acquired multidrug-resistant (MDR-TB) or extensively drug-resistant TB (XDR-TB), are on the rise in various parts of the world.

The use of insufficient anti-TB medication combinations or monotherapy can lead to the development of resistance in tuberculosis. Importantly, there may be a role for healthcare professionals in the emergence of multidrug-resistant tuberculosis. Actually, mishandling the prescription of chemotherapy, giving anti-tuberculosis medications, monitoring the patient, making decisions about additional treatment, and administering anti-TB medications incorrectly all directly lead to multi-drug-resistant tuberculosis. The global XDR-TB epidemic has grown to be extremely concerning. The only way to prevent the spread of MDR or XDR TB, which is a serious worldwide threat in the twenty-first century, is to provide appropriate treatment in accordance with a short regiment that is directly supervised for cases of TB that have been correctly classified.

The social aspect of tuberculosis (TB) is a crucial concern as it involves a multifaceted history and various interrelated elements that impact those afflicted both internally and externally. The disease is still highly stigmatized in many parts of the world. In light of this, the treatment of tuberculosis (TB) is complicated and calls for the use of psychological, medical, and particularly sociological approaches in addition to medical ones. This will help to improve TB management from the standpoint of collective medicine and increase non-affected individuals' acceptance of TB infected people's communities or neighborhoods. Programs that approach all of these factors will thus benefit from improved strategies that enable positive interactions between social actors involved in the intricate social matrix in which tuberculosis (TB) can occasionally be present in societies. By utilizing this, routine tasks like accurate diagnosis and treatment could be completed more quickly.

One challenge in the current context of TB particularly in developing countries is the access to reliable diagnostic tests, particularly those than allow to confirm species diagnostics as well to identify those isolates that are not fully susceptible to anti-mycobacterial first line drugs. However, today many diagnostic tests have been developed, but many of them are only used routinely in developed countries (e.g., IGRAs and molecular biology-based tests). Although is clear that DOTS (directly observed treatment strategy, short-course) programs have contributed in the successful treatment of TB, particularly because this strategy includes six major components that are: (i) pursue high-quality DOTS expansion and enhancement; (ii) address TB/HIV, MDR-TB (multi-drug resistant TB), and the needs of poor and vulnerable populations; (iii) contribute to health-system strengthening based on primary healthcare; (iv) engage all care providers; (v) empower people with TB, and communities through partnership; and (vi) enable and promote research; it is necessary to increase its coverage and usefulness particularly in those highly TB prevalent countries in the developing World in order to achieve the goals that have been established for 2015 in the Global Plan to Stop TB (2011–2015) of the World Health Organization and the Stop TB Partnership. The epidemiological burden of TB in developing countries can be measured directly from different global and national indicators and estimators, however, those mainly to be addressed should be incidence, prevalence, mortality, MDR-TB incidence, XDR-TB (extensively drug-resistant TB) incidence, case notifications, treatment outcomes and case detection rates.

Orientation and Directional Terms

Term	Definition	Illustration
Tuberculosis (TB)	Tuberculosis (TB) is an infectious disease that most often affects the lungs and is caused by a type of bacteria. It spreads through the air when infected people cough, sneeze or spit.	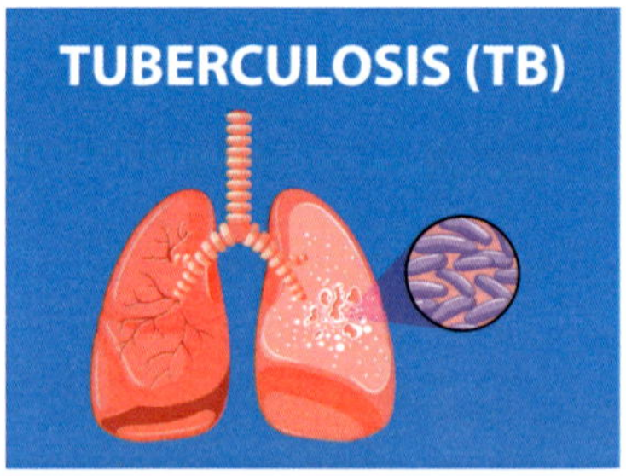
Latent Tuberculosis Infection (LTBI)	Latent tuberculosis infection (LTBI) is defined as a state of persistent immune response to stimulation by Mycobacterium tuberculosis antigens without evidence of clinically manifested active tuberculosis (TB) disease.	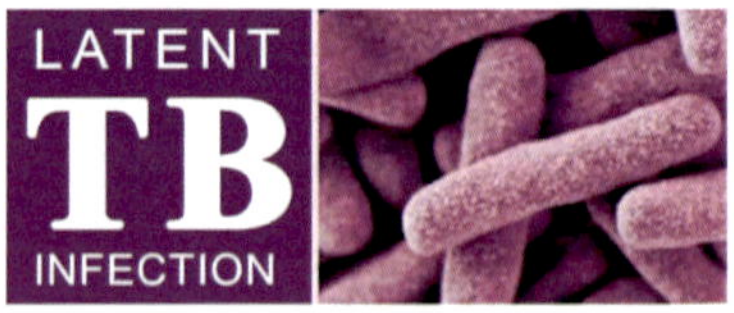
Immunosuppressant	Immunosuppressant is a class of medicines that inhibit or decrease the intensity of the immune response in the body. Most of these medications, are used to allow the body less likely to resist a transplanted organ i.e., kidney, heart and liver.	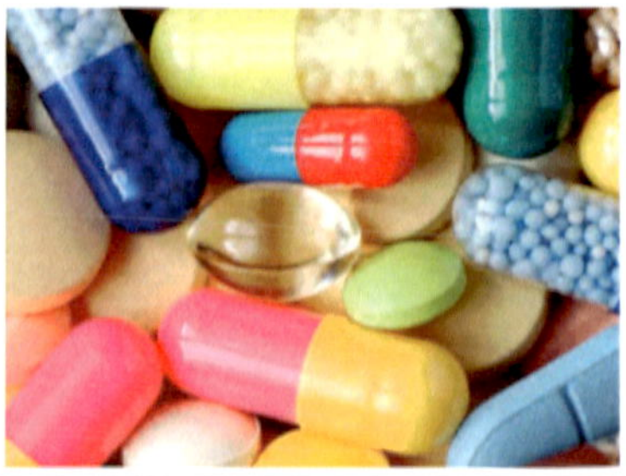
Extensively Drug-Resistant TB (XDR TB)	Extensively drug-resistant TB (XDR TB) is a rare type of multidrug-resistant tuberculosis (MDR TB) that is resistant to isoniazid, rifampin, a fluoroquinolone, and a second-line injectable (amikacin, capreomycin, and kanamycin) OR isoniazid, rifampin, a fluoroquinolone, and bedaquiline or linezolid.	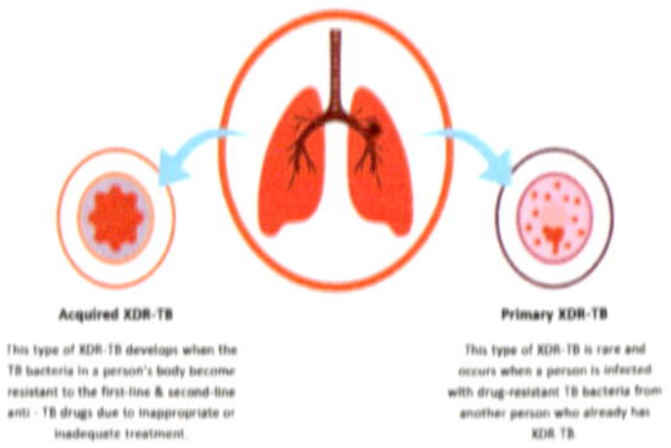
Multidrug-resistant TB (MDR TB)	Multidrug-resistant TB (MDR TB) is caused by TB bacteria that are resistant to at least isoniazid and rifampin, the two most potent TB drugs. These drugs are used to treat all persons with TB disease. TB experts should be consulted in the treatment of MDR TB.	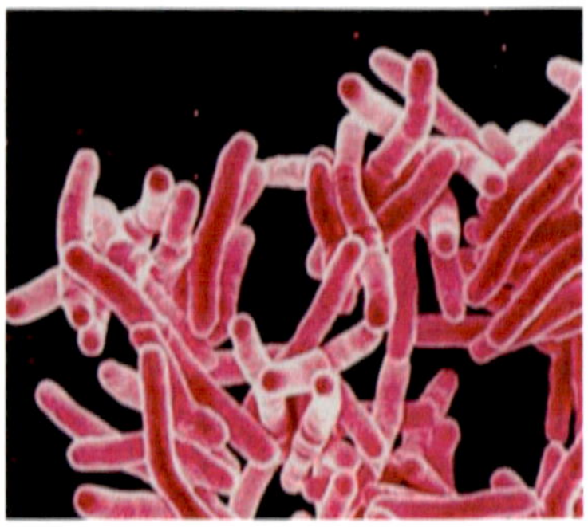

8.1. Tuberculosis in Developing Countries

The prevalence of HIV coinfection has increased in the majority of the world's countries, making tuberculosis a disease. TB was mostly endemic in developing nations and was losing ground globally until two to three decades ago. But ever since the AIDS pandemic began in June 1981, tuberculosis (TB) has become more prevalent, not just in these nations but also in developed nations in North America and Europe. In addition, the numerous issues that developing nations in Africa, Asia, and Latin America that deal with a high prevalence of tuberculosis must deal with are significant, particularly when these issues are compounded by coexisting conditions and diseases like HIV, comorbidities, poverty, and living in resource-constrained areas where diagnosis and treatment are not as timely as in other areas.

To accurately determine the true cost of disease in developing nations, improvements in epidemiology and public health concerning tuberculosis are imperative. An essential part of providing care for patients with tuberculosis (TB) and managing the illness is the recording and reporting of data. In order to track the TB epidemic's trends at the international, national, and subnational levels, as well as to track the treatment of individual patients and patient groups (cohorts) and guarantee continuity of care when patients are referred between healthcare facilities, data collection and reporting are essential. Additionally, programmatic efforts to control TB must be planned, funded, carried out, and evaluated, including forecasting the number of cases and the corresponding need for staff, medications, and laboratory supplies, as well as analyzing treatment outcomes.

The global burden of TB in the World is estimated at 8.8 million (range, 8.5–9.2 million) incident cases of TB (Table 8.1) for rates ranging from 123.7 to 133.9 cases/100,000 pop. (Table 8.1); however, this can be very different among the WHO Regions in the World, being higher in Africa where those estimates can reach 250.9 to 298.7 cases/100,000 pop (Table 8.1). Rates of incidence are important because can show the real populational problem of the disease. For example, in South East Asia there are more crude numbers of cases of TB, estimated at 3.5 million (range, 3.2–3.7 million) incident cases, however, the incidence rates are quite lower than in Africa, reaching 177.0 to 204.7 cases/100,000 pop (Table 8.1); (Figure 8.4).

Table 8.1. Estimated Epidemiological Burden of Incident TB, According Regions by the WHO in 2010 (World Health Organization 2011)

		Incidence(cases)			Incidence Rates (cases/100,000pop)		
Region	**Population**	**Best**	**Low**	**High**	**Best**	**Low**	**High**
Global burden	6,869,573,000	8,800,000	8,500,000	9,200,000	128.1	123.7	133.9
WHO African Region	836,970,000	2,300,000	2,100,000	2,500,000	274.8	250.9	298.7
WHO South-East Asia Region	1,807,594,000	3,500,000	3,200,000	3,700,000	193.6	177.0	204.7
WHO Eastern Mediterranean Region	596,747,000	650,000	580,000	730,000	108.9	97.2	122.3
WHO Western Pacific Region	1,798,335,000	1,700,000	1,500,000	1,800,000	94.5	83.4	100.1

WHO European Region	896,480,000	420,000	390,000	450,000	46.8	43.5	50.2
WHO Region of the Americas	933,447,000	270,000	250,000	280,000	28.9	26.8	30.0

Source: Diana M. Castañeda-Hernández and Alfonso J. Rodriguez-Morales. (2013). Epidemiological burden of tuberculosis in developing countries. InTech. doi: 10.5772/53363

The prevalence of TB for some countries is still difficult to estimate and in many cases are not reported and/or analyzed. According the WHO, for 2010 the prevalence was estimated at 12.0 million (range, 11.0–14.0 million) prevalent cases of TB (Table 8.2) for rates ranging from 160.1 to 203.8 cases/100,000 pop. (Table 8.2); however, this can be very different among the WHO Regions in the World, being higher in Africa where those estimates can reach 274.8 to 394.3 cases/100,000 population (Table 8.2).

Table 8.2. Estimated Epidemiological Burden of Prevalent TB, According Regions by the WHO in 2010 (World Health Organization 2011)

		Prevalence(cases)			Prevalence Rates (cases/100,000pop)		
Region	**Population**	**Best**	**Low**	**High**	**Best**	**Low**	**High**
Global burden	6,869,573,000	12,000,000	11,000,000	14,000,000	174.7	160.1	203.8
WHO African Region	836,970,000	2,800,000	2,300,000	3,300,000	334.5	274.8	394.3
WHO European Region	896,480,000	2,500,000	2,200,000	2,800,000	278.9	245.4	312.3
WHO Western Pacific Region	1,798,335,000	5,000,000	3,700,000	6,500,000	278.0	205.7	361.4
WHO Eastern Mediterranean Region	596,747,000	1,000,000	670,000	1,500,000	167.6	112.3	251.4
WHO Region of the Americas	933,447,000	330,000	260,000	410,000	35.4	27.9	43.9
WHO South-East Asia Region	1,807,594,000	560,000	430,000	720,000	31.0	23.8	39.8

Source: Diana M. Castañeda-Hernández and Alfonso J. Rodriguez-Morales. (2013). Epidemiological burden of tuberculosis in developing countries. InTech. doi: 10.5772/53363.

Regarding the deaths, WHO estimates indicate that around 1.1 million (range, 0.9–1.2 million) deaths from TB among HIV-negative people occurred and an additional 0.35 million (range, 0.32–0.39 million) deaths from HIV-associated TB were also reported (Table 8.3). Higher mortality rates are reported in Africa, ranging from 26.3 to 33.5 deaths/100,000., but very close to those reported by South East Asia, ranging from 20.5 to 35.4 deaths/100,000 (Table 8.3).

Table 8.3. Estimated Epidemiological Burden of Mortality Due to TB, According to Regions by the WHO in 2010 (World Health Organization 2011) (Excluding HIV-Positive Deaths)

		Mortality(deaths)			Mortality rates (deaths/100,000pop)		
Region	**Population**	**Best**	**Low**	**High**	**Best**	**Low**	**High**
Global burden	6,869,573,000	1,100,000	920,000	1,200,000	16.0	13.4	17.5
WHO African Region	836,970,000	250,000	220,000	280,000	29.9	26.3	33.5
WHO South-East Asia Region	1,807,594,000	500,000	370,000	640,000	27.7	20.5	35.4
WHO Eastern Mediterranean Region	596,747,000	95,000	74,000	120,000	15.9	12.4	20.1
WHO Western Pacific Region	1,798,335,000	130,000	120,000	150,000	7.2	6.7	8.3
WHO European Region	896,480,000	61,000	48,000	75,000	6.8	5.4	8.4
WHO Region of the Americas	933,447,000	20,000	17,000	23,000	2.1	1.8	2.5

Source: Diana M. Castañeda-Hernández and Alfonso J. Rodriguez-Morales. (2013). Epidemiological burden of tuberculosis in developing countries. InTech. doi: 10.5772/53363

Tuberculosis incidence in HIV-patients is a very relevant indicator worldwide for TB epidemiology and burden (Table 8.4). Africa presented the highest rates for HIV-Positive Incident TB cases, ranging from 98.0 to 117.1 cases/100,000 (Table 8.4).

Table 8.4. Estimated Epidemiological Burden of Mortality Due to TB, According Regions by the WHO in 2010 (World Health Organization 2011) (Excluding HIV Positive Deaths)

		HIV-Positive Incident TB Cases			Rates (Cases/100,000pop)		
Region	**Population**	**Best**	**Low**	**High**	**Best**	**Low**	**High**
Global burden	6,869,573,000	1,100,000	1,000,000	1,200,000	16.0	14.6	17.5
WHO African Region	836,970,000	900,000	820,000	980,000	107.5	98.0	117.1
WHO South-East Asia Region	1,807,594,000	190,000	140,000	230,000	10.5	7.7	12.7
WHO Region of the Americas	933,447,000	35,000	31,000	38,000	3.7	3.3	4.1
WHO European Region	896,480,000	20,000	19,000	22,000	2.2	2.1	2.5
WHO Eastern Mediterranean Region	596,747,000	12,000	9,800	15,000	2.0	1.6	2.5
WHO Western Pacific Region	1,798,335,000	35,000	26,000	45,000	1.9	1.4	2.5

Source: Diana M. Castañeda-Hernández and Alfonso J. Rodriguez-Morales. (2013). Epidemiological burden of tuberculosis in developing countries. InTech. doi: 10.5772/53363

Even more, difference in all these aspect can differ among countries and be higher. For example, in Colombia, TB is still a significant public health problem. Figure 8.3 shows the WHO profile for TB in Colombia for 2010.

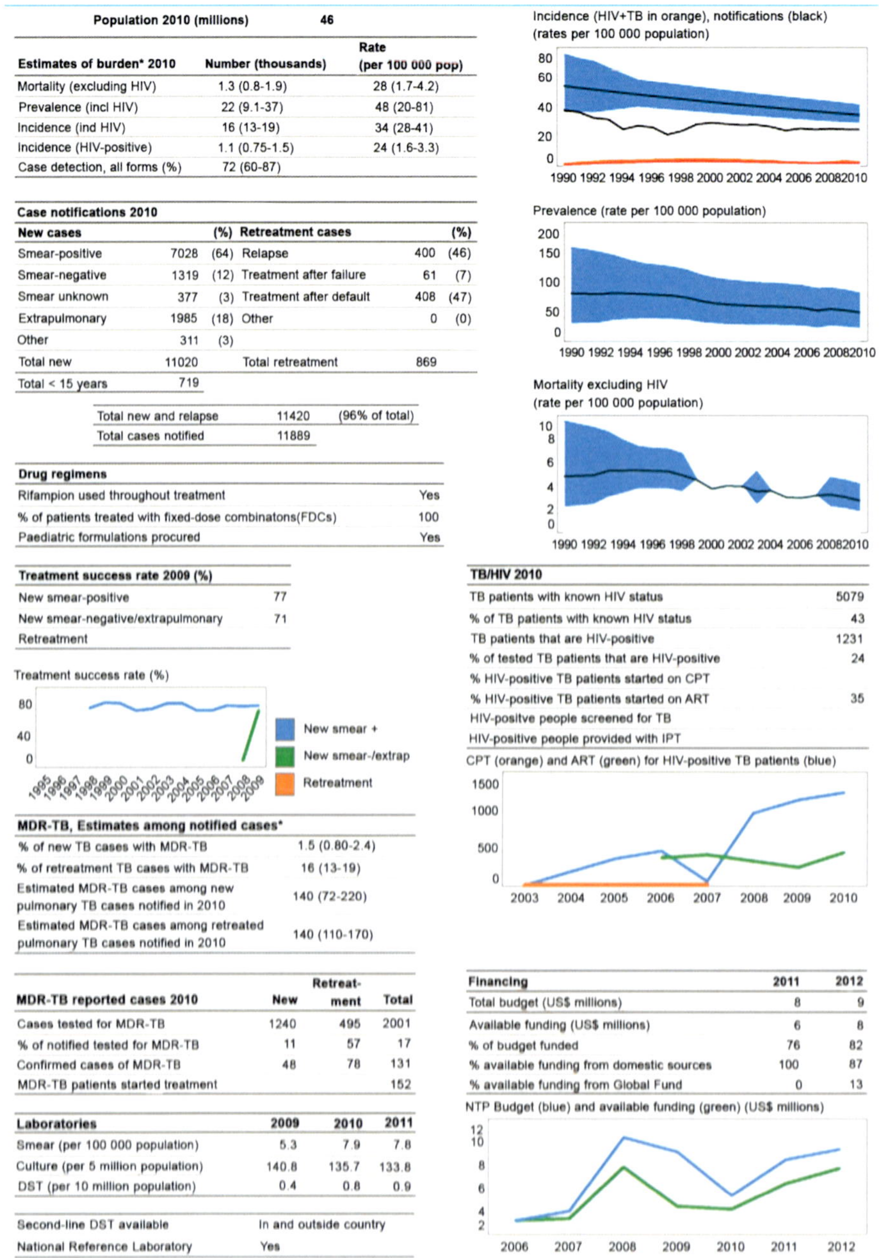

Population 2010 (millions)	46	

Estimates of burden* 2010	Number (thousands)	Rate (per 100 000 pop)
Mortality (excluding HIV)	1.3 (0.8-1.9)	28 (1.7-4.2)
Prevalence (incl HIV)	22 (9.1-37)	48 (20-81)
Incidence (ind HIV)	16 (13-19)	34 (28-41)
Incidence (HIV-positive)	1.1 (0.75-1.5)	24 (1.6-3.3)
Case detection, all forms (%)	72 (60-87)	

Case notifications 2010

New cases		(%)	Retreatment cases		(%)
Smear-positive	7028	(64)	Relapse	400	(46)
Smear-negative	1319	(12)	Treatment after failure	61	(7)
Smear unknown	377	(3)	Treatment after default	408	(47)
Extrapulmonary	1985	(18)	Other	0	(0)
Other	311	(3)			
Total new	11020		Total retreatment	869	
Total < 15 years	719				

Total new and relapse	11420	(96% of total)
Total cases notified	11889	

Drug regimens	
Rifampion used throughout treatment	Yes
% of patients treated with fixed-dose combinatons(FDCs)	100
Paediatric formulations procured	Yes

Treatment success rate 2009 (%)	
New smear-positive	77
New smear-negative/extrapulmonary	71
Retreatment	

MDR-TB, Estimates among notified cases*	
% of new TB cases with MDR-TB	1.5 (0.80-2.4)
% of retreatment TB cases with MDR-TB	16 (13-19)
Estimated MDR-TB cases among new pulmonary TB cases notified in 2010	140 (72-220)
Estimated MDR-TB cases among retreated pulmonary TB cases notified in 2010	140 (110-170)

MDR-TB reported cases 2010	New	Retreat-ment	Total
Cases tested for MDR-TB	1240	495	2001
% of notified tested for MDR-TB	11	57	17
Confirmed cases of MDR-TB	48	78	131
MDR-TB patients started treatment			152

Laboratories	2009	2010	2011
Smear (per 100 000 population)	5.3	7.9	7.8
Culture (per 5 million population)	140.8	135.7	133.8
DST (per 10 million population)	0.4	0.8	0.9

Second-line DST available	In and outside country
National Reference Laboratory	Yes

TB/HIV 2010	
TB patients with known HIV status	5079
% of TB patients with known HIV status	43
TB patients that are HIV-positive	1231
% of tested TB patients that are HIV-positive	24
% HIV-positive TB patients started on CPT	
% HIV-positive TB patients started on ART	35
HIV-positve people screened for TB	
HIV-positive people provided with IPT	

Financing	2011	2012
Total budget (US$ millions)	8	9
Available funding (US$ millions)	6	8
% of budget funded	76	82
% available funding from domestic sources	100	87
% available funding from Global Fund	0	13

Figure 8.3. *Tuberculosis epidemiological profile for Colombia according to the World Health Organization, 2010.*

Source: Diana M. Castañeda-Hernández and Alfonso J. Rodriguez-Morales. (2013). Epidemiological burden of tuberculosis in developing countries. InTech. doi: 10.5772/53363.

8.1.1. Tuberculosis Incidence in High Burden Developing Countries

As has been stated TB is highly endemic in many developing countries, particularly in Africa and Asia highest rates of TB are located. These 22 countries, summarizing 62.9% of the World population (4,321,966,000 pop) concentrated 81.5% of the incident cases of TB in the World (7,169,000 cases), reaching mean incidence rates higher than in the rest of the World, 165.9 cases/100,000pop (Table 8.5). However, in many of these countries, those numbers are higher. India (although considered not official data) in 2010 reported 2,300,000 incident cases (ranging from 2,000,000 to 2,500,000 cases) (Table 8.5), followed by China with 1,000,000 incident cases (ranging from 910,000 to 1,200,000 cases) (Table 8.5) and South Africa with 490,000 incident cases (ranging 400,000 to 590,000 cases) (Table 8.5). That, again rates are higher in this last country, South Africa, where for the same year were reported between 797.9 to 1176.9 cases/100,000. (7.9 to 11.8 cases/1,000 or 0.8 to 1.2 cases/100) (Table 8.5). For Asia, the country with the highest rates is Cambodia (374.9 to 509.3 cases/100,000.) (Table 8.5). For Latin America, the country with the highest rates (and the only one from that region in this list) is Brazil (35.9 to 51.3 cases/100,000.) (Table 8.5) (Figure 8.4).

Table 8.5. Estimated Epidemiological Burden of TB Incidence in the Countries with the Considered Higher Burden of TB, According to WHO in 2010 (World Health Organization 2011)

		Incidence (cases)			Incidence rates (cases/100,000pop)		
Countries	**Population**	**Best**	**Low**	**High**	**Best**	**Low**	**High**
South Africa	50,133,000	490,000	400,000	590,000	977.4	797.9	1176.9
Zimbabwe	12,571,000	80,000	61,000	100,000	636.4	485.2	795.5
Mozambique	23,391,000	130,000	87,000	170,000	555.8	371.9	726.8
Cambodia	14,138,000	62,000	53,000	72,000	438.5	374.9	509.3
Myanmar	47,963,000	180,000	160,000	210,000	375.3	333.6	437.8
DR Congo	65,966,000	220,000	190,000	250,000	333.5	288.0	379.0
Kenya	40,513,000	120,000	120,000	130,000	296.2	296.2	320.9
Philippines	93,261,000	260,000	210,000	310,000	278.8	225.2	332.4
Ethiopia	82,950,000	220,000	20,000	230,000	265.2	24.1	277.3
Pakistan	173,593,000	400,000	330,000	480,000	230.4	190.1	276.5
Bangladesh	148,692,000	330,000	270,000	400,000	221.9	181.6	269.0
Uganda	33,425,000	70,000	56,000	85,000	209.4	167.5	254.3
Vietnam	87,848,000	180,000	130,000	220,000	204.9	148.0	250.4
Afghanistan	31,412,000	59,000	49,000	71,000	187.8	156.0	226.0
India	1,224,614,000	2,300,000	2,000,000	2,500,000	187.8	163.3	204.1
Indonesia	239,871,000	450,000	370,000	540,000	187.6	154.2	225.1
UR Tanzania	44,841,000	79,000	75,000	85,000	176.2	167.3	189.6
Thailand	69,122,000	94,000	78,000	110,000	136.0	112.8	159.1
Nigeria	158,423,000	210,000	99,000	360,000	132.6	62.5	227.2

Russian Federation	142,958,000	150,000	130,000	180,000	104.9	90.9	125.9
China	1,341,335,000	1,000,000	910,000	1,200,000	74.6	67.8	89.5
Brazil	194,946,000	85,000	70,000	100,000	43.6	35.9	51.3
Subtotal	4,321,966,000	7,169,000	5,868,000	8,393,000	165.9	135.8	194.2
% from the global burden	62.9	81.5	69.0	91.2	-	-	-
Global burden	6,869,573,000	8,800,000	8,500,000	9,200,000	128.1	123.7	133.9

Source: Diana M. Castañeda-Hernández and Alfonso J. Rodriguez-Morales. (2013). Epidemiological burden of tuberculosis in developing countries. InTech. doi: 10.5772/53363.

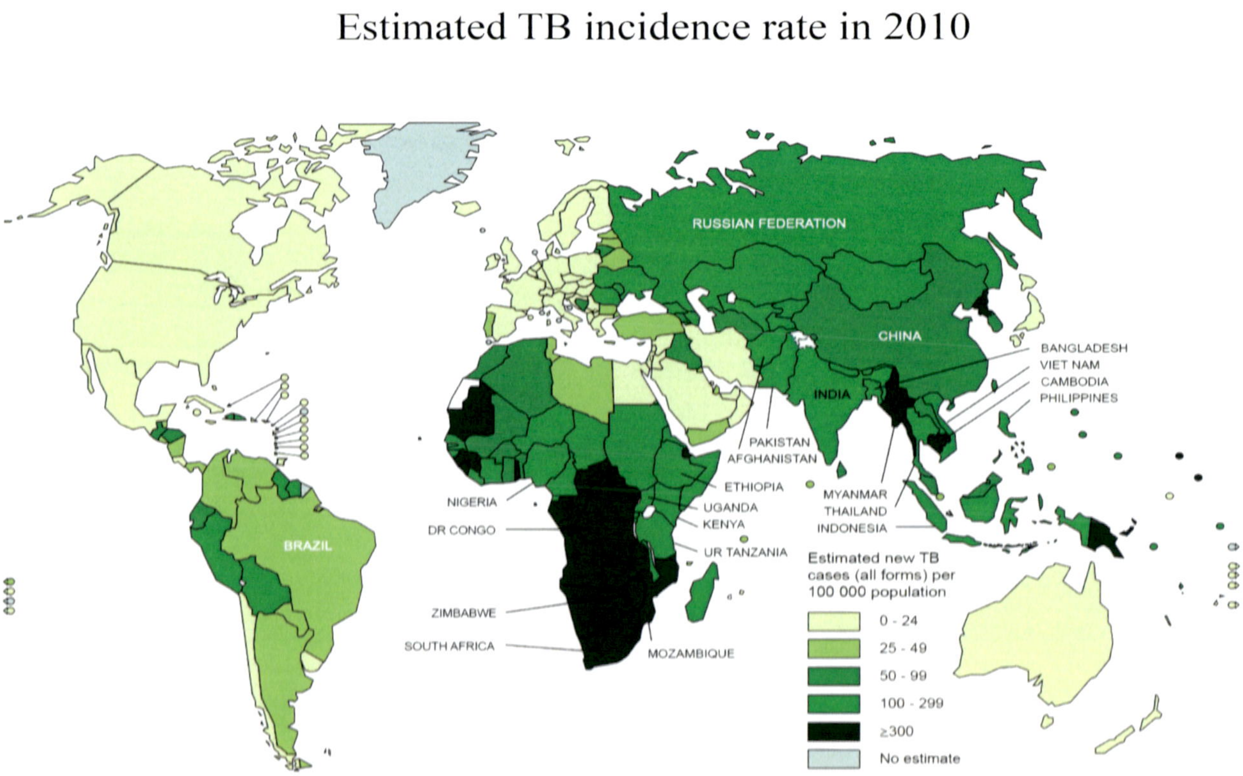

Figure 8.4. *Map of the World with the Tuberculosis incidence rates classified according to the World Health Organization, 2010.*

Source: Diana M. Castañeda-Hernández and Alfonso J. Rodriguez-Morales. (2013). Epidemiological burden of tuberculosis in developing countries. InTech. doi: 10.5772/53363.

8.1.2. Tuberculosis Prevalence in High Burden Developing Countries

For prevalence, a similar epidemiological situation is seen. These 22 countries, concentrated 83.1% of the prevalent cases of TB in the World (9,972,000 cases), reaching mean prevalence rates higher than in the rest of the World, 230.7 cases/100,000. (Table 8.6). However, in many of these countries, those numbers are higher. India (although considered not official data) in 2010 reported 3,100,000 prevalent cases (ranging from 2,000,000 to 4,600,000 cases) (Table 8.6), followed by China with 1,500,000 prevalent cases (ranging from 1,300,000 to 1,700,000 cases) (Table 8.6) and Indonesia with 690,000 prevalent cases (ranging 300,000 to 1,200,000 cases) (Table 8.6). Although that, again rates are higher in other countries, such as South Africa, where for the same year were reported between 359.0 to 1256.7 cases/100,000. (3.6 to 12.6 cases/1,000 or 0.4 to 1.3 cases/100) (Table 8.6). For Asia, the country with the highest prevalence rates is Cambodia (297.1 to 1061.0 cases/100,000.) (Table 8.6). For Latin America, the country with the highest rates (and the only one from that region in this list) is Brazil (17.4 to 82.1 cases/100,000.) (Table 8.6).

Table 8.6. Estimated Epidemiological Burden of TB Prevalence in the Countries with the Considered Higher Burden of TB, According to WHO in 2010 (World Health Organization 2011)

		Prevalence (cases)			**Prevalence Rates (cases/100,000pop)**		
Countries	**Population**	**Best**	**Low**	**High**	**Best**	**Low**	**High**
South Africa	50,133,000	400,000	180,000	630,000	797.9	359.0	1256.7
Cambodia	14,138,000	93,000	42,000	150,000	657.8	297.1	1061.0
DR Congo	65,966,000	350,000	160,000	560,000	530.6	242.5	848.9
Myanmar	47,963,000	250,000	180,000	310,000	521.2	375.3	646.3
Philippines	93,261,000	470,000	410,000	530,000	504.0	439.6	568.3
Mozambique	23,391,000	110,000	54,000	200,000	470.3	230.9	855.0
Bangladesh	148,692,000	610,000	280,000	1,000,000	410.2	188.3	672.5
Zimbabwe	12,571,000	51,000	23,000	80,000	405.7	183.0	636.4
Ethiopia	82,950,000	330,000	140,000	520,000	397.8	168.8	626.9
Pakistan	173,593,000	630,000	270,000	1,100,000	362.9	155.5	633.7
Afghanistan	31,412,000	110,000	51,000	180,000	350.2	162.4	573.0
Viet Nam	87,848,000	290,000	130,000	510,000	330.1	148.0	580.5
Indonesia	239,871,000	690,000	300,000	1,200,000	287.7	125.1	500.3
Kenya	40,513,000	110,000	49,000	180,000	271.5	120.9	444.3
India	1,224,614,000	3,100,000	2,000,000	4,600,000	253.1	163.3	375.6
Nigeria	158,423,000	320,000	110,000	690,000	202.0	69.4	435.5
Uganda	33,425,000	64,000	32,000	100,000	191.5	95.7	299.2
Thailand	69,122,000	130,000	55,000	210,000	188.1	79.6	303.8
UR Tanzania	44,841,000	82,000	39,000	130,000	182.9	87.0	289.9

Russian Federation	142,958,000	190,000	70,000	330,000	132.9	49.0	230.8
China	1,341,335,000	1,500,000	1,300,000	1,700,000	111.8	96.9	126.7
Brazil	194,946,000	92,000	34,000	160,000	47.2	17.4	82.1
Subtotal	4,321,966,000	9,972,000	5,909,000	15,070,000	230.7	136.7	348.7
% from global burden	62.9	83.1	53.7	107.6	-	-	-
Global burden	6,869,573,000	12,000,000	11,000,000	14,000,000	174.7	160.1	203.8

Source: Diana M. Castañeda-Hernández and Alfonso J. Rodriguez-Morales. (2013). Epidemiological burden of tuberculosis in developing countries. InTech. doi: 10.5772/53363.

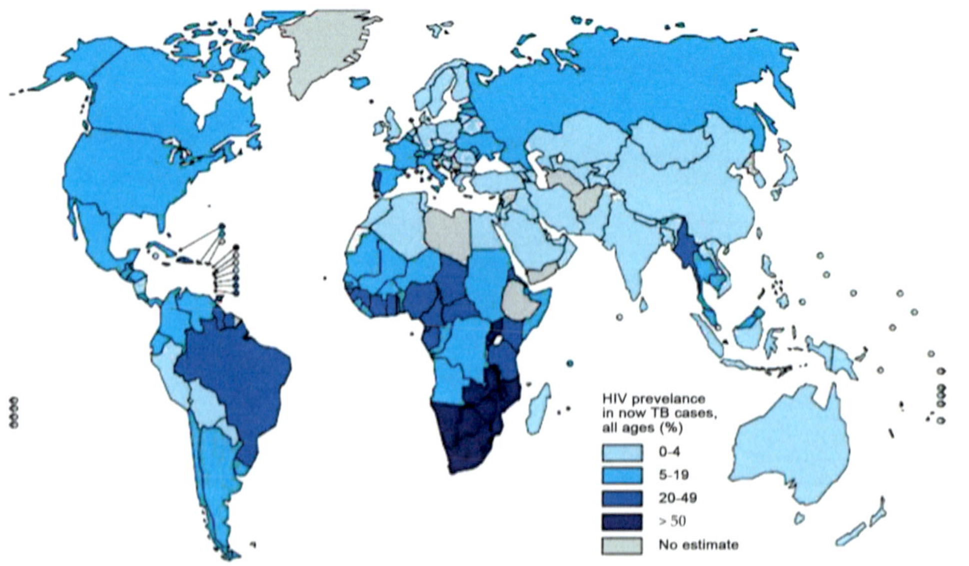

Figure 8.5. *Map of the World with the estimated HIV prevalence in new TB cases classified according to the World Health Organization, 2010.*

Source: Diana M. Castañeda-Hernández and Alfonso J. Rodriguez-Morales. (2013). Epidemiological burden of tuberculosis in developing countries. InTech. doi: 10.5772/53363.

8.1.3. Tuberculosis Mortality in High Burden Developing Countries

An analogous epidemiological scenario is observed for mortality. These 22 nations accounted for 78.0% of all TB-related deaths worldwide (857,800 deaths, ranging from 581,900 to 1,229,000 deaths), with mean mortality rates of 19.8 deaths per 100,000 people, which was higher than the global average. (Table 8.7). These numbers are higher in many of these countries, though. Table 8.7 shows that, despite not being official data, India reported 320,000 deaths in 2010 (between 210,000 and 470,000). Indonesia came in second with 64,000 deaths (between 42,000 and 91,000) and Bangladesh with 64,000 deaths (between 47,000 and 85,000). Despite this, rates are higher in other nations, like Cambodia, where 43,9 to 84,9 deaths per 100,000 people were reported in the same year (Table 8.7). The Democratic Republic of the Congo has the highest death rate in Africa, ranging from 40 to 68 deaths per 100,000 people) (Table 8.7). Brazil is the only country from Latin America on this list with the highest rates, ranging from 1 to 4 deaths per 100,000 people) (Table 8.7).

Table 8.7. Estimated Epidemiological Burden of TB Mortality in the Countries with the Higher Burden of TB, According to WHO in 2010 (World Health Organization 2011).

		Mortality (deaths)			**Mortality rates (deaths/100,000pop)**		
Countries	**Population**	**Best**	**Low**	**High**	**Best**	**Low**	**High**
Cambodia	14,138,000	8,600	6,200	12,000	60.8	43.9	84.9
DR Congo	65,966,000	36,000	27,000	45,000	54.6	40.9	68.2
South Africa	50,133,000	25,000	16,000	38,000	49.9	31.9	75.8
Mozambique	23,391,000	11,000	7,000	17,000	47.0	29.9	72.7
Bangladesh	148,692,000	64,000	47,000	85,000	43.0	31.6	57.2
Myanmar	47,963,000	20,000	12,000	31,000	41.7	25.0	64.6
Afghanistan	31,412,000	12,000	8,600	16,000	38.2	27.4	50.9
Ethiopia	82,950,000	29,000	23,000	35,000	35.0	27.7	42.2
Pakistan	173,593,000	58,000	39,000	84,000	33.4	22.5	48.4
Philippines	93,261,000	31,000	21,000	43,000	33.2	22.5	46.1
Viet Nam	87,848,000	29,000	19,000	43,000	33.0	21.6	48.9
Zimbabwe	12,571,000	3,400	2,100	5,100	27.0	16.7	40.6
Indonesia	239,871,000	64,000	42,000	91,000	26.7	17.5	37.9
India	1,224,614,000	320,000	210,000	470,000	26.1	17.1	38.4
Nigeria	158,423,000	33,000	11,000	68,000	20.8	6.9	42.9
Russian Federation	142,958,000	26,000	16,000	42,000	18.2	11.2	29.4
Kenya	40,513,000	6,900	4,900	9,400	17.0	12.1	23.2
Thailand	69,122,000	11,000	7,000	16,000	15.9	10.1	23.1
Uganda	33,425,000	5,100	3,300	7,300	15.3	9.9	21.8
UR Tanzania	44,841,000	5,800	4,700	6,900	12.9	10.5	15.4
China	1,341,335,000	54,000	52,000	56,000	4.0	3.9	4.2
Brazil	194,946,000	5,000	3,100	8,300	2.6	1.6	4.3
Subtotal	4,321,966,000	857,800	581,900	1,229,000	19.8	13.5	28.4
% from the global burden	62.9	78.0	63.3	102.4	-	-	-
Global burden	6,869,573,000	1,100,000	920,000	1,200,000	16.0	13.4	17.5

Source: Diana M. Castañeda-Hernández and Alfonso J. Rodriguez-Morales. (2013). Epidemiological burden of tuberculosis in developing countries. InTech. doi: 10.5772/53363.

8.2. Tuberculosis-HIV Incidence in High Burden Developing Countries

One of the primary issues that high-burden developing nations should address in light of the public health threat posed by tuberculosis is coinfection. With a concentration of 78.1% of all TB-HIV cases worldwide (859,600 cases, ranging from 636,200 to 1,128,900 cases), these 20 countries have mean TB-HIV rates of 20.4% per 100,000 people, which is higher than the global average (Table 8.8). These numbers are higher in many of these countries, though. Africa reported 300,000 cases of TB-HIV in 2010 (between 240,000 and 350,000), followed by Mozambique with 77,000 cases (between 53,000 and 110,000) and India (though not official data) with 110,000 cases (between 75,000 and 160,000) (Table 8.8). Despite this, rates in other nations are once more higher. The nation with the greatest TB-HIV rates is South Africa, where there are 478.7 to 698.1 cases per 100,000 people. (Table 8.8). Myanmar has the highest rates of tuberculosis and HIV in Asia (43–118 cases/100,000 people).) (Table 8.8). Brazil is the only country from Latin America on this list with the highest rates (5.1 to 14.4 cases/100,000 population) (Figure 8.5; Table 8.8).

Table 8.8. Estimated Epidemiological Burden of TB-HIV in the Countries with the Higher Burden of TB, According to WHO in 2010 (World Health Organization 2011)

		HIV-Positive Incident TB Cases			HIV-TB Rates (Cases/100,000 Population)		
Countries	**Population**	**Best**	**Low**	**High**	**Best**	**Low**	**High**
South Africa	50,133,000	300,000	240,000	350,000	598.4	478.7	698.1
Zimbabwe	12,571,000	60,000	47,000	76,000	477.3	373.9	604.6
Mozambique	23,391,000	77,000	53,000	110,000	329.2	226.6	470.3
Kenya	40,513,000	50,000	45,000	55,000	123.4	111.1	135.8
Uganda	33,425,000	38,000	30,000	46,000	113.7	89.8	137.6
Myanmar	47,963,000	37,000	21,000	57,000	77.1	43.8	118.8
UR Tanzania	44,841,000	30,000	28,000	31,000	66.9	62.4	69.1
Nigeria	158,423,000	51,000	25,000	87,000	32.2	15.8	54.9
Cambodia	14,138,000	4,000	3,400	4,700	28.3	24.0	33.2
DR Congo	65,966,000	18,000	13,000	24,000	27.3	19.7	36.4
Thailand	69,122,000	12,000	13,000	18,000	17.4	18.8	26.0

Brazil	194,946,000	18,000	10,000	28,000	9.2	5.1	14.4
India	1,224,614,000	110,000	75,000	160,000	9.0	6.1	13.1
Viet Nam	87,848,000	7,600	4,600	11,000	8.7	5.2	12.5
Indonesia	239,871,000	18,000	9,900	29,000	7.5	4.1	12.1
Russian Federation	142,958,000	8,100	6,800	9,400	5.7	4.8	6.6
China	1,341,335,000	18,000	10,000	28,000	1.3	0.7	2.1
Philippines	93,261,000	1,000	500	1,800	1.1	0.5	1.9
Pakistan	173,593,000	1,200	700	1,900	0.7	0.4	1.1
Bangladesh	148,692,000	700	300	1,100	0.5	0.2	0.7
Subtotal	4,207,604,000	859,600	636,200	1,128,900	20.4	15.1	26.8
% from the global burden	61.2	78.1	63.6	94.1	-	-	-
Global burden	6,869,573,000	1,100,000	1,000,000	1,200,000	16.0	14.6	17.5

Source: Diana M. Castañeda-Hernández and Alfonso J. Rodriguez-Morales. (2013). Epidemiological burden of tuberculosis in developing countries. InTech. doi: 10.5772/53363.

8.3. Multidrug Resistant Tuberculosis in High Burden Developing Countries

MDR (multidrug resistant) tuberculosis is a disease of public health concern. Its burden is a pertinent issue that needs to be addressed, especially in developing nations. Up to 26% of newly diagnosed cases of tuberculosis in certain countries may be multidrug-resistant (MDR-TB) (Figure 8.6).

Since a range of antituberculosis medications have been available for 30 years, MDR strains have emerged that essentially downplay the benefits of chemotherapy for tuberculosis. The strains with extensive drug resistance (XDR), which are typically resistant to four or five different drugs, are the most dangerous of them. The strain resistance's molecular mechanisms are taken into account. Different regions of the mycobacterial genome give rise to successive, usually independent resistance mutations that result in the formation of XDR and MDR strains. Furthermore, mycobacterial latency and tolerance in infected tissues have an impact on the development of resistant strains.

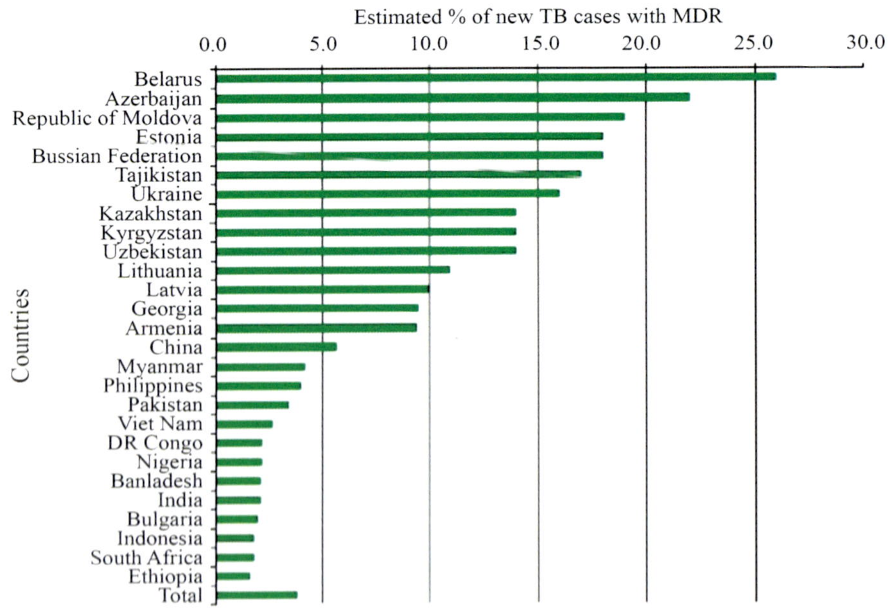

Figure 8.6. *Estimated proportion of TB cases that have MDR-TB.*

Source: Diana M. Castañeda-Hernández and Alfonso J. Rodriguez-Morales. 2013). Epidemiological burden of tuberculosis in developing countries. InTech. doi: 10.5772/53363.

The increasing emergence of multidrug-resistant (MDR) and extensively drug-resistant (XDR) tuberculosis (TB) in the era of human immunodeficiency virus (HIV) infection presents a major threat to effective control of TB. Drug resistance in *Mycobacterium tuberculosis* arises from spontaneous chromosomal mutations at low frequency. Clinical drug-resistant TB largely occurs as a result of man-made selection during disease treatment of these genetic alterations through erratic drug supply, suboptimal physician prescription and poor patient adherence. Molecular mechanisms of drug resistance have been elucidated for the major first- and second-line drugs rifampicin, isoniazid, pyrazinamide, ethambutol, the aminoglycosides and the fluoroquinolones. The relationship between drug resistance in *M. tuberculosis* strains and their virulence/transmissibility needs to be further investigated. Understanding the mechanisms of drug resistance in *M. tuberculosis* would enable the development of rapid molecular diagnostic tools and furnish possible insights into new drug development for the treatment of TB.

8.4. Tuberculosis in Colombia and in a City of the Country: Pereira

In Colombia for 2010 incident cases were 16,000 cases (ranging from 13,000 to 19,000 cases) for a rate of 34 cases/100,000 population (28 to 41 cases/100,000 population). Prevalence was estimated in 22,000 cases (9,100 to 37,000 cases) for a rate of 48 cases/100,000 population (ranging from 20 to 81 cases/100,000 population.). Mortality was estimated at 1,300 deaths (ranging from 800 to 1,900 deaths) for a mortality rate of 2.8 deaths/100,000 population. (1.7 to 4.2 deaths/100,000 population.). All these figures are excluding HIV cases. TB incidence in HIV-positive patients is 1,100 cases (ranging from 750 to 1,500 cases) for a rate of 2.4 cases/100,000 population. (ranging from 1.6 to 3.3 cases/100,000 population.).

One example of a location with a high TB burden is the Colombian city of Pereira. The Department of Risaralda's capital municipality is Pereira (Figure 8.7). Situated in a small valley that descends from a section of the western Andes Mountain chain, it is the focal point of the western region of the country. The city is an urban center in Colombia due to its strategic location in the coffee-producing region and its close proximity to Bogotá, Cali, and Medellín.

For 2011, Pereira municipality has an estimated population of 459,690. Official reported records for TB in Risaralda registered a disease incidence for 2010 of 25 cases per 100,000 population (which is above the national average rate of 24 cases per 100,000 population). Pereira is divided into 19 urban submunicipalities: Ferrocarril, Olímpica, San Joaquín, Cuba, Del Café, El Oso, Perla del Otún, Consota, El Rocío, El poblado, El Jardín, San Nicolás, Centro, Río Otún, Boston, Universidad, Villavicencio, Oriente and Villasantana. Additionally, also has rural townships which include Altagracia, Arabia, Caimalito, Cerritos, La Florida, Puerto Caldas, Combia Alta, Combia Baja, La Bella, Estrella, La Palmilla, Morelia and Tribunas. The municipality of Pereira has a diversified economy: the primary sector accounts for 5.7% of the domestic product, the secondary sector shows a relative weight of 26.2%, while the tertiary sector is the most representative with 68.1%. The GDP of Pereira grew by 3.7% in 2004. For 2010, Pereira reported 301 cases of TB (incidence rate of 65.85 cases per 100,000population). In Pereira, previously reported interventions have been developed and working intersectorially with the academia in order to increase the impact of activities in TB control.

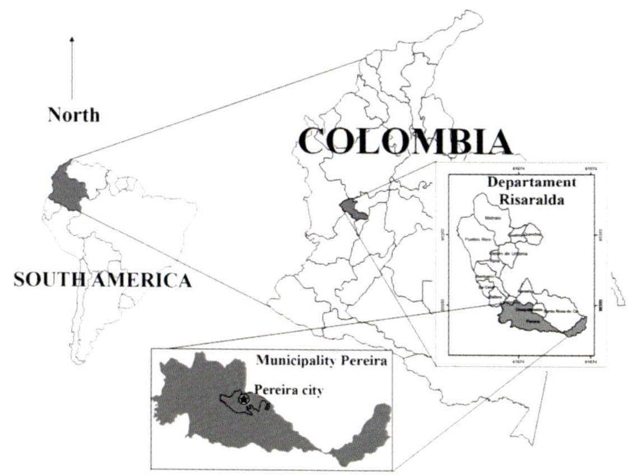

Figure 8.7. *Relative location of Pereira, Risaralda, Colombia, South America.*

Source: Diana M. Castañeda-Hernández and Alfonso J. Rodriguez-Morales. (2013). Epidemiological burden of tuberculosis in developing countries. InTech. doi: 10.5772/53363.

In the country, the strategic plan "*Colombia Libre de Tuberculosis para la Expansión y Fortalecimiento de la Estrategia Alto a la TB, 2010–2015*" (Colombia Free of TB for the Expansion and Enhancement of the Strategy Stop TB, 2010–2015), define as goal the achievement of notifications of new positive baciloscopy cases in more than 70% and a curation rate of at least 85%. In this context the routine surveillance allow to follow management and measurement of the impact of the realized actions by the control programs at municipal, departmental and national level, in order to generate interventions that contribute to achievement of the established goals to stop the advance of TB in the country.

In Pereira, control of TB among the homeless has found that between 2007 and 2010, 74 homeless persons with TB were evaluated, from a total of 1,470 registered homeless persons (from the Social Development Secretary of Pereira) (cumulated incidence=50.3

cases/1,000population., range 5.44 to 22.44; year 2010=16.32). Outcome condition was in 43.2% treatment self-withdrawal (range 36.4%-55.6%), therapeutical failure, 4.1% (0.0–9.1%), deaths, 2.7% (0.0%-8.3%), cured, 39.2% (33.3%-42.4%) and finished treatments, 10.8% (4.2%-25.0%). Comparing the 2010 TB incidence among homeless persons with that of the general population (0.6585/1,000population.) that is 76.45 times higher in that risk population. In the same way, the case fatality rate in 2010 was 2.5 times higher than in the general population (3.3%). These results have important implications in public health as well in the management and evolution of TB in these individuals, persistence of infection, drug resistance and potential transmission to those that can be around these populations.

Also, as part of the integrative control of TB in special populations, surveillance has included control in a prison. Evaluating TB among prisoners between 2010 and 2012, seven prisoners with TB (AFB+), from a total of 1,508 registered prisoners at the penitentiary were diagnosed (cumulated incidence=4.64 cases/1,000pop., 2.99 in 2010 and 2.13 in 2011). The mean age was 40.5 years old (100% males), and all had pulmonary disease. All of them received voluntary counseling and testing for HIV, one of them was HIV+. Three of them are under anti-TB treatment, 2 were transferred, 1 finished treatment and 1 was a therapeutical failure. Comparing the 2011 TB incidence among prisoners with that of the general population (0.67/1,000population) that was 3.19 times higher in that risk population. In 2010, the figure in Pereira was 0.66/1,000population, then 4.55 times higher in prisoners (Castañeda-Hernández DM et al 2012b). These results have important implications in public health as well in the management and evolution of TB in these individuals, persistence of infection, drug resistance and potential transmission to those that can be around these prisoners. This is in agreement with recent data indicating that TB incidence rates among prisoners can be as high as approximately 5 to 50 times higher than in the general population. In Brazil, this has been reported as high as 61.8 times higher for latent TB and 36.08 for active TB. Prisoners are at risk of rapidly progressing to a latent TB or having an active TB posterior a recent infection or reactivation due to latent coexisting pathologies, particularly HIV infection, IV drug use and poor nutritional status. It has been shown that workers in such facilities as well the community, are at risk. For these reasons, strategies oriented to bring an integrated, social, epidemiological, clinical, diagnostic and therapeutic management, are proposed and for the Americas, the Pan-American Health Organization (PAHO) guideline for TB control in population in prisons should be followed (OPS, 2008)

A Closer Look

Tuberculosis Control in Developing Countries

Tuberculosis (TB) remains a significant public health challenge, particularly in developing countries where factors such as poverty, overcrowding, limited access to healthcare, and high prevalence of HIV/AIDS contribute to its persistence. Controlling TB in developing countries requires a multifaceted approach that addresses both medical and socio-economic determinants of the disease, aiming to reduce transmission, improve diagnosis and treatment, and mitigate the social and economic impact on affected communities.

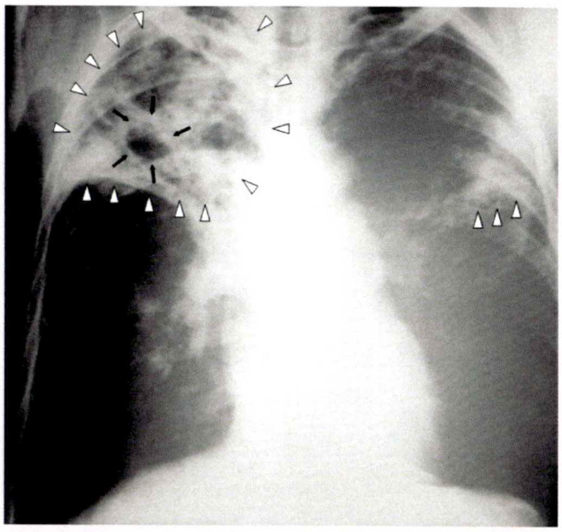

https://upload.wikimedia.org/wikipedia/commons/9/9c/Tuberculosis-x-ray-1.jpg.

One crucial aspect of TB control in developing countries is strengthening healthcare systems to ensure timely diagnosis and treatment of TB cases. This includes expanding access to TB diagnostic tools such as GeneXpert machines, which can rapidly detect TB and drug resistance, particularly in remote and resource-limited settings where conventional diagnostic methods may be unavailable or impractical. Additionally, training healthcare workers in TB case detection and management is essential to ensure that TB patients receive appropriate care and adhere to treatment regimens, thereby reducing the risk of transmission and the development of drug resistance.

Furthermore, TB control efforts in developing countries often involve implementing community-based interventions to reach marginalized populations and improve treatment outcomes. Community health workers play a crucial role in TB control by conducting active case finding, providing directly observed therapy (DOT) to ensure treatment adherence, and promoting TB awareness and prevention measures within communities. By engaging communities and leveraging existing networks, TB control programs can enhance access to care, reduce stigma associated with TB, and empower individuals to seek timely diagnosis and treatment.

In addition to medical interventions, addressing socio-economic determinants is essential for TB control in developing countries. Poverty, malnutrition, inadequate housing, and lack of access to education and healthcare services contribute to the burden of TB by increasing vulnerability to infection, delaying diagnosis and treatment, and hindering treatment adherence. Therefore, TB control programs must adopt a holistic approach that integrates social protection measures, poverty alleviation strategies, and efforts to improve living conditions and access to basic services. By addressing underlying socio-economic inequalities, TB control efforts can enhance resilience and reduce the risk of TB transmission within communities.

Moreover, TB control in developing countries requires collaboration and partnerships among governments, civil society organizations, international agencies, and the private sector. Multisectoral collaboration is essential for mobilizing resources, advocating for policy change, and implementing integrated approaches that address the complex challenges of TB control. By working together, stakeholders can leverage their respective strengths and expertise to scale up TB prevention, diagnosis, and treatment efforts, ultimately aiming to achieve the Sustainable Development Goal target of ending the TB epidemic by 2030.

Summary

- Tuberculosis (TB) is an infectious disease caused by different species of the genus *Mycobacteria*. Together with human immunodeficiency virus infection (HIV)/ Acquired Immunodeficiency Syndrome (AIDS) and malaria, tuberculosis is one of the biggest killers in the Word.
- Epidemiology of tuberculosis can be influenced by multiple not only clinical factors, but also demographical, geographical and social aspects at local or national levels, as the development of the country, currently measured by indicators such as the Human Development Index (HDI).
- Tuberculosis is a complex disease in terms of the multiple factors that are involved in its occurrence and persistence in the human societies. In first place there are factors associated with the bacillus (viability, transmissibility and virulence), with the host as a biological individual (immune status, genetic susceptibility, duration and intensity of exposure) as well, at the bacillus-host interaction (place of affection, severity of illness).
- Tuberculosis is a disease present, due the raise of HIV coinfection in most countries in the World. Until two to three decades ago, TB was decreasing in importance in the World and was predominantly endemic in developing countries.
- Multidrug resistant (MDR) tuberculosis is a public health problem. Its burden particularly in developing countries is a relevant issue to be addressed. In some countries, proportions as high as 26% of the new TB cases can be MDR-TB.
- The molecular mechanisms that make a strain resistant are considered. XDR and MDR strains result from successive and usually independent resistance mutations, which arise in various regions of the mycobacterial genome. In addition, the formation of resistant strains is affected by the phenomenon of tolerance and mycobacterial latency in infected tissues.
- The increasing emergence of multidrug-resistant (MDR) and extensively drug-resistant (XDR) tuberculosis (TB) in the era of human immunodeficiency virus (HIV) infection presents a major threat to effective control of TB.

References

1. Arbelaez, M. P., Nelson, K. E., & Munoz, A. (2000). BCG vaccine effectiveness in preventing tuberculosis and its interaction with human immunodeficiency virus infection. *International Journal of Epidemiology, 29*(6), 1085–1091.
2. Arenas-Suárez, N. E., García-Gutiérrez, A. M., Coronado-Ríos, S. M., Beltrán-Bocanegra, C. A., Acosta-Botero, S. M., Gómez-Marín, J. E., & Quintero-Álvarez, L. (2010). Prevalence of childhood tuberculosis in Armenia, Colombia. *Revista de Salud Pública (Bogotá), 12*(6), 1000–1009.
3. Black, G. F., Weir, R. E., Chaguluka, S. D., Warndorff, D., Crampin, A. C., et al. (2003). Gamma interferon responses induced by a panel of recombinant and purified mycobacterial antigens in healthy, non-mycobacterium bovis BCG-vaccinated Malawian young adults. *Clinical and Diagnostic Laboratory Immunology, 10*(4), 602–611.

4. Castañeda-Hernández, D. M., & Rodríguez-Morales, A. J. (2012a). Scientific research in tuberculosis: bibliometric assessment of the Colombian contributions to the literature. *Infectio, 16*(S1), 33.

5. Castañeda-Hernández, D. M., & Rodríguez-Morales, A. J. (2012b). Social Networking in Tuberculosis: Experience in Colombia. In A. J. Rodriguez-Morales (Ed.), *Current Topics in Tropical Medicine* (pp. 67–80). InTech.

6. Castañeda-Hernández, D. M., Rodríguez-Morales, A. J., & Sepulveda-Arias, J. C. (2012d). Importancia del uso de pruebas de medición de la liberación de interferon-gamma en la vigilancia epidemiológica de la tuberculosis. *Revista Médica de Chile, 140*(1), 128–129.

7. Chadha, S. S., Sharath, B. N., Reddy, K., Jaju, J., Vishnu, P. H., Rao, S., Parmar, M., Satyanarayana, S., Sachdeva, K. S., Wilson, N., & Harries, A. D. (2011). Operational challenges in diagnosing multi-drug resistant TB and initiating treatment in Andhra Pradesh, India. *PLoS One, 6*(11), e26659.

8. Curto, M., Scatena, L. M., de Paula Andrade, R. L., Palha, P. F., de Assis, E. G., et al. (2010). Tuberculosis control: patient perception regarding orientation for the community and community participation. *Revista Latino-Americana de Enfermagem, 18*(5), 983–989.

9. Dim, C. C., Dim, N. R., & Morkve, O. (2011). Tuberculosis: a review of current concepts and control programme in Nigeria. *Nigerian Journal of Medicine, 20*(2), 200–206.

10. Fernández, M., & Dickson González, S. M. (2007). Coloraciones especiales e impregnaciones argénticas. *Revista de la Sociedad Médico Quirúrgica Hospital de Emergencias Pérez de León, 38*(1), 8–10.

11. Ferro, B. E., Nieto, L. M., Rozo, J. C., Forero, L., & van Soolingen, D. (2011). Multidrug-resistant Mycobacterium tuberculosis, Southwestern Colombia. *Emerging Infectious Diseases, 17*(7), 1259–1262.

12. Francis, J., Reed, A., Yohannes, F., Dodard, M., & Fournier, A. M. (2002). Screening for tuberculosis among orphans in a developing country. *American Journal of Preventive Medicine, 22*(2), 117–119.

13. Franco-Paredes, C., Jones, D., Rodriguez-Morales, A. J., & Santos-Preciado, J. I. (2007a). Commentary: improving the health of neglected populations in Latin America. *BMC Public Health, 7*, 11.

14. Franco-Paredes, C., Von, A., Hidron, A., Rodriguez-Morales, A. J., & Tellez, I. (2007b). Chagas disease: an impediment in achieving the Millennium Development Goals in Latin America. *BMC International Health and Human Rights, 7*, 7.

15. Galimi, R. (2011). Extrapulmonary tuberculosis: tuberculous meningitis new developments. *European Review for Medical and Pharmacological Sciences, 15*(4), 365–386.

16. Garcia-Rodriguez, J. F., Alvarez-Diaz, H., Lorenzo-Garcia, M. V., Marino-Callejo, A., Fernandez-Rial, A., & Sesma-Sanchez, P. (2011). Extrapulmonary tuberculosis: epidemiology and risk factors. *Enfermedades Infecciosas y Microbiología Clínica, 29*(7), 502–509.

17. Ginsberg, A. M. (2000). A proposed national strategy for tuberculosis vaccine development. *Clinical Infectious Diseases, 30*(Suppl 3), S233–S242.

18. Glaziou, P., Floyd, K., & Raviglione, M. (2009). Global burden and epidemiology of tuberculosis. *Clinics in Chest Medicine, 30*(4), 621–636, vii.

19. Gotuzzo, E. (2011). Xpert MTB/RIF for diagnosis of pulmonary tuberculosis. *Lancet Infectious Diseases, 11*(11), 802–803.

20. Hoek, K. G., Van, R. A., van Helden, P. D., Warren, R. M., & Victor, T. C. (2011). Detecting drug-resistant tuberculosis: the importance of rapid testing. *Molecular Diagnosis & Therapy, 15*(4), 189–194.

21. Marais, B. J., & Schaaf, H. S. (2010). Childhood tuberculosis: an emerging and previously neglected problem. *Infectious Disease Clinics of North America, 24*(3), 727–749.

22. Murcia-Aranguren, M. I., Gómez-Marin, J. E., Alvarado, F. S., Bustillo, J. G., de Mendivelson, E., Gómez, B., León, C. I., Triana, W. A., Vargas, E. A., & Rodríguez, E. (2001). Frequency of tuberculous and non-tuberculous mycobacteria in HIV infected patients from Bogota, Colombia. *BMC Infectious Diseases, 1*, 21.

23. Orcau, A., Cayla, J. A., & Martinez, J. A. (2011). Present epidemiology of tuberculosis. Prevention and control programs. *Enfermedades Infecciosas y Microbiología Clínica, 29*(Suppl 1), 2–7.

24. Prozorov, A. A., Zaĭchikova, M. V., & Danilenko, V. N. (2012). Mycobacterium tuberculosis mutants with multidrug resistance: history of origin, genetic and molecular mechanisms of resistance, and emerging challenges. *Genetika, 48*(1), 5–20.

25. Robledo, J., Mejia, G. I., Paniagua, L., Martin, A., & Guzmán, A. (2008). Rapid detection of rifampicin and isoniazid resistance in Mycobacterium tuberculosis by the direct thin-layer agar method. *International Journal of Tuberculosis and Lung Disease, 12*(12), 1482–1484.

26. Rodríguez-Morales, A. J., & Castañeda-Hernández, D. M. (2012). Relationships between morbidity and mortality from tuberculosis and the Human Development Index (HDI) in Venezuela, 1998-2008. *International Journal of Infectious Diseases, 16*(9), e704–e705.

27. Rodríguez-Morales, A. J., Lorizio, W., Vargas, J., Fernández, L., Durán, B., Husband, G., Rondón, A., Vargas, K., Barbella, R. A., & Dickson, S. M. (2008). Malaria, Tuberculosis, VIH/SIDA e Influenza Aviar: ¿Asesinos de la Humanidad? *Revista de la Sociedad Médico Quirúrgica Hospital de Emergencias Pérez de León, 39*(1), 52–76.

28. Solari, L., Gutiérrez, A., Suárez, C., Jave, O., Castillo, E., Yale, G., Ascencios, L., Quispe, N., Valencia, E., & Suárez, V. (2011). Cost analysis of rapid methods for diagnosis of multidrug resistant tuberculosis in different epidemiologic groups in Perú. *Revista Peruana de Medicina Experimental y Salud Pública, 28*(3), 426–431.

29. Tamaru, A., Nakajima, C., Wada, T., Wang, Y., Inoue, M., Kawahara, R., Maekura, R., Ozeki, Y., Ogura, H., Kobayashi, K., Suzuki, Y., & Matsumoto, S. (2012). Dominant incidence of multidrug and extensively drug-resistant specific Mycobacterium tuberculosis clones in Osaka Prefecture, Japan. *PLoS One, 7*(8), e42505.

30. Torres, J., Sardón, V., Soto, M. G., Anicama, R., Arroyo-Hernández, H., Munayco, C. V. (2011). Cluster of multidrug-resistant tuberculosis cases in a school of the district of Ica, Peru. *Revista Peruana de Medicina Experimental y Salud Pública, 28*(3), 497–502.

31. Vargas, J., Gamboa, C., Negrin, D., Correa, M., Sandoval, C., et al. (2005). Disseminated Mycobacterium mucogenicum infection in a patient with idiopathic CD4+ T lymphocytopenia manifesting as fever of unknown origin. *Clinical Infectious Diseases, 41*(5), 759–760.

32. Zhang, Y., & Yew, W. W. (2009). Mechanisms of drug resistance in Mycobacterium tuberculosis. *International Journal of Tuberculosis and Lung Disease, 13*(11), 1320–1330.

Chapter 9

ENVIRONMENTAL AND OCCUPATIONAL EPIDEMIOLOGY

Contents

Introduction

Environmental and occupational epidemiology is a branch of epidemiology that focuses on studying the impact of environmental and occupational factors on human health. In this field, researchers investigate how various exposures in the environment or workplace contribute to the development of diseases and health conditions within populations.

In environmental epidemiology, the emphasis is on understanding how exposures to pollutants, chemicals, radiation, and other environmental factors affect human health. Researchers study the links between environmental contaminants and diseases such as respiratory illnesses, cancer, neurological disorders, and reproductive issues. They utilize epidemiological methods to assess the associations between exposure levels and health outcomes across different populations, often employing techniques such as cohort studies, case-control studies, and meta-analyzes. On the other hand, occupational epidemiology examines the health effects of exposures encountered in the workplace. This includes exposure to hazardous substances like asbestos, heavy metals, solvents, and biological agents, as well as physical hazards such as noise, heat, and ergonomic stressors. Occupational epidemiologists investigate the incidence of work-related diseases, injuries, and deaths, aiming to identify high-risk occupations and industries and develop strategies for prevention and control.

Both environmental and occupational epidemiology play crucial roles in informing public health policies, regulations, and interventions aimed at reducing exposures and protecting human health. By identifying and quantifying the health risks associated with environmental and occupational factors, epidemiologists contribute to efforts to promote healthier environments, safer workplaces, and improved overall well-being for individuals and communities.

Orientation and Directional Terms

Term	Definition	Illustration
Water Pollution	Water pollution is the contamination of water bodies by directly or indirectly discharging chemicals, pollutants and wastes without adequate treatment.	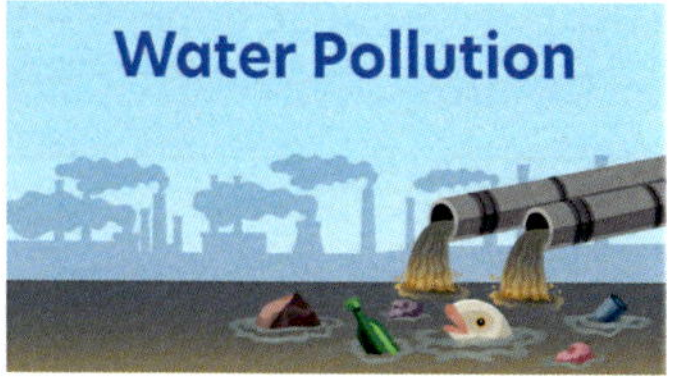
Psychosocial Environment	Psychosocial environment refers to the combination of psychological and social factors that influence an individual's mental well-being and behavior within a particular context or setting. It encompasses various aspects such as social relationships, cultural norms, economic conditions, family dynamics, community support, and other environmental factors.	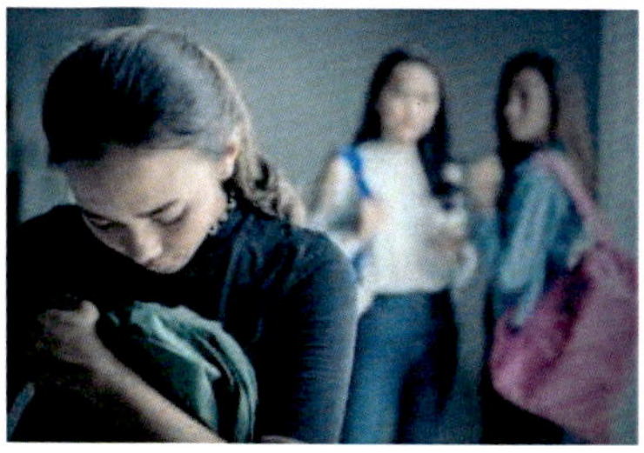
Environmental Tobacco Smoke (ETS)	Environmental tobacco smoke (ETS), also known as secondhand smoke or passive smoke, refers to the combination of smoke exhaled by smokers and smoke emitted from burning tobacco products like cigarettes, cigars, or pipes. When non-smokers are exposed to ETS, they involuntarily inhale the toxic chemicals and particles present in the smoke.	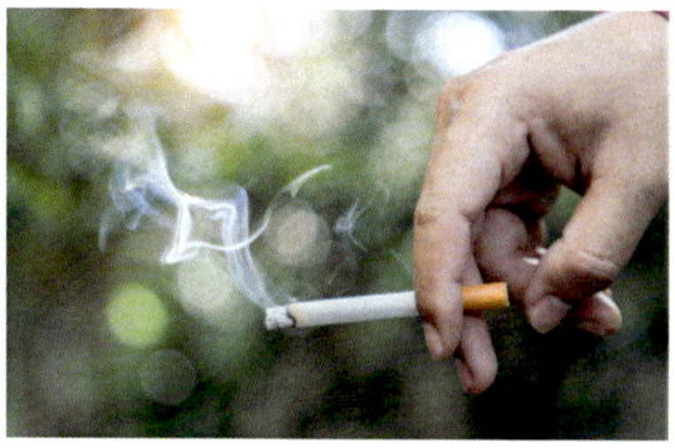
Environmental Risk Assessment	Environmental risk assessment is a systematic approach for identification, evaluation, mitigation and control of hazards that could occur as a result of failures in process, procedures, or equipment.	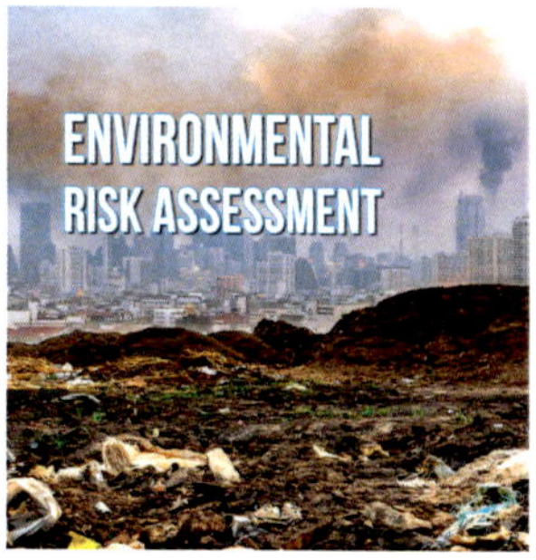
Environmental Health	Environmental health is a discipline that examines human health effects from exposure to harmful agents in the environment. The 'environment' may include the outdoors, home, workplace, or public buildings.	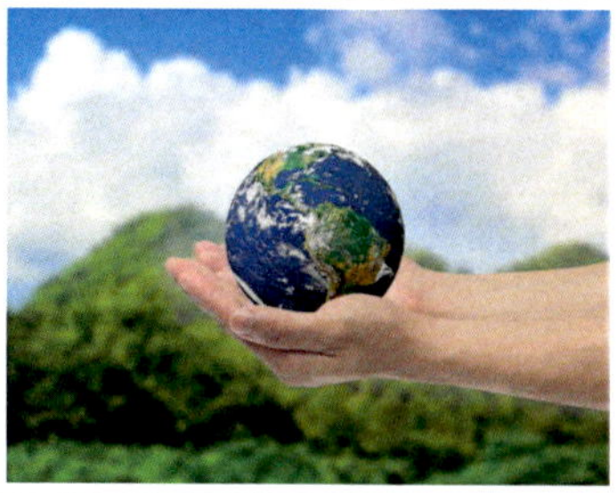

9.1. Definition of Environmental Epidemiology

The study of health and disease distribution, determinants, morbidity, injury, disability, and mortality in populations is the focus of epidemiology. Epidemiologic research is utilized in the management of health issues within populations. One of the fundamental fields that studies the relationships between environmental risks and health outcomes is epidemiology. The study of illnesses and health issues that affect the population and are connected to environmental factors is known as environmental epidemiology. The exposures, which are typically caused by occupational and ambient environments and are often out of the individual's control, can generally be regarded as involuntary. This definition of environmental epidemiology states that the relationship between environmental factors (exposures) and health outcomes is investigated using conventional epidemiologic techniques. The study of air and water pollution, the use of chemicals and physical agents in the workplace, and the psychosocial environment are a few examples of the topics covered.

It is possible to examine smoking-related risks as an exposure dimension that an individual can control or not. As an illustration of the former, environmental epidemiology would not typically be concerned with studies on the health effects of smoking among smokers. However, since nonsmokers and vulnerable groups like children cannot control whether they are exposed to environmental tobacco smoke, there would be concern over populations being exposed to secondhand cigarette smoke.

Therefore, the traditional focus of environmental epidemiology has been on health effects associated with the deterioration of our food, water, and air. A greater focus has been placed on the physical and chemical effects on the environment as a result of the 20th century's advancements in environmental sanitation and the management of biological organisms that cause disease. Lead toxicity, diesel exhaust particulates, pesticide and halogenated compound exposures are a few of the agents and environmental factors that are being studied. Polychlorinated biphenyls (PCBs) are in the final category. They can affect the reproductive system, pose a risk as possible carcinogens, and become more concentrated in food due to biological processes.

Environmental epidemiology continues to be concerned with the relationship between environmental exposures and their unknown hazards, but it now takes a broader approach, identifying and quantifying previously unrecognized exposures to known hazardous agents, estimating an individual's exposure to environmental hazards, assessing the risks associated with exposures, and evaluating exposure prevention procedures. Similar to this, the objectives of epidemiologic research in the related field of occupational health include describing exposure-response gradients, figuring out how occupational hazards might have negative effects, identifying workers who are at risk, and contributing to initiatives aimed at preventing diseases linked to the workplace.

9.1.1. Contributions of Epidemiology to Environmental Health

Epidemiology aids the environmental health field through:

- Concern with populations
- Use of observational data
- Methodology for study designs
- Descriptive and analytic studies

The study of environmental health problems benefits greatly from the application of epidemiology because: (1) many environmental exposures and health effects occur at the population level; (2) natural experiments and observational techniques are appropriate epidemiologic methods; (3) study designs used in epidemiologic research can be directly applied to the study of environmental health issues; and (4) epidemiology facilitates the development of hypotheses and the investigation of causal relationships.

9.1.1.1. Concern with Populations

One distinctive feature of epidemiology—which is sometimes referred to as population medicine—is that it studies the entire population, in contrast to clinical medicine's customary focus on the individual. For instance, epidemiologic research on lung disease may look at the prevalence of lung cancer mortality within counties or within census tracts, which are local geographic divisions. Researchers may wish to look into whether the death rate from lung cancer is higher in areas where "smokestack" industries are concentrated than in areas where air pollution is either relatively low or nonexistent. The doctor's other strategy would be to focus on the identification and management of lung cancer in particular patients.

9.1.1.2. Use of Observational Data

Because of ethical concerns like possible harm to subjects, researchers are frequently forbidden from using experimental methods when examining the prevalence of health and disease in human populations. Epidemiology is essentially an observational science that uses naturally occurring situations to study the occurrence of disease, which makes it partially suited to studies of the health of populations.

9.1.1.3. Methodology for Study Designs

Epidemiologic research in the field of environmental health typically attempts to depict the prevalence of disease occurrence in the population or to connect disease outcomes to particular exposures. The field of environmental epidemiology employs cross-sectional, ecologic, case-control, and cohort study designs to investigate diseases caused by environmental factors in the population. These techniques, for instance, are helpful in and directly related to the field of risk assessment. According to Smith, "the interpretation of epidemiological studies and their application to estimating the potential health risks to populations from known or estimated environmental exposures" constitute the epidemiologic input to environmental risk assessment."

9.1.1.4. Two Classes of Epidemiologic Studies: Descriptive and Analytic

The representation of disease incidence in populations based on person, place, and time variables is known as descriptive epidemiology. Demographic traits like age, sex, and race/ethnicity are examples of person variables. Place variables refer to geographical locations, such as a particular country or countries, regions inside a country, and locations where disease patterns may be localized. A decade, a year, a month, a week, or a day can occasionally be used as variables. Epidemiologists consider descriptive studies to be a basic method that helps define the patterns and processes by which disease strikes populations.

An example of a pattern derived from descriptive studies is disease clustering, which refers to "A closely grouped series of events or cases of a disease or other health-related phenomena with well-defined distribution patterns in relation to time or place or both. The term is normally used to describe aggregation of relatively uncommon events or diseases, e.g., leukemia, multiple sclerosis." Analytic epidemiology investigates theories about the relationship between exposures and health outcomes that are causal (etiologic). Etiologic studies are organized analyzes of the disease's natural history and causation. The significance of low-level exposures has been investigated, and more refinement in exposure-effect relationships is sought, which has led to the need for increasingly complex analytical techniques in these studies. Analytical epidemiology develops and assesses causal models that use exposure and outcome variables in tandem.

In epidemiologic research, exposure variables can include exposure to air pollution, toxic substances, or possible carcinogens. Other situations could involve exposure to biological agents or energy sources like noise, temperature extremes, ionizing and nonionizing radiation, etc. A valid assessment of the level of exposure in a population is necessary for the validity of an environmental epidemiologic research study. In epidemiologic studies, the outcome variable is typically a particular disease, cause of death, or health issue. For epidemiologic research to be of high quality, accurate clinical evaluations of outcomes like lung cancer are essential.

Analytic epidemiology uses naturally occurring circumstances or events as a starting point for testing causal hypotheses. When subsets of the population experience varying degrees of exposure to a putative causal factor, in a scenario that resembles an actual experiment in which human subjects would be randomly assigned to groups, these naturally occurring events are called natural experiments.

9.2. Types of Studies in Environmental Epidemiology

Studies on environmental epidemiology can be broadly divided into two groups: descriptive and analytical, which are not mutually exclusive. Although both types of studies can be used for either purpose, analytical studies are typically most helpful for testing hypotheses and descriptive studies for generating hypotheses. A study's classification as either hypothesis-generating or hypothesis-testing primarily depends on the order of earlier investigations and the current body of knowledge (i.e., whether a hypothesis being examined was proposed by a prior study) rather than the study's design. Sometimes more accurate evaluations of etiologic factors and dose-response relationships are possible thanks to recent advancements in descriptive research.

9.2.1. Descriptive Studies

Descriptive studies include case reports, surveillance systems, ecological studies, and cluster studies.

9.2.1.1. Case Reports

A case report is a descriptive study of a single person or small group in which the individual(s)'s clinical evaluations and histories are thoroughly examined to investigate any potential relationships between an observed effect and a particular environmental exposure. These reports may suggest whether further research on a larger group of individuals with comparable health issues and exposures should be conducted. They also require minimal financial or human resources outside of those used in clinical medicine. However, the lack of controls, uncertainty about exposure time and dose, and lack of context regarding the disease in unexposed individuals often limit the usefulness of case reports. They are most likely to be helpful in cases where the illness is rare and mostly or mostly caused by a single type of exposure. Despite these restrictions, a large number of recognized human environmental toxins (e.g., asbestos, radon, methyl mercury, and tobacco smoke) were initially brought to light in case studies and series created by knowledgeable medical professionals. When private doctors and other sources report clusters of cases to public health agencies, they frequently have to look into them. Even though case reports might not reveal brand-new disease causes, if the illness or the exposure is relatively uncommon, they are more likely to highlight particular theories and biologically significant correlations.

9.2.1.2. Surveillance Systems

These systems offer comprehensive data on designated populations, enabling the execution of epidemiologic analyzes. The general goal of surveillance systems is to capture all detected instances of a given condition in a defined population, either completely or almost completely. As a result, trends over time and between populations or geographic regions can be examined, and they can be used to estimate the background incidence and prevalence of adverse effects.

Surveillance systems can detect changes in the number of deaths resulting from particular diseases, which can lead to the recommendation or testing of theories regarding environmental exposures. For instance, the United States' age-adjusted stomach cancer rates have been declining over time, which has led to the emergence of theories regarding dietary changes in the general population as well as variations in the use of refrigeration and food preservatives that may account for these trends. Similar to this, rates of endometrial carcinoma in women over 65 decreased as postmenopausal estrogen use fell in the United States. This finding supported the conclusion from case-control studies that postmenopausal estrogen use raised the risk of endometrial cancer. In a different case, surveillance data from the National Center for Health Statistics revealed a possible correlation between a decline in gasoline-lead levels and a decline in blood-lead levels in US children.

Studying the connections between disease patterns and changes in environmental factors has become possible as public health organizations have broadened the scope of surveillance systems. It is anticipated that the prevalence of surveillance systems will rise due to improving statistical techniques, growing data quality, and falling costs. The Agency for Toxic Substances and Disease Registry (ATSDR) has developed many surveillance systems to track the health of individuals who may have been exposed to chemicals like dioxin and trichloroethylene. As of right now, those systems have produced no results. These exposure registries must include enough people over long enough periods of time for diseases of interest to manifest in sufficient numbers to show that a problem exists or that it is unlikely to exist, and they must be large enough to raise serious concerns if the results are to be valuable.

9.2.1.3. Ecologic Studies

Ecologic studies investigate, in population groups as opposed to individuals, the statistical relationship between disease and estimated exposures. They incorporate aggregated data or estimates of exposure, such as factory emissions in a certain region, closeness to waste sites, or levels of air or water pollution, with information from vital records, hospital discharges, or disease registries. Observed correlations might lend credence to additional research. Ecologic studies have significant flaws, including assigning group exposure levels to each participant, failing to account for individual confounding variables, using inevitably imprecise estimates of exposure, and possibly missing pertinent exposure during the onset of the disease. While some population groups in ecologic studies may resemble "cohorts," they do not have the individual data necessary for a cohort study to analyze them. Making inaccurate conclusions about groups or individual members of the groups based on data is known as the "ecologic fallacy."

An increase in ecologic studies has been made possible by several advancements, such as the creation of surveillance systems, enhanced environmental exposure databases (e.g., by ASTDR), as well as the expanded accessibility of advanced instruments like geographic information systems. As techniques for estimating exposure advance, the significance of ecologic studies could grow. When appropriate substitutes for exposure levels and pertinent confounding factors can be developed, the ecological fallacy can be mitigated or surmounted.

Ecologic studies, despite their interpretive challenges, have yielded valuable insights into causal relationships. For instance, correlations between geographic differences in natural fluoride levels and rates of tooth decay led to the discovery that fluoride could prevent dental caries. Similar correlations have been found between the rates of cancer and cardiovascular disease among immigrants and their recently acquired compatriots, indicating the possible involvement of dietary and other changes. These studies may be able to produce more accurate indicators of the relationships between risk factors and disease with additional refinement of the parameters of interest. Research examining health issues in connection to stationary environmental exposure sources has frequently depended on labor-intensive methods, like in-person interviews, or far more broad classifications, like ZIP code or town of residence. The latter approach has the obvious drawbacks of misclassifying actual residences and including individuals who live far from the site and have limited exposure opportunities in the exposed category. Better geographic-location data has helped to partially address this issue by being added to state and federal lists of possible environmental exposure sources (e.g., Superfund sites), as well as by making more comprehensive geographic coding of US census data accessible to the general public.

The availability of better mapping software and this extra data have significantly enhanced our capacity to connect health data, like cancer incidence, with a person's residence close to an environmental exposure source. To study different measures of distance and direction, disease cases and controls can be quickly and easily located in relation to an environmental source with the use of effective geographic coding. Census data can also provide information on the population and demographics of the area.

9.2.1.4. Cluster Studies

A descriptive study of the population in a small group, occupational setting, or geographic area where the rate of a particular adverse effect is significantly higher than anticipated is called a cluster study. Furthermore, it is common for the group to be defined after the fact—that is, after the "cluster" comes to light, the group is expanded to include it. As a result, clusters typically suffer from small sample sizes. Cluster studies suffer from a major tautology: information that suggests a relationship between a particular exposure and a particular health outcome is typically used to test the hypothesis; after that, exposure and risk-factor information may be produced for individuals who are defined as belonging to the study group and, typically, a control group. For instance, comparing the measured rates of cardiac birth defects in a specific geographic area with those from outside the area can "test" a reported cluster of these defects that happens close to a hazardous-waste site. Methodologically and statistically, this is a very unreliable approach because the sample under study has not been chosen at random. However, the method can be helpful in developing hypotheses for further research with additional data, as well as in situations where the relative risk is very high. Clusters of diseases were found in particular workplaces, which led to the initial identification of many occupational hazards. Cluster analysis may also be used to determine the presence of other environmental diseases.

9.2.2. Analytic Studies

Analytical studies, in contrast to descriptive studies, are typically more expensive and labor-intensive and are based on more individually detailed data from individuals that can be used to control for confounding. Analytical studies may be able to explore hypotheses regarding possible causes of disease or identify and measure risk factors that increase the likelihood that a particular disease will occur with the help of information from medical records, clinical or laboratory investigations, questionnaire results, or direct measures or estimates of exposures. Additional specific hypotheses can also come from analytical studies, which frequently result in a series of studies with the more recent ones aiming to disprove the theories put forth by the earlier ones.

The classic designs of analytical studies are case-control and cohort studies. In addition, 2 "hybrid" designs—nested case-control studies and case-cohort studies—can be based on identified cohorts.

9.2.2.1. Case-Control Studies

In case-control studies, the exposures of subjects with a particular adverse effect or disease are compared to those of controls, who do not have the effect or disease; controls typically belong to the same population as the cases. The design of case-control studies has been extensively studied in the literature. This includes the presentation of measures of effect, typically the odds ratio, statistical methods for analysis, confounding correction, and control selection. Retrospective data collection is typically necessary for these kinds of investigations. They might experience recall bias, i.e., the propensity of individuals with a particular disease to recall potential causes more easily than those without it. However, compared to large cohort studies, where the costs of gathering significant exposure data from every member of the cohort may be prohibitive, case-control studies frequently allow for the collection of histories of exposure to a wide range of factors and more effective confounding control. As new methods of characterizing exposure through the use of biologic markers are developed, case-control studies are likely to be conducted more frequently, following the development that has occurred in other areas of epidemiology over the last 20 years.

9.2.2.2. Cohort Studies

These studies pinpoint a population referred to as a cohort, or occasionally multiple cohorts with various exposure types of interest. A control group may occasionally experience no exposure. The purpose of the cohort study is to assess correlations between the exposure(s) and one or more cohort health outcomes. Cohort studies involve the identification of individuals with varying exposures to a suspected risk factor, followed by an observation period (usually years rather than weeks or months) for the occurrence of specific health effects. Measured and correlated with estimated exposure levels are the disease of interest's occurrence rates.

There are two types of cohort studies: prospective and retrospective, each with pros and cons. A retrospective (or historical) cohort study links exposures that happened in the past to an entire set of outcomes that have already been seen in a defined population; exposure and outcome data must be available at the time the study is conducted. Prospective cohort studies offer the potential for more accurate measurements because they follow individuals after measuring their current exposure directly. However, they may also suffer from bias in end point determination or subject loss to follow-up. Additionally, it might be necessary to wait for a long time to pass—perhaps even until the follow-up period surpasses the latent period between exposure and effect—or until enough outcome events take place.

Lab tests or questionnaires can be used in cohort studies to measure exposure and outcome. Comparing multiple outcomes to the exposure data at the same time is one advantage over case-control studies. However, the frequency of the various outcomes taken into account will determine the power to test associations, which in turn will depend on the number of participants.

A particular kind of cohort study looks for relationships between environmental exposures and time trends in outcome measures. These studies can be broadly classified into three groups: studies where the outcome is estimated or measured relatively infrequently; studies where the outcome variables are associated with intermittent variations in exposure; and studies where the long-term time trends in health outcome measures or estimates are associated with fluctuations in monitored or estimated exposures. The first class is observed in certain cardiovascular studies where annual assessments of health status are conducted. Both continuous and binary outcome measures are common. Additional examples include studies that link air pollution exposure to the development of chronic bronchitis and prospective cohort studies that track children's exposure to lead and cognitive development from conception to birth.

The second broad class looks at responses that are short-lived or episodic to exposures. This includes studies that relate patterns of asthma to peaks in air pollution. Time-series research, which is frequently carried out in the social sciences, is comparable to the third broad class. These studies collect exposure and outcome measures over periods of months or even years, sometimes daily.

There is a correlation between short-term changes in environmental exposures and short-term fluctuations in those outcomes. Studies on variations in hospital admission, peak respiratory flow, respiratory symptoms, and daily mortality, for example, can be connected to variations in ambient air pollution. The multifactorial nature of the results in the majority of these studies implies that each environmental variable's explanatory power is typically low. To prevent potential confounding, this has required relatively large samples and careful modeling.

9.2.2.3. Nested Case-control Studies

With the exception of the fact that only a sample of controls—individuals who are free of the illness—are thoroughly examined, these studies resemble standard cohort studies. Usually, they use older cases from a defined cohort that has been followed long enough to have enough outcome events, but they also use a random sample of cohort members who could have become cases but had either passed away or not developed the disease at the time the appropriate cases were diagnosed. Usually, controls and cases are matched based on one or more potential confounders (e.g., age, sex, and smoking status) that the researcher is not interested in looking into. In the event that the disease of interest manifests, a person chosen as a control might turn into a case. Because of tighter experimental control, nested case-control studies can be designed to have nearly as much statistical power as the cohort study from which they are derived, and they can be used to draw more accurate conclusions about the relationships between exposure and disease. If it is possible to restrict the controls' exposure determination to a sample, these studies might also be significantly more cost-effective.

9.2.2.4. Case-cohort Studies

In this design, the cohort's exposure experience is represented by a random sample taken from the entire cohort. The exposure experience of this subcohort is compared with that of the cases (who arise from the total cohort and may or may not be individuals in the subcohort who become cases) once the cohort has been followed long enough to accumulate enough cases for analysis. When compared to a cohort study, this design also offers cost savings in terms of exposure data acquisition; however, surveillance of the entire cohort is still required to detect cases that arise.

9.3. Toxicologic Concepts Related to Environmental Epidemiology

The terms dose–response curve, threshold, latency, and synergism, which are from toxicology, characterize exposure to hazardous agents.

9.3.1. Dose–Response Curve

The term "dose-response relationship" describes a particular kind of correlative relationship between an exposure (e.g., a hazardous substance) and result (e.g., a biological result, like cell death). This relationship is mapped out by a dose-response curve, which is employed to evaluate the impact of chemical or toxic substance exposure on an organism (e.g., a test subject). Figure 9.1 displays a typical dose-response curve. The response is displayed along the y-axis, while the dose is indicated along the x-axis. The response may represent the effect in a single subject or be expressed as the percentage of exposed animals exhibiting a specific effect. The sigmoid-shaped dose-response curve is a cumulative percentage response curve as well. There is a flat area at the beginning of the curve, indicating that an increase in dosage has no effect at low levels. The subthreshold phase is another name for this. Once the threshold is crossed, the curve rises sharply before entering a linear phase where the response increases in proportion to the dose. The curve flattens out upon reaching the maximum response. One of the markers used to determine whether a suspected exposure has a causal impact on a health outcome is a dose-response relationship.

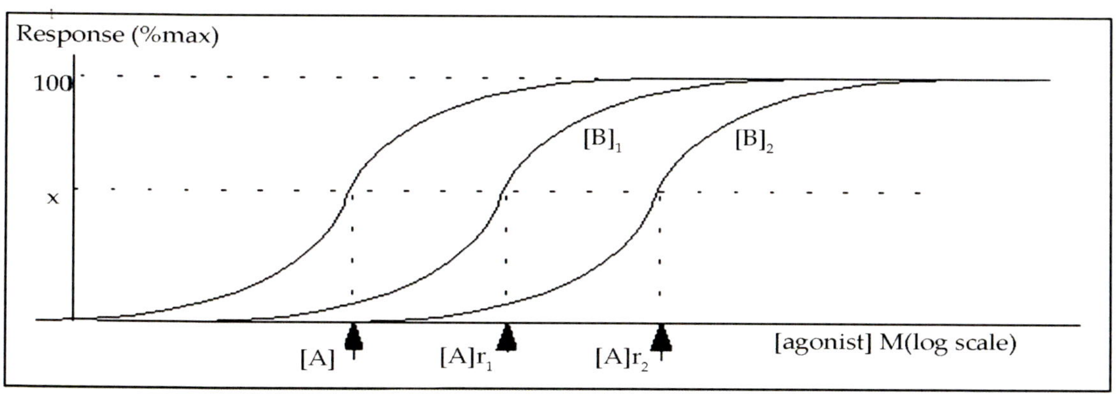

Figure 9.1. *Illustration of the dose–response curve.*

Source: By Dylan2106 – Own work, CC BY-SA 4.0, https://commons.wikimedia.org/w/index.php?curid=3354690.

9.3.2. Threshold

The lowest dose at which a specific response might manifest itself is referred to as the threshold. Whether exposure to toxic chemicals at low (subthreshold) levels is sufficient to cause any kind of health response is unknown, especially in the case of long-term exposure. It is challenging to evaluate the effects of low-level exposures on the population. However, a number of occupational health experts express growing concerns about the long-term consequences of low-level exposure to toxic substances at work. While some researchers speculate that low-level exposures could have pathologic effects, other researchers hold a perspective known as hormesis, which holds that low-level exposures could have protective effects on subsequent high-level exposures. Hormesis is debatable, and some experts think it might reject accepted science.

9.3.3. Latency

The interval of time between an initial exposure and a quantifiable response is referred to as latency. When it comes to agents that are extremely toxic, the latency period can be anywhere from a few seconds to several decades. For instance, there can be a 40-year latency period between the initial asbestos exposure and the subsequent development of mesothelioma, a rare type of cancer. Detecting hazards is a methodologically challenging problem because many of the health events that are studied in environmental research have a lengthy latency. It may be difficult for the epidemiologist to distinguish between exposures that are significant for a disease of interest and those that are not since numerous exposures—often at low levels—may have taken place during the latency period.

9.3.4. Synergism

A scenario known as synergism occurs when the total effect of multiple exposures exceeds the sum of their individual effects. As an illustration, consider the way smoking and asbestos work together to cause lung cancer. Selikoff and colleagues published a seminal study on the risk of lung cancer in asbestos insulation workers. 370 workers in all were the subject of a 1963–1967 study. Compared to the U.S white population as a whole, this occupational group had a seven- to eight-fold higher incidence of lung cancer. But it became clear that asbestos exposure was not the only explanation. Among the 283 workers who smoked, 24 died of lung cancer, a 92-fold increased risk compared to the 87 workers who did not smoke or were not exposed to asbestos at work. No deaths from lung cancer were noted among the nonsmoking workers.

9.3.4.1. Types of Agents

Table 9.1 provides a partial list of possible agents in the context of multiple sclerosis that can be found in the home, workplace, and outside environments. Below is a discussion of these agents' nature and importance. While there are thousands of potential environmental disease agents, the following general categories comprise: hazardous chemicals, metals (particularly heavy metals [e.g., Lead], dusts, molds, allergens, ionizing radiation, electric and magnetic radiation, and e.g., asbestos, coal dust, and silica), as well as mechanical and physical energy.

Table 9.1. Effects of Environmental Materials

Environmental and Microbial Toxins, Drugs, Organic Solvents and Heavy Metals	Beneficial Effect	Debilitating Effect
1. Environmental and Geographical Factors		
• Geographic latitude		Yes
• Sun exposure as a vitamin D source	Yes	
• Circadian disruption and sleep restriction		Yes
2. Toxic Effects of Lifestyle Habits		
• Smoking		Yes
• Obesity and fatty acids intake		Yes
• Ketogenic diet	Yes	
3. Toxic Effects of Food, Diet and Gut Microbiota		
• Coffee	Yes	
• Alcoholic beverages and fish		yes
• High sodium intake		Yes
• Vitamins	Yes	
• Probiotics	Yes	
4. Toxic Effects of Microbes		
• Epstein Barr virus (EBV) infection		Yes
• Bacterial toxins include staphylococcal, nasopharyngeal normal flora		Yes
• Clostridium perfringens epsilon toxin" ε-toxin,"		Yes
• Pertussis toxin (PTX) and botulinum toxins	Yes	? Yes
• Aspergillosis		Yes
• Mycotoxin ochratoxin A		Yes
• Candida species		Yes
5. Chemicals, Organic Solvents and Heavy Metals		
• Pesticides and mothballs		Yes
• Occupational chemical exposure		Yes
• Heavy metals (mercury, lead, arsenic)		Yes
• Copper	Yes	
• Zinc	Yes	Yes
6. Drugs		
• ShK, a toxin from the sea anemone (*Stichodactyla helianthus*) and scorpion venom	Yes	

• Snake venoms	Yes	
• *Thalassophryne nattereri* Brazilian fish venom	Yes	
• Glatiramer acetate, fingolimod (FTY720), mitoxantrone, IFN-β, fumaric acid esters and corticosteroids	Yes	
• Tetanus toxoid vaccination, antibiotics, antihistamines and antifungal agents	Yes	

Source: Hachim MY, Elemam NM, Maghazachi AA. The beneficial and debilitating effects of environmental and microbial toxins, drugs, organic solvents and heavy metals on the onset and progression of multiple sclerosis. Toxins. 2019; 11(3):147. https://doi.org/10.3390/toxins11030147

9.3.5. Chemical Agents

Chemicals are necessary for modern society to function, but their use raises questions about potential short- and long-term health effects. Chemical agents can be encountered by humans in the workplace and at home from a variety of sources. Additionally, there are more opportunities to be exposed to chemicals as their use grows exponentially. Numerous possible negative effects of chemical agents on human health have been investigated, including (e.g., pulmonary disorders, immediate skin irritation, acute toxicity, and long-term consequences like cancer).

Chemical exposure can occur from a variety of sources, such as paints, pesticides, automotive chemicals, household cleaners, and foods. Chemical additives that extend shelf life, maintain quality, improve taste and appearance, and boost nutritional content are found in our food. Bisphenol A (BPA) is a chemical that is used to make epoxy resins and polycarbonate plastics. It can be found in certain plastic types and food and drink packaging. The general public is becoming more and more concerned about the possible negative consequences of widespread exposure to BPA.

Detergents, air fresheners, air disinfectant soaps, and many more household products contain chemicals. Certain brands of engine and body cleaners for cars, as well as related goods, include corrosive and volatile solvents. Many paint and solvent varieties release vapors that could be dangerous if breathed or come into close contact with the skin. Other potential sources of chemical exposure at home include building materials that release vapors containing formaldehyde. Last but not least, a number of pesticides that are frequently used to eradicate weeds, rodents, and insects are extremely harmful to both people and animals.

9.3.6. Pesticides

Pesticides are substances (e.g., insecticides, herbicides, and rodenticides) used to control pests. The four major classes of insecticides are organophosphates, organocarbamates, pyrethroids, and organochlorides (also known as organochlorines), which include dichlorodiphenyltricloroethane (DDT), lindane, and chlordane. Polychlorinated biphenyls and dioxins are also from the organochloride family. Direct exposure to pesticides may follow mishandling, improper disposal in landfills, releases from chemical plants, accidents, or spills; indirect pesticide exposure may result from groundwater contamination through agricultural use of pesticides.

The vapors from pesticides can drift onto agricultural fields, exposing nearby community members as well as workers. Nearly 3,000 cases of agricultural pesticide drift exposures between 1998 and 2006 were examined by researchers. The majority of those exposed were exposed at work; the other half lived in the neighborhood. The distribution of acute health effects linked to pesticide drift cases is shown in Figure 9.2.

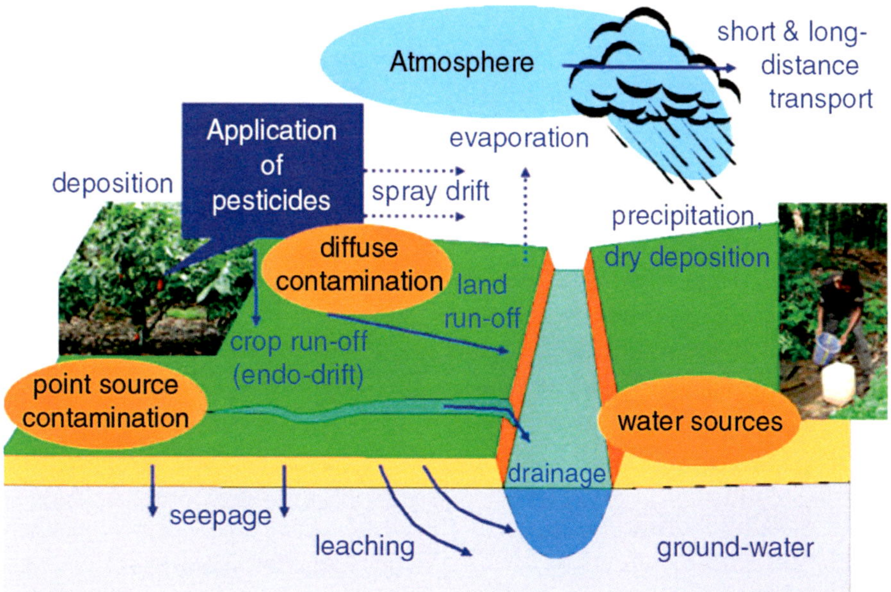

Figure 9.2. *Health effects associated with pesticide drift (n = 2,945). Percentages do not add up to 100% because of multiple mentions.*

Source: By Roy Bateman at English Wikipedia, CC BY-SA 3.0, https://commons.wikimedia.org/w/index.php?curid=11923365.

9.3.7. Asbestos

In the past, asbestos was frequently used in construction, shipbuilding, automobile brake linings, insulation, and other industries, which led to widespread contamination of public spaces like homes, schools, and buildings. Billions of tons of asbestos were applied to building sites and added to consumer goods prior to the United States restricting its use in the 1980s. The mineral is no longer as widely used in consumer goods as it formerly was, even though a court ruling in 1991 approved its numerous applications.

Classic epidemiologic studies determined that asbestos exposure was associated with asbestosis, malignant mesothelioma, and lung cancer. The research of Selikoff stands out as a pioneering effort to explore the epidemiology of asbestos-related health effects. Selikoff et al. reported unexpectedly high death rates due to cancer of the lung or pleura; mesothelioma; and cancer of the stomach, colon, or rectum among building trade insulation workers who had relatively light exposure to asbestos.

9.3.8. Metallic Compounds

Metallic compounds that pose an environmental hazard include aluminum, arsenic, antimony, beryllium, cadmium, chromium, lead, mercury, nickel, and tin. This section highlights three of these: arsenic, mercury, and lead.

9.3.8.1. Arsenic

When arsenic is pure, it is a crystalline metalloid, which is an element that can combine with other substances and has characteristics halfway between those of a metal and a nonmetal. For instance, arsenic can be found in the environment as inorganic compounds made of sulfur, oxygen, or chlorine combined with arsenic. Organic forms of arsenic are created when the element combines with carbon and hydrogen, which are present in plants and animals. Arsenic is a poisonous substance that is found in soils and water and is a byproduct of the refining of gold and other metals. Its toxicity varies depending on its chemical form. Prior to World War II, doctors treated syphilis with Salvarsan, an arsenic-based preparation, until antibiotics became available. Arsenic is currently used in some conventional medicines and leukemia chemotherapy, among other medical applications. Previously, arsenic-based preservatives were used by lumber mills to treat wood; however, on December 31, 2003, this practice was outlawed for dimensional lumber intended for residential use. Arsenic is currently used in semiconductor devices made by high-tech businesses.

Food contamination with arsenic has resulted in numerous documented cases of severe arsenic poisoning. 6,000 people were killed by arsenic-contaminated beer in England in 1900, and thousands more were poisoned by soy sauce and dry milk contaminated with arsenic in Japan in the middle of the 20th century. Certain groups of workers in mining and smelters, as well as agricultural workers who come into contact with pesticides, are particularly vulnerable to arsenic exposure (Figure 9.3).

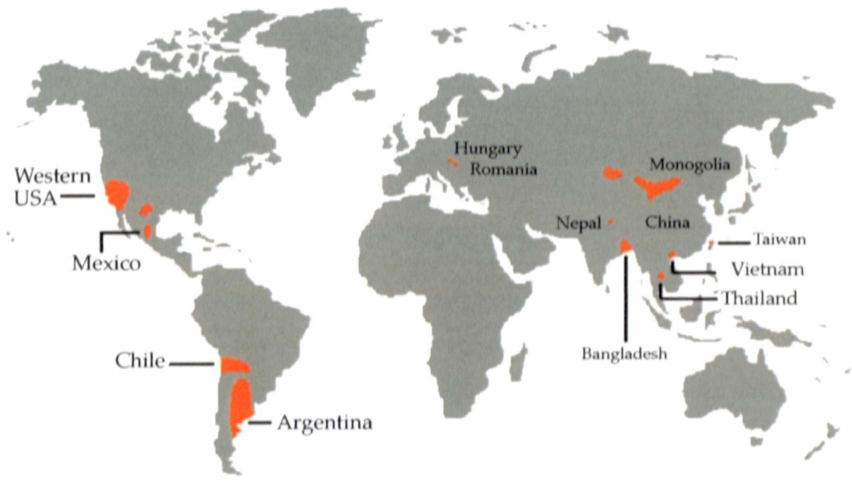

Figure 9.3. *Arsenic contamination.*

Source: By Eishiya – Own work, CC BY-SA 4.0, https://commons.wikimedia.org/w/index.php?curid=65015893.

The body of research indicates that arsenic is carcinogenic. When consumed or inhaled, it can cause skin and lung cancer. It has also been connected to internal cancers, including liver, kidney, and bladder cancers. Areas where drinking water naturally contains high concentrations of naturally occurring arsenic (e.g., Taiwan and Argentina) have higher mortality rates from bladder cancer. It has been documented that there is a dose-response relationship between bladder cancer and drinking water containing inorganic arsenic. Nevertheless, more analytical epidemiologic research would be beneficial in elucidating the relationship, as many of the studies that report this association have used ecologic study designs.

9.3.8.2. Mercury

Mercury is a highly toxic naturally occurring chemical that has been used in dental amalgams, as an agricultural fungicide, and as a medical treatment for syphilis. Around 3,000 cases of neurologic disease were reported in Minamata Bay, Japan, in 1956 as a result of methyl mercury contamination of fish. This was an environmental disaster. The neurological disorder, which was later named Minamata disease, was characterized by drowsiness, poor vision, numbness in the extremities, and deafness. It was incurable and frequently resulted in death. The plastics factory's releases of mercury compounds into the bay were identified as the cause. Some local waterways have been contaminated by mercury as a result of past mining operations (e.g., California).

Nowadays, consumers are advised to avoid certain species of ocean fish (e.g., swordfish and canned albacore) that may contain high levels of mercury. Aquatic organisms that live in the ocean and other bodies of water bioaccumulate contaminants such as mercury, pesticides, and PCBs. Subsequently, these contaminants pass up the food chain resulting in concentrations in top predator fish that are much higher than in the water in which they live. As a public health measure, the EPA issues advisories (recommendations) not to eat fish caught in certain U.S. freshwater lakes and rivers. More than 80% of advisories in 2010 were for mercury contamination. The EPA issued mercury advisories for 16.4 million acres of lakes and 1.1 million miles of rivers during 2010 (Figure 9.4).

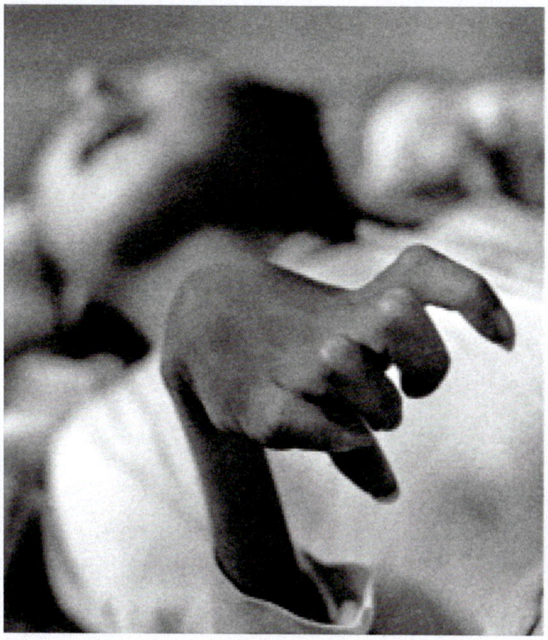

Figure 9.4. *The hand of Tomoko Kamimura, who had Minamata disease.*

Source: Fair use, https://en.wikipedia.org/w/index.php?curid=20131705.

9.3.9. Electric and Magnetic Fields

Nonionizing radiation is a term used to describe energy forms such as electric and magnetic fields. High-voltage electric lines, microwaves, stoves, clocks, electric blankets, toasters, and cell phones are a few examples of devices that produce electric and magnetic fields. Childhood cancers and residential proximity to high-tension wires have been linked, according to epidemiologic research. London and others carried out a case-control study examining the relationship between measured magnetic or electric fields, wiring configuration, and childhood leukemia risk in Los Angeles (e.g., facilities for the overhead transmission and distribution of electricity). They found a correlation between the wiring arrangement and the risk of childhood leukemia, but not between the measured magnetic and electric fields. A second case-control study looked into all Swedish residents under 16 who had resided on land 300 meters away from high-tension power lines over a 25-year period. The Swedish Cancer Registry yielded a total of 142 cancer cases, including 33 cases of central nervous system tumors and 39 cases of leukemia. Historical magnetic field exposure models were employed. Higher levels of magnetic field exposure were associated with an increased estimated relative risk of childhood leukemia. Additional studies did not discover any conclusive link between power lines and childhood leukemia. In relation to additional cancer-causing consequences of electromagnetic radiation exposure, studies carried out in the U.S and Norway revealed a higher chance of male breast cancer—a rare form of the disease—among male electricians who might be exposed to electromagnetic fields (Figure 9.5).

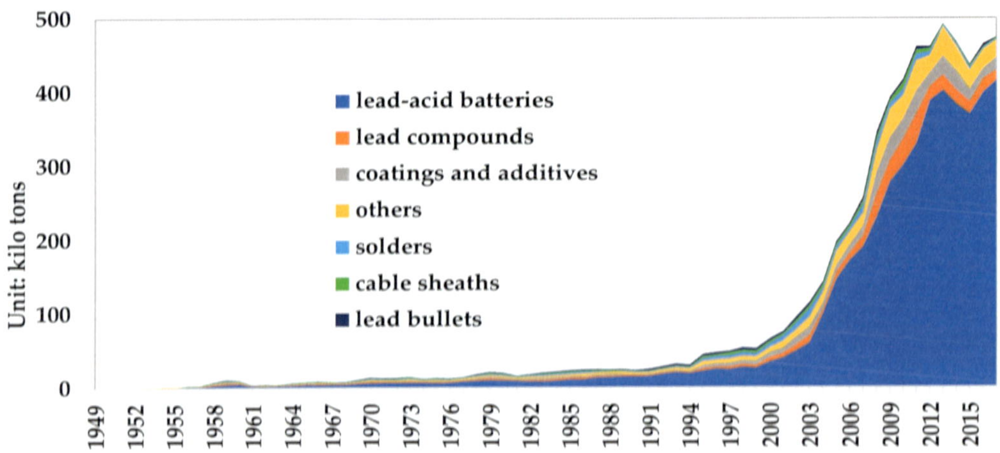

Figure 9.5. *Consumption structure of refined lead from 1949 to 2017. (Data source: China Nonferrous Industry Association; Beijing Antaike Information Co., Ltd.).*

Source: Yang J, Li X, Xiong Z, Wang M, Liu Q. Environmental pollution effect analysis of lead compounds in China based on life cycle. International Journal of Environmental Research and Public Health. 2020; 17(7):2184. https://doi.org/10.3390/ijerph17072184.

Despite its many methodological difficulties, the field of epidemiologic inquiry offers a wealth of opportunities to address a significant public policy issue. The accurate assessment of electromagnetic radiation exposure in homes and other settings is one of the methodologic concerns. It is debatable whether electromagnetic fields are linked to conditions like depression, heart disease, suicide, or breast cancer. Given the growing prevalence of cell phones, some researchers have looked into the connection between radiofrequency field exposure and cancer, specifically brain tumors. Despite worries about the potential for cell phone use to cause cancer, one of the main health effects of using them appears to be car accidents brought on by careless drivers who do not pay attention to the road while using a phone.

9.3.9.1. Ionizing Radiation

Ionizing radiation, a more intense form of energy than nonionizing radiation, consists of either particle energy (e.g., highly energetic protons, neutrons, and α and β particles) or electromagnetic energy (e.g., γ-rays and X-rays). U.S. radiation sources comprise two main categories: natural radiation, which is responsible for the majority of the annual radiation exposure of the human population, and synthetic radiation. Natural radiation consists of radon, cosmic rays from outer space, and radiation from geologic sources. Synthetic sources are medical X-rays and agents used in nuclear medicine, consumer products, nuclear generators, and nuclear weapons explosions.

Examples of topics in the field of ionizing radiation of interest to epidemiologists are:

- Health effects associated with ionizing radiation from nuclear facilities and disposal of nuclear waste.
- Long-term consequences of exposure to radiation from nuclear weapons detonated as part of aboveground testing or used during warfare. For example, radiation from atomic bombs dropped in Japan was associated with increases in the risk of breast cancer, especially if exposure occurred between the ages of 10 and 19 years.
- Intentional exposure of the population to ionizing radiation through terrorists' detonation of dirty bombs. In this scenario, terrorists would use conventional explosives to disperse radioactive materials. Emergency response agencies would need to have a protocol in place to deal with such an act. Although the radiation from a terrorist act would be confined to a limited geographic area, this event would cause panic among the general population.
- Health effects associated with low-level exposures as in the case of patients who receive X-rays and diagnostic nuclear medicine tests. The dose of radiation received from medical tests is generally low and carries more benefits than risks. Nevertheless, the possibility for adverse health effects exists.
- Adverse impacts of occupational exposure to ionizing radiation. Important epidemiologic research questions include the effects of occupational exposure upon pregnant women and health outcomes associated with continuous long-term exposures at low levels.

9.3.10. Allergens and Molds

Allergens are substances that cause allergic reactions in people who are susceptible to them. They can be found in the environment and in the ambient air. People can exhibit a wide range of sensitivity and responses if they are susceptible. The allergenic stimulus could be fur, pollen, or any of a wide range of other environmental materials. From dermatitis, asthma, itchy eyes, and other uncomfortable sensations to anaphylactic shock, allergic reactions can cause a variety of symptoms.

Mold is ubiquitous in the environment and thrives in moist conditions. Molds can cause health effects in sensitive people, such as respiratory system irritation, which can manifest as coughing and wheezing. Some people who are allergic to mold may experience more severe symptoms. Patients with weakened immune systems may experience life-threatening lung infections. Other major health effects, such as infantile memory loss and pulmonary hemorrhage, have not been proven, despite being mentioned in some research.

Robert Friis once looked into a community outbreak of respiratory disease symptoms while working for the local health department. The symptoms were thought to be caused by an allergy to molds that were growing in a specific housing tract. Upon visiting the area, it became evident that many of the opulent homes had tastefully designed sunken living rooms. The sunken areas flooded following heavy rains, staying permanently saturated with water. On the surrounding walls and carpets, multicolored molds proliferated and resisted removal efforts. A few of the inmates started to lament the rise in colds, respiratory ailments, and allergy symptoms. However, serologic testing and questionnaire studies conducted by the health department did not show any rise in illness or symptoms beyond what would be typically expected. Researchers came to the conclusion that, in this case, there was no statistically significant link between lung diseases and other conditions they looked at and mold exposure.

9.4. Limitations and Deficiencies of Environmental Epidemiology

The following three factors are essential for a successful epidemiologic investigation of environmental exposures: (1) direct and accurate estimates of the exposures that each study population member has received; (2) accurate and direct assessment of each member's disease status; and (3) appropriate statistical summarization and analysis of each individual data pertaining to exposure and disease. Limitations are added to epidemiologic studies to the extent that these requirements are not fulfilled. Long latency periods and rare occurrences, which are features of many diseases linked to environmental exposure, are additional limiting factors (Table 9.2).

Table 9.2. Actions Triggered by the Notification of a Suspected Mpox Case

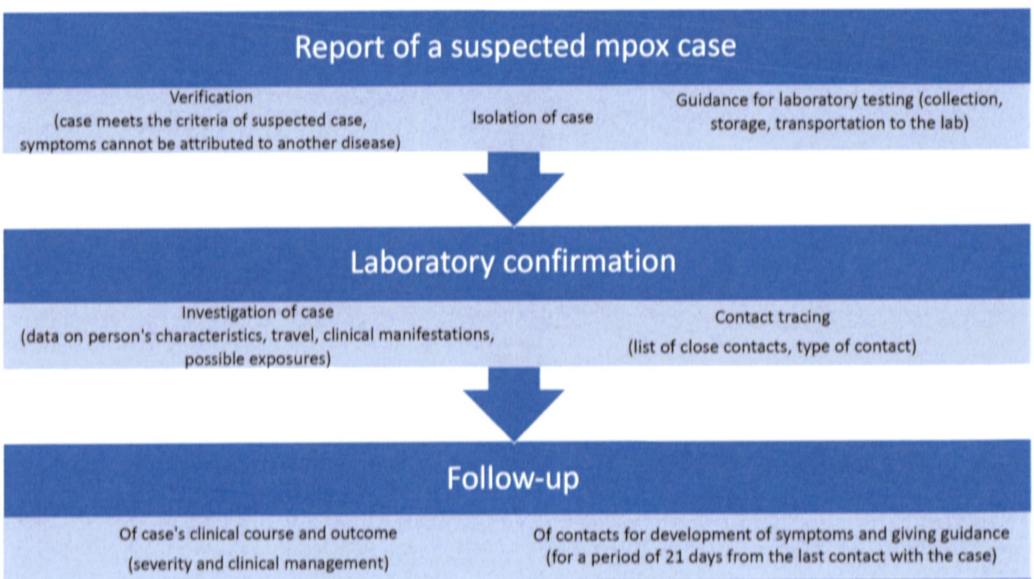

Source: Mellou K, Tryfinopoulou K, Pappa S, Gkolfinopoulou K, Papanikou S, Papadopoulou G, Vassou E, Kostaki E-G, Papadima K, Mouratidou E, et al. Overview of mpox outbreak in Greece in 2022–2023: Is it over? Viruses. 2023; 15(6):1384. https://doi.org/10.3390/v15061384.

9.4.1. Long Latency Periods

One factor that restricts the capacity to draw conclusions about causality from epidemiologic research is the long latency period phenomenon. The latency period is the amount of time that passes between first coming into contact with an agent that causes disease (e.g., exposure to environmental risks, and the onset of an illness or its symptoms in the host.

It should be noted that depending on the measure employed, such as screening tests and observation of clinical signs and symptoms, the occurrence of disease can be conceptualized in a variety of ways. Diseases that are caused by the environment, like cancer, can take years to manifest. The ability of the epidemiologist to conclusively determine the effects of exposure is diminished by these protracted latency periods. Asbestos-related illnesses are among the examples; these frequently don't show symptoms for years after first exposure.

9.4.2. Low Incidence and Prevalence

The rarity of some diseases, which are the focus of environmental epidemiologic studies, is another research constraint. One instance is the prevalence of cancer in children, which has been studied in connection to environmental variables like hazardous chemicals.

Just one-twentieth of adult incidence of cancers occurs in children, with rates for white males and females aged 0 to 14 years being 143.9 per million and 126.9 per million, respectively, and for white males and females of all ages being 330.4 and 277.0 per 100,000, respectively. One is less able to estimate exposure-disease associations precisely when diseases are uncommon. Additionally, the researcher might be forced to use less potent research designs, like case-control and descriptive studies.

9.4.3. Difficulties in Exposure Assessment

Several authorities have stressed the requirement for accurate assessment of exposures in epidemiologic studies of environmental health. Rothman points out that "Atop the list of methodologic problems is the problem of exposure assessment, a problem that extends through all of epidemiologic research but is a towering obstacle in environmental epidemiology." Gardner points out that "Epidemiological methods of investigation are incomplete without good quality exposure data to parallel information on health. The need for monitoring environmental and biological exposure is paramount to the successful interpretation of results and implementation of any required preventive programs."

Causation is evident for high exposure levels to toxic agents that result in distinct and noticeable effects right away. Two such incidents are the 1986 Chernobyl nuclear reactor disaster in the former Soviet Union and the 1984 release of toxic gases in Bhopal, India. Furthermore, the focus of current research has changed, despite the fact that previous generations of studies led to the control of intense environmental exposures that were strongly correlated with disease outcomes. Current research looks at low exposure levels that might be linked to low risk levels.

Epidemiologic researchers face challenges when dealing with low-level environmental exposures because they find it difficult to apply standard laboratory methods used to determine exposure levels. As a result, scientists are unable to conclusively determine whether exposure to a specific agent has occurred. Not only can multiple exposures be mixed in the ambient environment, but exposure levels can also be erratic. The following are some examples of exposure measurements used in environmental epidemiology: ozone readings in the community, samples of toxic fumes from manufacturing plants, and housing tract distances from high-tension power lines that emit electromagnetic radiation. Because they are all indirect measures of exposure and don't give specific information about how much exposure a person may actually receive, all of these measurements are prone to error. As mentioned, using proxies—which are stand-ins for direct measurements—is a popular technique for approximating exposure. The previously mentioned separation between a housing tract and the source of an environmental hazard is an illustration of such a metric. These surrogate or proxy measures are typically too nebulous to provide a definitive estimate of exposure.

9.4.4. Nonspecific Effects

A specific health outcome is one that is typically linked to a single, specific exposure. An outcome that lacks specificity may have multiple correlations with varying degrees of environmental exposure. Numerous factors influence most diseases and conditions that are believed to be linked to exposure to the environment. As a result, it is unlikely that any specific environmental exposure will be linked to a particular result. Our exposure to hundreds of chemicals in the environment makes determining our level of exposure even more difficult. These chemicals are frequently combined, making it difficult to determine how much exposure occurred. Any of these chemical exposures may result in outcomes that are comparable to one another.

9.5. Occupational Health and Safety

The highest level of social, mental, and physical wellbeing among employees across all professions is known as occupational health. It is the area of medicine that addresses every facet of occupational health and safety. It places a lot of emphasis on primary level hazard prevention. In essence, occupational health is seen as preventive medicine. Concerns about welfare, safety, and health at work are referred to as occupational health. The overall goal of occupational health and safety (OHS) laws, standards, and programs is to improve working conditions for employees, coworkers, families, clients, and other stakeholders. Better business practices, a stronger brand, high morale, and employee peace of mind are all guaranteed by the improved occupational health and safety regulations.

Addressing a variety of workplace hazards, such as chemical, physical, biological, and psychosocial ones as well as ergonomic problems and accidents, is the focus of occupational health and safety. The purpose of the occupational health and safety standards is to require that jobsite hazards be eliminated, reduced, or replaced. Programs for occupational health and safety should also incorporate resources that lessen the impact of potential risks. Encouraging a safe and healthy work environment is the aim of the occupational health and safety program. In addition, OSH aims to safeguard members of the general public who might be impacted by exposure to work-related substances or by the work environment itself.

The World Health Organization states that occupational health encompasses all aspects of worker health and safety, with a particular emphasis on the primary prevention of hazards. A state of total physical, mental, and social well-being has been described as health; it is not just the absence of illness or disability. The goal of occupational health, a multidisciplinary area of medicine, is to enable people to perform their jobs in a way that poses the least risk to their health. The three main goals of occupational health are as follows: first, it preserves and enhances workers' health and ability to work; second, it improves the workplace to make it safer and healthier; and third, it fosters the growth of workplace cultures that support workers' health and safety at work, as well as a positive social climate, smooth operations, and potential increase in productivity.

Encouraging and maintaining the highest level of physical, mental, and social wellbeing for every employee in every organization is the primary goal of occupational health and safety. The protection of employees in their employment from risks resulting from factors adverse to their health, and the prevention of workers leaving due to health issues caused by their working conditions the establishment and upkeep of a work environment tailored to each employee's individual physiological and psychological needs. Modernization and industrialization have a background impact on the public health of the entire population through environmental hazards. The personal health of individuals, particularly those of those who work in industrial settings where they are exposed to workplace hazards, is also directly and frequently negatively impacted. Accidents and injuries at work have a significant impact on society's general health. Even so, some professions continue to be extremely risky because of aspects of the workplace itself, a lack of tools and technology, or a lack of suitable regulations and worker protection.

Personal injury and trauma may rekindle interest in occupational health as a public health concern given the recent focus on public health research and policies. Depending on the size of the organization, different healthcare plans will offer different levels of occupational health and safety. It can be given by a part-time physician with training in occupational health and nursing, or by a variety of specialists such as occupational therapists, physiotherapists, hygienists, and experts in ergonomics. In addition to supporting health promotion and education initiatives, the occupational health service may collaborate with your employer to implement policies and guarantee compliance with health and safety regulations.

9.5.1. Types of Occupational Health Issues

Occupational health issues cover a broad spectrum of conditions that affect individuals in the workplace. These issues can manifest physically, mentally, and socially, impacting the overall well-being of workers. Understanding and addressing these concerns is crucial for creating a safe and healthy work environment. In this comprehensive exploration, we'll delve into various types of occupational health issues, categorizing them based on their nature and impact.

1. Physical Injuries:

i. **Musculoskeletal Disorders (MSDs):** Musculoskeletal disorders are prevalent occupational health issues characterized by pain, inflammation, or damage to the muscles, joints, tendons, ligaments, and other components of the musculoskeletal system. Common examples include carpal tunnel syndrome, tendonitis, and lower back pain. These conditions often result from repetitive movements, awkward postures, or overexertion in the workplace.

ii. **Accidents and Trauma:** Workplace accidents can lead to traumatic injuries. These incidents may involve slips, trips, falls, machinery malfunctions, or collisions. The consequences range from minor cuts and bruises to severe injuries, impacting physical health and well-being.

2. Respiratory Issues

i. **Occupational Asthma:** Asthma triggered or exacerbated by exposure to workplace allergens such as dust, fumes, or chemicals is known as occupational asthma. Workers in industries like manufacturing, agriculture, or healthcare may be at risk. Symptoms include wheezing, shortness of breath, and chest tightness.

ii. **Occupational Lung Diseases:** Inhaling specific particles or substances at work can lead to various occupational lung diseases. Examples include pneumoconiosis (e.g., coal worker's pneumoconiosis), caused by prolonged exposure to coal dust, and asbestosis, resulting from asbestos exposure.

3. Chemical and Biological Exposures:

i. **Chemical Exposures:** Exposure to hazardous chemicals in the workplace can result in a range of health issues. Chemical substances may cause skin irritation, respiratory problems, or long-term health effects. Employees in industries such as manufacturing, construction, or laboratories are particularly vulnerable.

ii. **Biological Exposures:** Some workplaces involve exposure to biological agents like bacteria, viruses, fungi, or other microorganisms. Healthcare workers, laboratory technicians, and those in agricultural settings may face the risk of infections or allergic reactions due to biological exposure.

4. Psychosocial and Mental Health Issues

i. **Work-Related Stress:** High levels of stress in the workplace can have detrimental effects on mental health. Factors such as excessive workload, tight deadlines, or a hostile work environment contribute to work-related stress. Long-term stress can lead to burnout and impact both mental and physical well-being.

ii. **Depression and Anxiety:** Chronic workplace stress, coupled with other factors such as job insecurity or interpersonal conflicts, may contribute to the development of depression and anxiety among employees. Addressing these mental health issues is crucial for promoting overall well-being.

iii. **Burnout:** Burnout is a state of chronic workplace stress that results in physical and emotional exhaustion. It often stems from prolonged periods of high stress, unrealistic expectations, or a lack of support. Burnout can negatively impact job performance, personal relationships, and mental health.

5. Noise-Related Issues

i. **Noise-Induced Hearing Loss:** Prolonged exposure to high levels of noise in the workplace can lead to permanent hearing damage. Industries such as manufacturing, construction, and aviation pose a higher risk of noise-induced hearing loss. Protective measures such as earplugs or noise-canceling headphones are essential in mitigating this risk.

6. Ergonomic Issues

i. **Repetitive Strain Injuries (RSIs):** Repetitive strain injuries result from repetitive motions or sustained awkward postures. Common in office settings, manufacturing, and assembly lines, RSIs can lead to pain, inflammation, and functional impairments. Proper ergonomics and regular breaks can help prevent these injuries.

ii. **Poor Ergonomics:** Inadequate workplace design and ergonomics can contribute to discomfort, musculoskeletal issues, and reduced productivity. Addressing ergonomic concerns involves designing workstations that support proper body mechanics and providing ergonomic tools and furniture.

7. Occupational Dermatitis

i. **Contact Dermatitis:** Occupational dermatitis is inflammation of the skin caused by contact with irritants or allergens in the workplace. Common culprits include chemicals, solvents, or certain plants. Individuals in healthcare, manufacturing, and cleaning professions are at higher risk.

8. Occupational Infectious Diseases

i. **Healthcare-Associated Infections:** Healthcare workers face the risk of acquiring infections in the workplace due to close contact with patients, contaminated surfaces, and exposure to bodily fluids. Infections such as MRSA or influenza can pose a significant threat to healthcare professionals.

ii. **Zoonotic Diseases:** Workers in industries involving close contact with animals, such as agriculture or veterinary services, may be at risk of contracting zoonotic diseases. These illnesses can transfer from animals to humans and include conditions like brucellosis or Q fever.

9. Radiation Exposure

i. **Ionizing Radiation:** Workers in industries like nuclear power, radiology, or certain research settings may be exposed to ionizing radiation. Prolonged exposure can lead to adverse health effects, including an increased risk of cancer. Strict safety measures and protective equipment are essential to mitigate this risk.

10. Workplace Violence

i. **Physical Assault or Threats:** Workplace violence can manifest as physical assault, threats, or harassment. Employees may face violence from clients, colleagues, or other individuals in the workplace. Workplace violence prevention programs, security measures, and employee training are crucial for maintaining a safe environment.

9.5.2. Prevention of Occupational Diseases

Prevention of occupational diseases in general may be discussed under the following five headings as per the classical approach of preventive medicine.

9.5.2.1. Health Promotion

Like any other segment of population, workers in different occupations should have positive health. Measures recommended are as follows.

- Pre-employment or preplacement examination, both medical and general, for adapting the job to the worker and the worker to the job. The worker should be assigned the job in which he fits. If he gets job satisfaction, he will give better output and will keep fit physically and mentally. Thus a man with potential hernia should not be assigned the job of weight lifting and a person with color blindness or poor vision should not be employed as a driver.
- Carrying out periodic health checkup and giving advice on nutrition, oral hygiene, rest and recreation.
- Promotion of mental health: Workers' problems at home or at the job should be studied and solved. Otherwise, they may develop emotional difficulties which may reduce work output and may make the worker prone to

accidents.

- Health education: Each worker should be educated in healthy habits such as washing and cleaning and should be educated to avoid hazards attached to his job.
- Provision of healthy physical environment is important. This includes good lighting and ventilation, effective temperature, washing and toilet facilities, and cleanliness at place of work.
- Provision of welfare facilities such as insurance against loss of job, illness and disablement, MCH and family welfare services, creeche, place for having rest, changing clothes and having meals and then first aid.

Recreation grounds and clubs.

- Limiting long hours of work, provision for rest between work periods and liberalization of leave rules.
- Provisions of good housing.

9.5.2.2. Specific Protection

This is done through specific measures which are partly medical in nature but, to a large extent they are related to engineering measures.

- *Medical Measures*
  - Immunization and other specific measures against biological agents such as BCG vaccination against tubercle bacillus, use of shoes against hookworms, etc.
  - Protection of the body against physical agents has already been dealt with. Protection against chemical agents is done by:
  - Protecting skin by suitable clothing, gloves, shoes, barrier cream, etc., and by washing hands and body with soap and water
  - Preventing inhalation by use of face masks
  - Preventing ingestion by not taking food at the place of work, washing hands properly before taking food and rinsing of mouth.
  - § Health education: The worker is educated about the particular occupational risks and about the use of protective measures.
- **Engineering Measures**
  - Designing and construction of work place having enough space, light, ventilation and comfortable temperature.
  - Proper designing, layout, maintenance and regular check of machines. Machines may be encased or enclosed if feasible. They should have minimum projecting parts.
  - Modifications of machines and processes to minimize their hazards.
  - Training and education of workers.
  - Appropriate measures to minimize the production and spread of harmful agents (e.g., local exhaust system for dusts).
  - Cleanliness of work rooms and premises.
  - Research on offensive and hazardous machines, materials and processes.

It should be noted that pollutants such as smoke, wastewater, noise, etc., are produced by all industries. Costly and complex equipment must be installed in order to control pollution. The social costs of pollution, however, are much greater. These include ill health and the resulting decline in life expectancy and productivity, the burden on healthcare systems, building deterioration, land degradation, and the impact on plants and animals that lead to irreversible imbalances. Not only are these expenses unavoidable, but they also exceed the cost of installing pollution control technology.

9.5.3. Early Diagnosis and Treatment

Depending on the type of work, an occupational physician and other members of the team should make up the occupational health team. The group should conduct recurrent surveys, schedule routine physical examinations, look into any occupational illnesses or injuries, and suggest preventative and control strategies. Any illness or injury, whether acute or chronic, that the occupational health team discovers or learns about through other sources needs to be properly and quickly treated. If required, the worker's position might need to be modified.

9.5.4. Disability Limitation

Any employee who has even the slightest degree of disability as a result of an occupational hazard should be placed in a different, suitable job that may not involve that specific hazard right away. Additional targeted actions might also be required.

- **Rehabilitation:** If an employee has been handicapped after injury or illness, he should be given a suitable job to prevent psychological trauma and to ensure his productivity as a worker.

9.6. Special Features of Environmental and Occupational Epidemiology

Epidemiology is used in environmental and occupational fields to establish:

- Etiology
- Natural history
- The health status of a population
- The value of interventions and health services.

The geographic basis of environmental epidemiology is one of its unique characteristics. Pollution of the air, water, and soil is typically linked to sources that have specific geographic locations. Thus, mapping exposures or environmental levels can be a helpful tool in epidemiological research. Individual exposure measurements are very hard to assemble, so approximations and modeling are frequently needed in environmental epidemiology studies to quantify exposures. Numerous studies on the health effects of air pollution have combined air quality modeling with geographic information system (GIS) analysis. The number of days when nitrogen dioxide concentrations surpass various cut-off points and the number of exposed individuals in various city regions based on census data are two examples of exposure assessment.

9.6.1. Setting Safety Standards

In environmental and occupational epidemiology, dose-effect and dose-response relationships are especially significant since they serve as the basis for establishing safety regulations. The relationship between dose and effect can be used to determine which effect needs to be prevented most. The dose-response relationship indicates the highest dose that would be considered acceptable once a decision is made regarding an acceptable response level. Using this method, WHO has created a number of guidelines for air and water quality as well as health-based maximum occupational exposure limits. Guidelines for determining the radioactive contamination of food were also developed in response to the nuclear power plant accident at Chernobyl. Since there are often too few data to establish an accurate standard for a given environmental factor, the safety standard is instead based on educated guesses or real-world experience. To provide more details on dose-response relationships, more epidemiological research is required.

9.6.2. Measuring Past Exposure

The utilization of trade union or company records to identify individuals who have previously been exposed to a particular type of work or hazard is a unique characteristic of many etiological studies in occupational epidemiology. Such records can be used to conduct retrospective cohort studies. In this way, a number of correlations between workplace risks and health outcomes have been found.

9.6.3. Healthy Worker Effect in Occupational Studies

Studies on occupational epidemiology frequently only include physically fit men. Therefore, compared to the corresponding age group in the general population, the exposed group of workers has a lower overall mortality rate. When comparing the mortality rate of a group of workers to the general population, it is important to consider the healthy worker effect, which refers to the lower mortality. Typically, rates among healthy workers range from 70% to 90% of the overall population. The presence of sick and disabled individuals in the non-working population, who typically have higher death rates, accounts for the discrepancy.

A Closer Look

Studies in Environmental Epidemiology

Studies in environmental epidemiology investigate the complex relationship between environmental exposures and health outcomes within populations, aiming to identify environmental risk factors, quantify their impact on health, and inform strategies for disease prevention and environmental health protection. These studies utilize epidemiological methods to examine the distribution of diseases associated with environmental exposures, assess exposure-response relationships, and evaluate the effectiveness of interventions to mitigate environmental health risks.

2016 EPI: Environmental Health Objective

Environmental Performance Index (EPI)

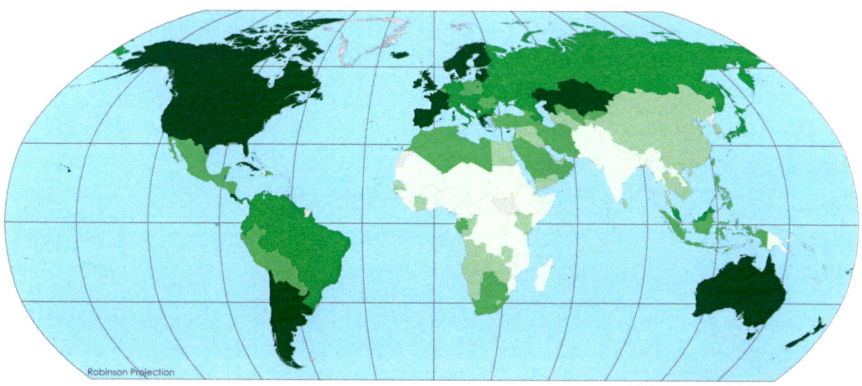

The 2016 EPI builds on measures relevant to the goal of reducing environmental stresses to human health, which are grouped into one policy objective named environmental health. Environmental health scores are based on three constituent policy categories: health impacts, air quality, and water and sanitation. All indicators and composite indices in the EPI are normalized as a 0–100 proximity-to-target score, with 100 representing "at target" and 0 being furthest from the target.

Environmental Health Scores
- 25.11–54.47
- 54.48–71.61
- 71.62–81.19
- 81.20–88.32
- 88.33–98.71
- no EPI score

One key focus of environmental epidemiology is investigating the health effects of air pollution, including particulate matter, ozone, nitrogen dioxide, sulfur dioxide, and other pollutants emitted from industrial activities, transportation, and other sources. Epidemiological studies have linked air pollution exposure to a wide range of adverse health outcomes, including respiratory diseases, cardiovascular diseases, cancer, and adverse birth outcomes. By assessing the health impact of air pollution and identifying vulnerable populations, environmental epidemiologists inform air quality standards, regulatory policies, and public health interventions aimed at reducing pollution levels and protecting public health.

Moreover, environmental epidemiology examines the health effects of water and soil contamination, hazardous waste sites, industrial chemicals, pesticides, and other environmental contaminants. Epidemiological studies have identified associations between exposure to environmental toxins and various health outcomes, including neurological disorders, developmental disabilities, reproductive disorders, and cancer. By evaluating exposure pathways, biomarkers of exposure, and health outcomes, environmental epidemiologists contribute to the development of risk assessment methodologies, environmental monitoring programs, and policies to prevent exposure to harmful contaminants and mitigate their health effects.

Additionally, environmental epidemiology investigates the health impacts of climate change, including extreme weather events, heatwaves, floods, droughts, and changes in temperature and precipitation patterns. Epidemiological studies have demonstrated associations between climate-related factors and a wide range of health outcomes, including heat-related illnesses, vector-borne diseases, food and waterborne diseases, and mental health disorders. By assessing the health risks associated with climate change and identifying vulnerable populations, environmental epidemiologists inform adaptation strategies, public health preparedness efforts, and policies to address climate-related health threats.

Environmental epidemiology plays a critical role in understanding the cumulative effects of multiple environmental exposures and the interaction between environmental and social determinants of health. Epidemiological studies examine the combined impact of air pollution, water contamination, socioeconomic deprivation, and other factors on health outcomes, highlighting the importance of addressing multiple determinants of health to reduce health disparities and promote health equity. By integrating epidemiological evidence with social, behavioral, and environmental data, environmental epidemiologists contribute to the development of comprehensive strategies for environmental health protection and disease prevention.

Summary

- Environmental and occupational epidemiology are specialized branches that focus on understanding how environmental and workplace exposures influence human health. These fields play critical roles in identifying and mitigating health risks associated with environmental pollutants, hazardous substances, and occupational hazards.
- Environmental epidemiology investigates how exposure to environmental factors such as air and water pollutants, hazardous chemicals, radiation, and climate change impacts human health.
- Epidemiologists in this field study populations exposed to specific environmental hazards to assess their health outcomes. They employ various study designs, including cohort studies and case-control studies, to identify associations between environmental exposures and diseases such as respiratory disorders, cancers, neurological conditions, and reproductive issues.
- Occupational epidemiology focuses on assessing health risks associated with workplace exposures, occupational hazards, and work-related practices. This field examines how factors like exposure to chemicals, physical hazards (e.g., noise, vibration), biological agents (e.g., viruses, bacteria), ergonomic conditions, and psychosocial stressors affect the health of workers.
- The term descriptive epidemiology refers to the depiction of the occurrence of disease in populations according to classification by person, place, and time variables. Examples of person variables are demographic characteristics such as sex, age, and race/ethnicity. Place variables denote geographic locations including a specific country or countries, areas within countries, and places where localized patterns of disease may occur.
- Environmental and occupational epidemiology often intersect, as many environmental exposures can originate from workplace activities or industrial processes. Both fields face challenges such as identifying low-level exposures' health effects, assessing cumulative risks from multiple exposures, addressing disparities in exposure burdens among different socioeconomic groups, and anticipating health impacts from emerging environmental and occupational hazards. Advances in exposure assessment techniques, biomonitoring, and data analytics are crucial for overcoming these challenges and improving risk assessment accuracy.

References

1. Bohlin, N. I. (1967). A statistical analysis of 28,000 accident cases with emphasis on occupant restraint value. *SAE Transactions, 76*, 2981–2994.
2. Canfield, R. L., Henderson, C. R., Cory-Slechta, D. A., Cox, C., Jusko, T. A., & Lanphear, B. P. (2003). Intellectual impairment in children with blood lead concentrations below 100 μg/L. *New England Journal of Medicine, 348*, 1517–1526.
3. Dora, C., & Racioppi, F. (2003). Including health in transport policy agendas: The role of health impact assessment analyses and procedures in the European experience. *Bulletin of the World Health Organization, 81*, 399–403.

4. Kjellström, T., Lodh, M., McMichael, T., et al. (2006). Air and water pollution; burden and strategies for control. In D. T. Jamison, J. G. Breman, A. R. Measham, G. Alleyne, M. Claeson, D. B. Evans, et al. (Eds.), *Disease Control Priorities in Developing Countries* (pp. 817–832). New York: Oxford University Press.
5. Künzli, N., Kaiser, R., Medina, S., Studnicka, M., Chanel, O., Filliger, P., et al. (2000). Public health impact of outdoor and traffic-related air pollution: A European assessment. *Lancet, 356*, 795–801.
6. Meyer, P. A., Pivetz, T., Dignam, T. A., Homa, D. M., Schoonover, J., & Brody, D. (2003). Surveillance for elevated blood lead levels among children in the United States, 1997–2001. *MMWR Surveillance Summaries, 52*, 1–21.
7. Scoggins, A., Kjellstrom, T., Fisher, G., Connor, J., & Gimson, N. (2004). Spatial analysis of annual air pollution exposure and mortality. *Science of the Total Environment, 321*, 71–85.
8. Smith, K. R., Corvalán, C. F., & Kjellstrom, T. (1999). How much ill health is attributable to environmental factors? *Epidemiology, 10*, 573–584.
9. Sunyer, J., & Grimalt, T. (2006). Global climate change, widening health inequalities and epidemics. *International Journal of Epidemiology, 35*, 213–216.

Chapter

EPIDEMIOLOGY TO EVALUATION AND POLICY

10

Contents

Introduction

Epidemiology is the cornerstone of public health, serving as the scientific discipline that investigates the patterns, causes, and effects of health and disease within populations. It encompasses a broad range of methodologies to understand the distribution and determinants of health-related states or events, allowing for the development of effective strategies for disease prevention and health promotion. Epidemiologists employ various study designs, including observational studies and clinical trials, to explore the relationships between exposures (such as environmental factors, behaviors, and genetics) and outcomes (such as diseases or health conditions) in populations.

Once epidemiological evidence is gathered, evaluated, and analyzed, it serves as the basis for informing public health policy and practice. Evaluation is a crucial step in this process, involving the assessment of interventions, programs, and policies to determine their effectiveness, efficiency, and impact on public health outcomes. Through rigorous evaluation, policymakers and public health practitioners can identify successful strategies, modify approaches as needed, and allocate resources efficiently to address the most pressing health challenges facing communities.

Policy development in public health relies heavily on epidemiological evidence and evaluation findings to guide decision-making processes. Epidemiologists play a vital role in translating research findings into actionable policy recommendations by synthesizing complex data, identifying emerging health threats, and advocating for evidence-based interventions. By collaborating with policymakers, community stakeholders, and other relevant partners, epidemiologists contribute to the development of policies that promote population health and address disparities, ultimately improving the well-being of individuals and communities worldwide.

Orientation and Directional Terms

Term	Definition	Illustration
Etiological Epidemiology	Etiological epidemiology is a discipline that studies the causal factors of disease. For ethical and logistical reasons, most etiological studies are observational case/control studies or exposed/non-exposed cohorts.	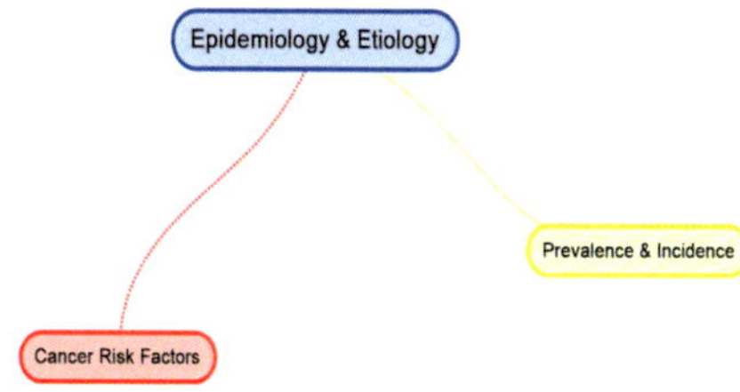
Health Services	Health services consist of medical professionals, organizations, and ancillary healthcare workers who provide medical care to those in need.	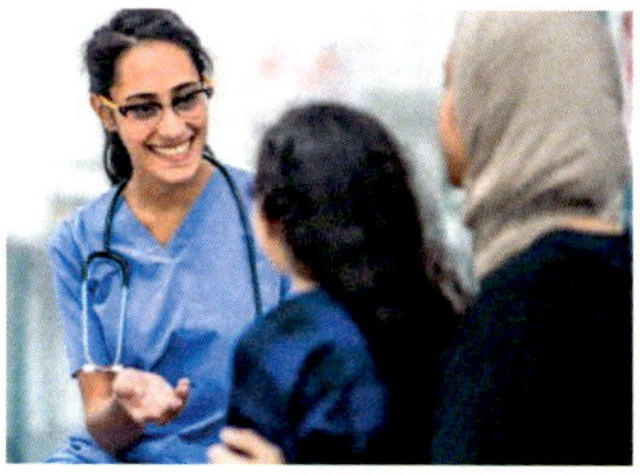
Medicare	Medicare is a federal health insurance program in the United States that primarily provides coverage for people aged 65 and older, as well as for certain younger individuals with disabilities and people with end-stage renal disease (ESRD).	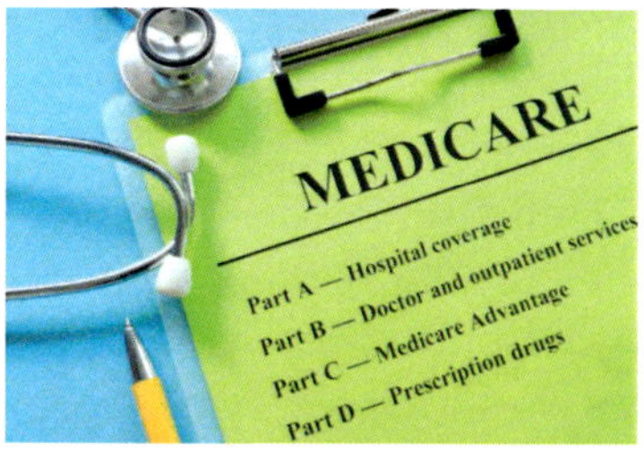
Prenatal Care	Prenatal care is when you get checkups from a doctor, nurse, or midwife throughout your pregnancy. It helps keep you and your future baby healthy.	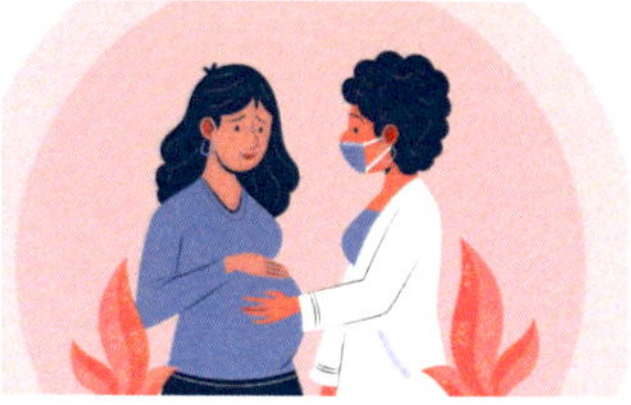
Health Indicators	Health indicators are quantifiable characteristics of a population that researchers use as supporting evidence for describing the health of a population.	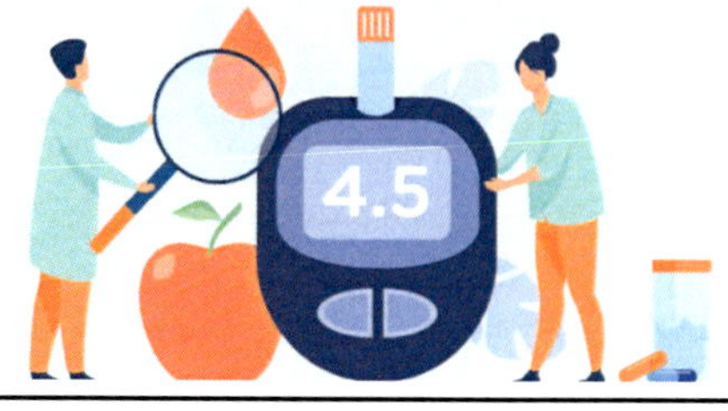

10.1. Using Epidemiology to Evaluate Health Services

Applying epidemiological concepts and techniques to evaluate the efficacy, accessibility, quality, and efficiency of healthcare delivery systems is known as "using epidemiology to evaluate health services."

10.1.1. Studies of Process and Outcome

- **Studies of Process:** First, it's important to understand the differences between process and outcome studies. Process implies that we make decisions about what makes for quality care. Usually, a panel of experts makes this kind of decision. After that, we can evaluate a clinic or healthcare provider by looking over pertinent documents or by making in-person observations to ascertain the degree to which the treatment offered satisfies recognized standards. We can ascertain, for instance, what proportion of patients have had their blood pressure checked. The issue with these process measures is that they don't tell you whether the patient is doing better or not. For instance, taking the patient's blood pressure doesn't guarantee that it's within normal range. Second, since process evaluations rely on expert opinion, the standards by which they are conducted may also evolve over time in response to shifts in expert opinion. For instance, in the 1940s, placing premature infants in 100% oxygen was considered the accepted standard of care for them. To ensure that these levels were kept, incubators were observed. However, high oxygen concentrations were later regarded as inappropriate after studies showed that they were a major factor in the development of retrolental fibroplasia, a type of blindness that occurs in infants who were born prematurely.
- **Studies of Outcome:** The term "outcome" refers to how well a patient responds to the treatment they receive. The area of study for epidemiology is health outcomes. While death and morbidity have historically been the primary metrics of interest, patient satisfaction, quality of life, level of dependence and disability, and other comparable measures have become more and more relevant in the last few years due to the growing interest in outcomes research.

10.1.2. Efficacy, Effectiveness, and Efficiency

Three terms that are often encountered in the literature dealing with the evaluation of health services are efficacy, effectiveness, and efficiency.

- **Efficacy:** In our ideal "laboratory" setting, where we test new drugs on a cohort of patients who consent to be hospitalized and monitored while receiving therapy, does the agent or intervention "work"? Alternatively, a group of willing subjects is used to test a vaccine. Therefore, efficacy is a metric in a scenario where all variables are managed to optimize the agent's effect.
- **Effectiveness:** Is the agent still effective if we administer it in a "real-life" setting? For instance, in a

community where a vaccine is being tested, a large number of people might not show up to receive the shot. Alternatively, an oral medication may taste so bad that people refuse to take it, rendering it ineffective even though it has been shown to be effective in controlled settings with compliance guaranteed.

- **Efficiency:** If an agent is proven to be effective, what is the cost-benefit ratio? Is there a more cost-effective way to accomplish our objectives? Cost encompasses not only financial costs but also pain, discomfort, disability, absenteeism, and social stigma.

If a healthcare measure has not been demonstrated to be effective, there is little point looking at efficiency, for if it is not effective, the cheapest alternative is not to use it at all. At times, of course, political and societal pressures may drive a program even if it is not effective.

10.1.3. Measures of Outcome

We can move on to assessing effectiveness if a measure's efficacy has been established, or if the relevant preventative and intervention strategies have been proven to be successful. First and foremost, the measure needs to be clearly quantifiable, meaning that its effect can be expressed in quantitative terms. These are the guidelines that should guide us in choosing an appropriate outcome measure to serve as an index of effectiveness. Second, it should be reasonably simple to define and diagnose the outcome measure. It would be unwise to rely on an invasive procedure to determine any benefits if the measure was to be used in a population study. Third, the measure that is chosen needs to be standardized for research purposes. Fourth, the condition for which an intervention is being evaluated must be one that the population being served (as well as the comparison population) is at risk. To test the efficacy of a sickle cell screening program, for instance, in a white population in North America would be absurd.

Table 10.1. Criteria for Establishing Additional Centrally Managed, State Vaccination Structures

Factors Increasing the Need to Establish Centrally Managed Government Vaccination Structures Beyond Regular Primary Care Infrastructure	
Pandemic conditions (N = 23) *	• Limited availability of vaccines paired with high demand (fair distribution challenges, need for prioritization of select population groups, lack of ability to provide all outpatient practices with vaccines) • Need for tighter control and follow-up (limited knowledge about side-effect profiles of novel vaccines, accuracy of vaccination coverage data, detection of vaccination gaps, evolving virulence, and infection rates, need for security, quality and standardization, cushioning of delivery irregularities) • Political and public pressure (symbolism of activity, need to comply with public and political will, ability to provide information)

Product properties and logistics (N = 15) *	• Complex storage and transport conditions (Galenics/vaccine stability, cold-chain maintenance, complex preparation) • Vial contents (multi-dose vials instead of pre-filled syringes)
Local circumstances and capacities (N = 16) *	• Overstretched resources of regular outpatient healthcare structures • Low local physician density • Weak public health service • Rural vs. urban infrastructure/large distance to closest vaccination site

Source: Danek S, Achelrod D, Wichmann O, Schwendicke F. The Role of vaccination centers in a national mass immunization campaign—policymaker insights from the german covid-19 pandemic vaccine roll-out. Vaccines. 2023; 11(10):1552. https://doi.org/10.3390/vaccines11101552.

The kind of outcome endpoint we choose ought to be contingent upon the question we pose. Even though it might seem obvious, this isn't always the case. A vaccine program's potential endpoints for assessing efficacy are listed in Table 10.1. Any conclusion we decide on should be made clear so that readers of our findings report can form their own opinions about the suitability of the chosen measure and the caliber of the data. Based on the clinical and public health aspects of the disease under consideration, we can determine whether the chosen measure is indeed appropriate.

Table 10.2 lists potential metrics that could be used to evaluate how well a children's throat culture program is working. Since they are generally simple to count and can be used to support requests for program budget increases the following year, metrics such as the volume of services rendered, number of cultures taken, and number of clinic visits have long been preferred.

These measurements, however, are process measurements and do not provide any information regarding the efficacy of an intervention. Thus, we go on to the other options shown in this table. Once more, the answer to a given question should determine the best course of action. A specific question is required. Merely asking about the program's quality is insufficient.

Table 10.2. Collection of Possible Preparedness Measures for the Rapid Establishment of Crisis Response Structures Mentioned by Experts (Not Exhaustive)

Operational Readiness Measures for the Rapid Establishment of Crisis Response Structures	
Processes	• **Evaluate processes** employed during the COVID-19 pandemic • **Create and update** blueprints, checklists and **contingency plans** • **Outline sample process chains and structures**, e.g., clear responsibilities, especially with regard to the demarcation of state governments vs. the federal government, communication chain, registration and documentation • **Create templates** for public tenders and sample models

Locations/ properties	• **Designate adequate locations** and prioritize the order of use • Plan with **more flexible structures** (large structures such as exhibition halls are not absolutely necessary) • **Reserve space within the public health service** (small vaccination centers) • **Cooperate** with the city and municipality council for the selection of properties
Staff	• **Create profile archetypes** with typical qualifications and responsibilities • **Train management staff** (also pre-crisis) • **Train professional preparedness teams** • **Identify potential staffing pools**, e.g., list of retired doctors, event and catering industry, trade shows, hospitality • **Strengthen health skills** of emergency/crisis response teams as well as the general public • **Conduct emergency drills**
Materials/ technology	• **Establish a state material warehouse** for storage of • Universally usable material, e.g., partitions, chairs, tables, sirens, ... • Medical materials, e.g., personal protective equipment, vaccination kits (syringes, needles, ...), vaccines (e.g., smallpox vaccine against a background of monkeypox) • Storage of technical equipment (i.e., computers, tablets, ...) not recommended due to rapidly changing technological standards

Source: Danek S, Achelrod D, Wichmann O, Schwendicke F. The role of vaccination centers in a national mass immunization campaign—policymaker insights from the German COVID-19 pandemic vaccine roll-out. Vaccines. 2023; 11(10):1552. https://doi.org/10.3390/vaccines11101552.

10.1.4. Comparing Epidemiologic Studies of Disease Etiology and Epidemiologic Research Evaluating Effectiveness of Health Services

A potential relationship between a putative cause (the independent variable) and one or more detrimental health effects (the dependent variable) is examined in traditional epidemiologic studies of disease etiology. While doing this, we consider additional variables that could alter or complicate the relationship, such as healthcare. In health services research, the health service is the main variable, and the expected outcome (dependent variable) is the decrease in unfavorable health effects in the event that the treatment modality is successful. Environmental and other factors that could affect the relationship are also considered in this case. Thus, the potential relationship between an independent and dependent variable, as well as the impact of other factors on the relationship, are the subjects of both health services research and etiologic epidemiologic research. It follows that many of the study designs covered in this discussion, along with the methodological issues and potential biases that often accompany these kinds of studies, are shared by epidemiologic and health services research (Figure 10.1).

The New APC Model: 12 Principles

1. APC models produce Estimable Functions that *describe* the data and provide an *explanation*.
2. The New APC Model decomposes the data into **identifiable** functions of age, period, and cohort including six key parameters $\Theta \equiv (\mu, (\alpha_L - \gamma_L), (\pi_L + \gamma_L), \theta_\alpha, \theta_\pi, \theta_\gamma)$ and three sets of higher-order deviations for age, period, and cohort, respectively: $\check{\gamma}_{a_*}, \check{\gamma}_{p_*}$, and $\check{\gamma}_{c_*}$.
3. Net Drift $(\pi_L + \gamma_L)$ – analogue of the *EAPC* – is the single most important APC parameter.
4. Age-specific time trends aka Local Drifts are identifiable:

   $$(\pi_L + \gamma_L)_{a_*} = (\pi_L + \gamma_L) - 2\theta_\gamma(a_* - \bar{a}_*) + \mathcal{S}(L_P^\Delta, C)\mathcal{E}_C\check{\gamma}_{c_*}$$

   $\mathcal{E}_C$ orders the $\check{\gamma}_{c_*}$ from youngest to oldest and $\mathcal{S}(L_P^\Delta, C)$ calculates a sliding slope through P consecutive birth cohorts. Hence, Local Drifts are a **consequence** of birth cohort effects.
5. Net Drift is equal to the average of the Local Drifts:

   $$(\pi_L + \gamma_L) = \sum_{a=1}^{A} (\pi_L + \gamma_L)_{a_*(a)}$$
6. Global Curvature for Cohort θ_γ is the second most important APC parameter.
   - If $\theta_\gamma \neq 0$, then $(\pi_L + \gamma_L)$ **cannot** be equal to the time trend in every age group.
     - *You should always examine Local Drifts.*
7. Global Curvature for Period θ_π is the third most important APC parameter.
8. In the presence of Net Drift, the cross-sectional age curve (CAC), which has an average gradient equal to the CAT $(\alpha_L - \gamma_L)$, does **not** describe the age-associated natural history.
9. The natural history **is** characterized by the longitudinal age curve (LAC), which has an average gradient equal to the LAT $(\alpha_L + \gamma_L) \equiv (\alpha_L - \gamma_L) + (\pi_L + \gamma_L)$.
10. Even if $\theta_\gamma \approx 0$ and $\check{\gamma}_{c_*} \approx 0$, birth cohort effects could be operating through the Net Drift.
11. Even If $\theta_\pi \approx 0$ and $\check{\pi}_{p_*} \approx 0$, period effects could be operating through the Net Drift.
12. Even if the Net Drift $(\pi_L + \gamma_L) = 0$ it is possible that $\pi_L = -\gamma_L$.
    - *You can never rule out calendar period or birth cohort trends.*

Figure 10.1. *The new age-period-cohort model: 12 principles.*

Source: Rosenberg PS and Miranda-Filho A (2024) Advances in statistical methods for cancer surveillance research: an age-period-cohort perspective. Front. Oncol. 13:1332429. doi: 10.3389/fonc.2023.1332429.

10.1.5. Evaluation Using Group Data

Evaluation studies frequently make use of readily available data, such as hospitalization and mortality statistics. These kinds of data can be found in a variety of sources, some of which may differ significantly from one another. For instance, the National Hospital Discharge Survey (NHDS) and the National Health Interview Survey (NHIS) provide data on short-term hospital stay discharge rates in the United States, which are displayed in Figure 10.2.

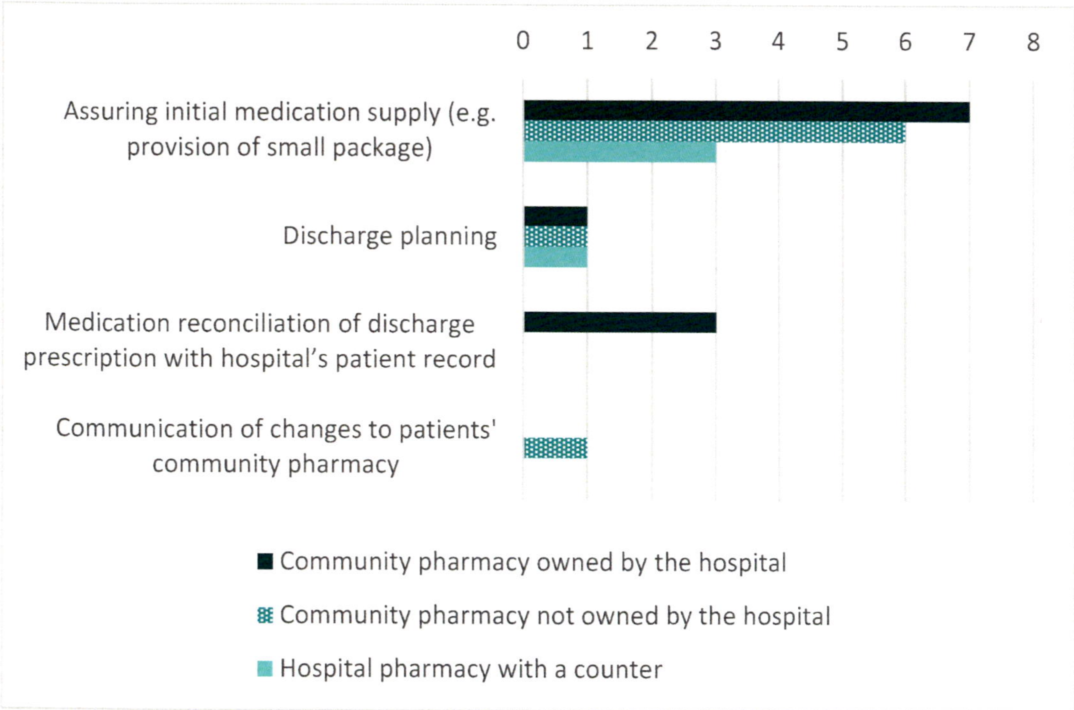

Figure 10.2. *Frequency of predefined roles of the pharmacies that were collaborating with hospitals and that were accessible to patients at hospital discharge.*

Source: Studer H, Boeni F, Hersberger KE, Lampert ML. Pharmaceutical discharge management: implementation in Swiss hospitals compared to international guidelines. Pharmacy. 2021; 9(1):33. https://doi.org/10.3390/pharmacy9010033.

The rates vary in magnitude even though the trends are similar. Hospital records of patients released from short-stay nonfederal hospitals are used by the NHDS. Personal interviews are used by the NHIS, and individuals frequently forget about previous hospital stays. Discharges from federal hospitals—the majority of which are Veterans Administration hospitals—are also included in the NHIS. Both hospitalized and admitted patients pass away; these two categories are excluded from the NHIS and are included in the NHDS. Patients who stay in the hospital for less than a day are counted as discharges under the NHDS, but not the NHIS. The key takeaway is that, in order to evaluate any modality of healthcare, we need to recognize and comprehend the features of each data source that will be consulted, including what or who is excluded or included, what variables are used to collect the data, and how the data are categorized. Next, we evaluate the significance of these attributes and the reliability of the collected data, while also looking into potential biases. The issues might not be crucial if our interest is in trends or changes over time, but they might be significant if our focus is on absolute values.

10.1.5.1. Outcomes Research

The term "outcomes research" has become more widely used in recent years to refer to studies that compare the effects on health or economic outcomes of two or more healthcare interventions or modalities, such as treatments, healthcare organization structures, insurance coverage types and amounts, and provider reimbursement. Morbidity and mortality as well as indicators of functional status, quality of life, and patient perceptions of their health, including symptom recognition and patient satisfaction, may be included in the health endpoints. Economic measures may reflect direct or indirect costs and can include hospitalization rates, outpatient and emergency room visits, lost days of work, child care, and days of restricted activity. Consequently, epidemiology is one of several disciplines needed in outcomes research.

Large data sets that were derived from large populations are frequently used in outcomes research. Many of the data sets used were frequently initially initiated for administrative or fiscal purposes rather than for any research goals, even though in recent years some of the larger data sets have been developed from cohorts that were originally set up for different research purposes. To investigate an interesting question, it is common practice to link multiple sizable data sets, each containing information on a variety of variables. Large data sets have the advantage of referring to real-world populations, which minimizes the problem of "representativeness" or "generalizability." Additionally, analysis can usually be finished and results produced fairly quickly because the data sets are already there when the research is started. Furthermore, except in cases where smaller subgroups are investigated, sample size is usually not an issue due to the large data sets used. Because of these factors, using pre-existing data sets often comes with less expense than collecting new data from scratch.

The data may not be well suited for research purposes and for providing an answer to the particular research question addressed in the study, as they were frequently originally collected for fiscal and administrative reasons. This is one of the study's drawbacks. Even though the data were first collected for research purposes, our understanding of the subject may have expanded since then, and new research questions might have emerged that were not even considered at the time the data were first collected. Generally speaking, data might be lacking. There could be a dearth of information on the independent and dependent variables. Clinical information, such as the severity of the disease and the specifics of the interventions, may be lacking in the data, and there may be discrepancies in the diagnostic coding. Since the research that is currently being done was frequently not even possible when the data were generated, information about potential confounders may be insufficient or nonexistent. Researchers occasionally use variables that are included in the data set but may not accurately reflect the variable of interest to create surrogate variables for the missing variables because some variables that are relevant and significant today were not included in the original data set. The degree to which these surrogate variables accurately represent the important missing variable varies, though. The validity of the conclusions drawn may thus be questioned for all of these reasons. Large data sets can also present another significant issue: the investigator may, consciously or unconsciously, stray from the question he had intended to answer in favor of one that is less interesting to him but for which the variables required to conduct the study are present in the data set because the necessary variables may be absent in the available data set. As a result, the data set might be given the freedom to choose the research questions that are investigated in the study, as opposed to the researcher making this decision. Ultimately, researchers distance themselves from the subjects of their studies by using massive data sets. Large computerized databases have tended to replace in-person interviews and patient record reviews over time. These data sources almost never allow for the exploration of the subjects' many personal traits or the evaluation of their applicability to the questions posed. Prenatal care is one area where evaluation studies frequently draw upon already-existing data sources. The use of birth certificates serves as an example of the issues previously discussed. Due to their accessibility and ability to provide specific medical care information, like the trimester in which prenatal care was started, these records are frequently used. However, compared to birth certificates for women with low-risk pregnancies, those with high-risk pregnancies frequently have missing data. Additionally, there may be regional and global variations in the quality of the data provided on birth certificates, which could impede any attempts at comparison.

A study by Gornick et al. is an illustration of outcomes research with big data sets of Americans who are Medicare beneficiaries. Since almost all elderly people in the United States receive Medicare health coverage, it is assumed that if a study population is restricted to those with Medicare coverage, other variables, such as financial barriers to care, will remain constant across various groups, such as ethnic subpopulations. Nonetheless, there are still significant differences in the use of many Medicare services between Whites and Blacks. The authors looked at how Medicare beneficiaries' use of services and mortality were impacted by their income and race. They did this by combining Medicare administrative data for 26.3 million beneficiaries 65 years of age or older from 1993 with 1990 census data on median income broken down by zip code. They computed black to white ratios and age- and sex-adjusted rates of various diagnoses and procedures based on income and race. They also calculated age-adjusted mortality rates.

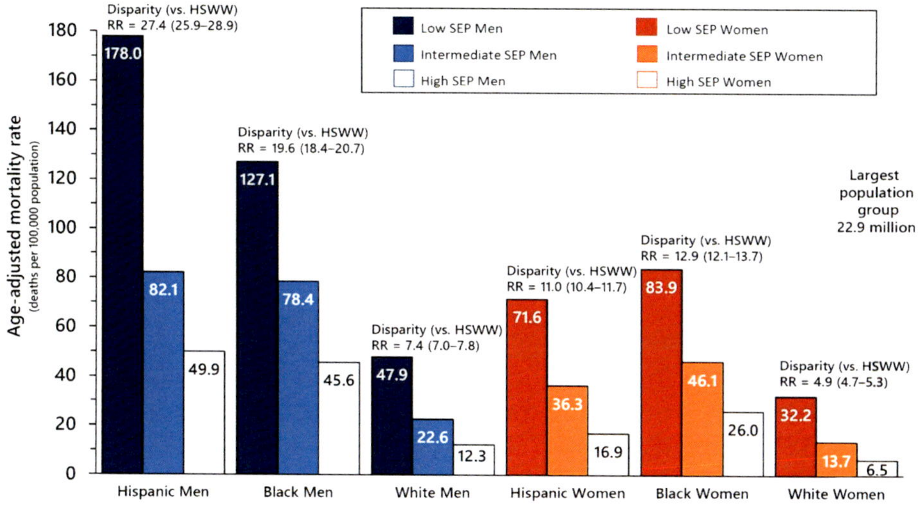

Figure 10.3. *COVID-19 Death Rates by Socioeconomic Position (SEP), Gender, and Race/Ethnicity with High-SEP White Women (HSWW) as the Referent Group for Disparity Rate Ratios ** among adults 25–64 Years Old, United States 1 January 2020 to 31 December 2020.*

Source: Pathak EB, Menard JM, Garcia RB, Salemi JL. Joint effects of socioeconomic position, race/ethnicity, and gender on COVID-19 mortality among working-age adults in the United States. International Journal of Environmental Research and Public Health. 2022; 19(9):5479. https://doi.org/10.3390/ijerph19095479.

Age-adjusted mortality for black men was higher than for white men (black: white mortality ratio = 1.19), and for black women it was higher than for white women (black: white mortality ratio = 1.16), as Figure 10.3 illustrates. With the exception of black women, the highest income group in each of these subgroups had the lowest mortality rates, while the lowest income group had the highest.

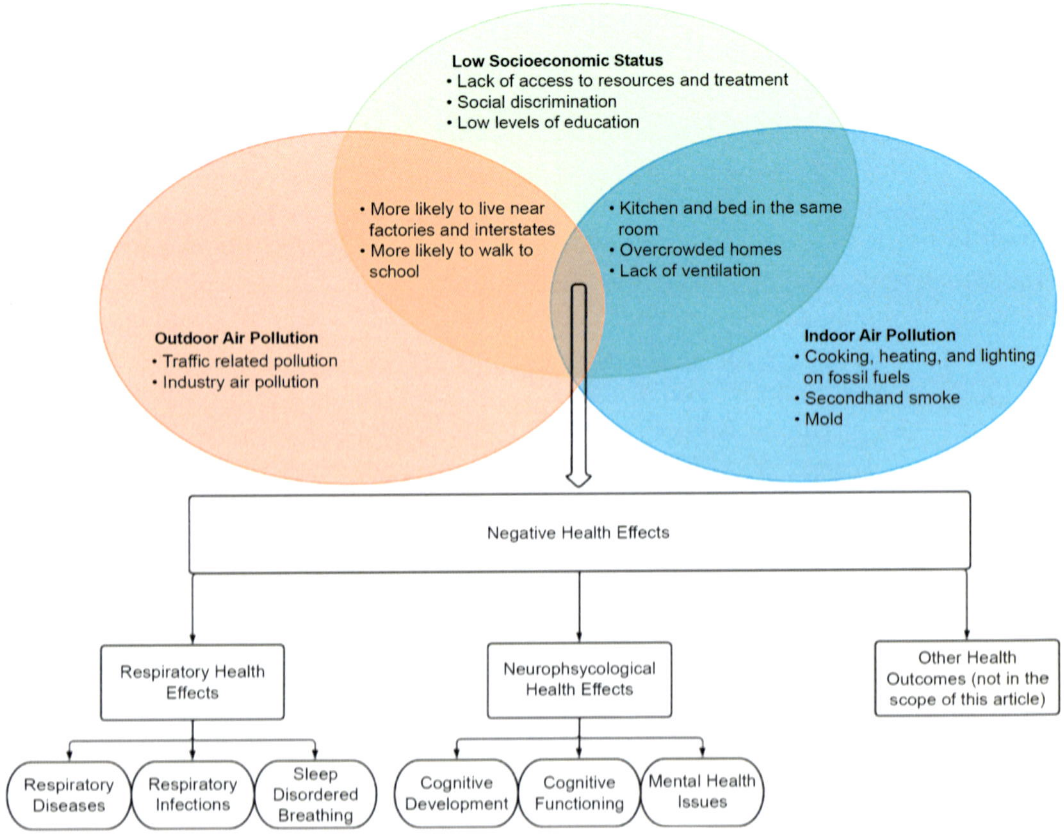

Figure 10.4. *Environmental injustice. The detrimental intersection of outdoor and indoor air pollution with socioeconomic status and its consequences for children's health.*

Source: *Mathiarasan S, Hüls A. Impact of environmental injustice on children's health—interaction between air pollution and socioeconomic status. International Journal of Environmental Research and Public Health. 2021; 18(2):795. https://doi.org/10.3390/ijerph18020795.*

Many treatments and diagnoses were looked at. For instance, there were significant racial and economic differences in mammography use. White people were more likely than Black people to get a mammogram, but the less wealthy had fewer mammograms than the wealthier individuals in both groups. Blacks compared to Whites had significantly higher rates of partial or total amputations of lower extremities (black: white ratio = 3.64). The least wealthy people had the highest rates of amputations among both Blacks and Whites. These findings indicate that these beneficiary groups may be more susceptible to treatments linked to subpar management of long-term illnesses like diabetes (Figure 10.4).

10.1.5.2. Potential Biases in Evaluating Health Services Using Group Data

Furthermore, biases have a special bearing on certain fields and subjects of study. Studies examining how prenatal care affects birth outcomes, for instance, are vulnerable to a number of significant potential biases. Whether prenatal care lowers the risk of prematurity and low birth weight is a common question in these studies, and it is measured by the number of prenatal visits. This kind of analysis could be biased in a number of ways. When all else is equal, a woman who gives birth early will, for instance, have fewer prenatal visits (i.e., because the pregnancy lasted shorter, she could not have been "at risk" for prenatal visits for as long). Since the gestation period was shorter, the outcome would be an artifactual relationship between prematurity and fewer prenatal visits. Bias, though, can also work the other way around. As long as she continues her pregnancy until the last trimester, a woman who starts prenatal care in the latter stages of her pregnancy will not give birth prematurely. As a result, there would be an observed correlation between fewer prenatal visits and a lower risk of an early, premature delivery. Women who have previously experienced medical issues might also be so nervous that they attend more prenatal appointments, but this puts them at higher risk of a negative outcome. The possible biases can therefore run either way. If these women are at high risk and cannot be prevented, there may be a clear correlation between more prenatal visits and unfavorable outcomes.

Lastly, the bias in these studies is frequently self-selection; that is, women who decide to start prenatal care early in their pregnancy tend to be more well-educated, come from affluent backgrounds, and have more positive views about healthcare. As a result, a group of women who are already less likely to experience unfavorable birth outcomes choose to receive prenatal care earlier. This means that, even in cases where early prenatal care has no real health benefits, there may be an apparent correlation between it and a decreased chance of an unfavorable pregnancy outcome.

10.1.5.3. Two Indices Used in Ecologic Studies of Health Services

Avoidable mortality is one metric used in ecologic studies to assess health services. The premise of avoidable mortality analyzes is that the rate of "avoidable deaths" ought to be inversely correlated with the accessibility, availability, and standard of healthcare in various geographical areas. Therefore, in an ideal world, avoidable mortality would be a gauge of how well care is provided in a given area. Plotting changes over time and drawing comparisons with other regions are both possible. Regrettably, for many of the conditions recommended for avoidable mortality analyzes, the requisite data are not available. Furthermore, the conclusions drawn from the lack of available data on confounders may be debatable.

The use of health indicators is a second strategy. This method involves charting changes in the incidence of certain sentinel conditions over time and comparing the results with data for other populations, with the idea being that these conditions represent the overall quality of healthcare. The observed alterations and distinctions are then connected to shifts in the health services industry and utilized to draw conclusions regarding causality. It can be challenging to determine the requirements that must be satisfied for a particular condition to be recognized as a reliable health indicator.

10.1.6. Evaluation Using Individual Data

Because of the limitations inherent in studies using group data, that is, studies in which we do not have data on both healthcare (exposure) and health outcomes for each individual, studies using individual data are generally preferable. If we wish to compare two populations, one receiving the care being evaluated and one not receiving it, we must ask the following two questions in order to be able to derive inferences about the effectiveness of care:

1. Are the characteristics of the two groups comparable—demographically, medically, and in terms of factors relating to prognosis?
2. Are the measurement methods comparable (e.g., diagnostic methods and the way disease is classified) in both groups?

Prognostic stratification is a critical issue to consider when using epidemiology to study outcomes for health service evaluation. To address these issues, such outcome studies must perform a prognostic stratification by carefully characterizing the individuals studied based on disease severity and studying case mix. If a change in health outcome is observed after a certain type of care has been delivered, can we necessarily conclude that the change is due to the healthcare provided, or could it be a result of differences in prognosis based on comorbidity—preexisting disease which may or may not be specifically related to the disease being studied, in severity, or in other associated conditions that bear on prognosis?

10.1.6.1. Randomized Designs

By using randomization, selection bias that arises from the patient's self-selection or the healthcare provider's selection of the patient is eliminated. Typically, study participants are paired with a particular type of care or left without any care at all (Fig. 10.5). Randomizing patients to receive no care is typically not considered for a variety of reasons, both pragmatic and ethical (Figure 10.5).

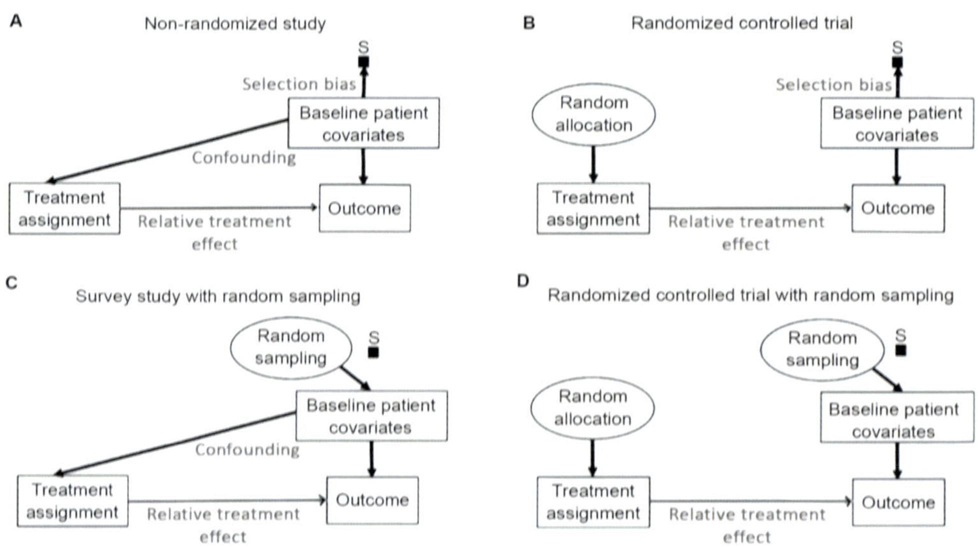

Figure 10.5. *Design of control trials.*

Source: Msaouel P, Lee J, Thall PF. Interpreting randomized controlled trials. Cancers. 2023; 15(19):4674. https://doi.org/10.3390/cancers15194674.

Let's look at one study that compared various healthcare delivery methods using a randomized design. For the care of stroke patients, early, structured, hospital-based management has been highly recommended. But there aren't many data from carefully executed controlled trials to contrast hospital care with specialized home care (domiciliary care). Additionally, a specialist stroke team that can offer care wherever in the hospital where stroke patients may be treated is an alternative to the hospital's stroke units. This is a practical consideration because space constraints and other administrative and financial concerns may prevent all hospitals from providing care for stroke patients in a specialized unit.

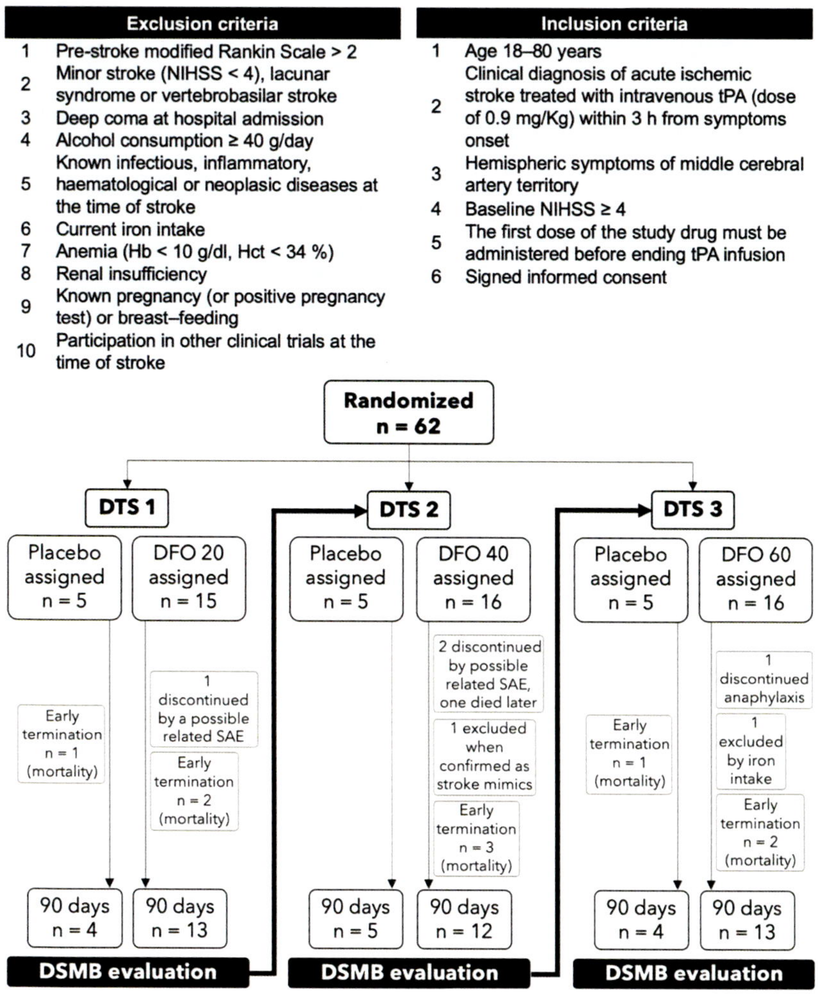

Figure 10.6. *Profile of an inclusion and exclusion criteria and CONSORT flow diagram of the three-dose tier sub-studies (DTS). In each DTS early termination cases due to mortality, discontinuation due to serious adverse events (SAE) possibly related to treatment, and patients excluded are indicated.*

Source: Millán M, DeGregorio-Rocasolano N, Pérez de la Ossa N, Reverté S, Costa J, Giner P, Silva Y, Sobrino T, Rodríguez-Yáñez M, Nombela F, et al. Targeting pro-oxidant iron with deferoxamine as a treatment for ischemic stroke: Safety and optimal dose selection in a randomized clinical trial. Antioxidants. 2021; 10(8):1270. https://doi.org/10.3390/antiox10081270.

Kalra and colleagues carried out a randomized, controlled trial to compare the effectiveness of three forms of care in order to determine the optimal organizational structure for the care of stroke patients (Fig. 10.6). Patients were randomly assigned to one of three groups: (1) care from a multidisciplinary team led by a stroke physician in a hospital stroke unit; (2) care from a multidisciplinary team with experience managing strokes; or (3) care from a specialized team at home. At 3, 6, and 12 months following the start of a stroke, the outcome—mortality or institutionalization—was evaluated. By using intention-to-treat, data were examined. Patients receiving treatment in the stroke unit had a lower risk of death or institutionalization at each of the three time points compared to patients receiving domiciliary care or treatment from the stroke team. Figure 10.6 displays the combined survival for the three groups. The research backs up the treatment of stroke patients in specialized stroke units.

An intriguing and somewhat unexpected finding of this study is that patients who were randomized to receive domiciliary care—that is, care at home—had a higher survival rate than those who were randomized to receive hospital-based stroke team treatment.

This observation could be explained by the fact that patients in the domiciliary care group were transferred from domiciliary care to a stroke unit when their conditions worsened or they developed new issues. Since an intention-to-treat analysis was performed, which examines outcomes in accordance with the initial randomization, these patients were still included in the analysis of the domiciliary care group. Because of the intention-to-treat analysis, these patient outcomes would typically be better than those of the domiciliary care group if they had benefited from care in the stroke unit.

A 10-year follow-up of a randomized controlled trial of care in a stroke rehabilitation unit was carried out by Drummond and associates. They discovered that even ten years after the stroke, management in a stroke rehabilitation center improved survivorship. Although the precise causes are unknown, the authors speculate that one possibility is that early disability reduction is linked to long-term survival.

10.1.6.2. Nonrandomized Designs

Randomized trials are not appropriate for all healthcare interventions for a number of reasons. First of all, these trials are frequently exceedingly costly and logistically challenging. It is not practical to put every healthcare measure through randomized evaluations because there are so many that are used at any given time. Second, studies that evaluate health services may be thought to have ethical issues. In particular, many patients and healthcare professionals may consider randomization to be an inappropriate procedure. Third, because programs and health issues change over time, randomized trials frequently take a long time to finish. As a result, by the time the study's results are finally collected and examined, they might not be totally applicable. For these reasons, a large number of researchers in the field of healthcare are searching for different methods that could at least produce some data. One such method, outcomes research, was covered above and typically refers to the use of data from nonrandomized studies, which frequently make use of sizable amounts of preexisting data.

10.1.6.2.1. Before–After Design (Historical Controls)

Comparing individuals who received care prior to the program's establishment (or before the healthcare measure became available) with those who received care from the program following its establishment (or after the measure became available) is one potential study design to evaluate a program if randomization is not possible or will not be used for any reason. What are the issues with this before-after design? To start, there are often differences in the completeness and quality of the data collected during the two periods. When developing a new health service delivery model, it's common practice to assess the program using a comparison group of individuals who received treatment in the past, prior to the program's launch. Because of this, information about individuals who joined the program after its inception might have been gathered using a carefully thought-out research tool, but information about previous patients might only be accessible through medical records that were created at the time and utilized for administrative or clinical functions. Therefore, in the event that a difference in outcome is noticed, we might not be able to determine whether this difference is due to program effects or variations in the quality of the data collected during the two time periods. Second, even in the event that a difference is observed—for instance, a decrease in mortality—we are unable to determine whether this is the result of the program or of other variables that may have evolved over time, such as housing, food, other lifestyle factors, or other health services.

Third, there is a selection issue. It is frequently challenging to determine whether, in terms of other variables that might affect outcome, the population studied after a program was established is genuinely similar to that observed before the program was established. That being said, this does not imply that before-and-after studies are worthless. However, it does imply that these kinds of studies are rarely definitive in proving the efficacy of a health service; rather, they merely offer a suggestion.

A study evaluating the effect of the Medicare Prospective Payment System (PPS) on care quality in the U.S employed a before-and-after design. The PPS's strictly regulated length of hospital stays and cost-cutting incentives raised concerns that the quality of care might have suffered as a result, which led to the study. Since the PPS was implemented nationwide, a prospective cohort design was not possible, hence the before-after design was chosen. Data from nearly 17,000 Medicare patients hospitalized in 1981–1982—prior to the PPS's implementation—were compared to data from patients admitted in 1985–1986—post-PPS. Five diseases were assessed for quality of care: hip fractures, congestive heart failure, myocardial infarction, pneumonia, and cerebrovascular accident. The degree of patient illness at hospital admission was taken into account when adjusting the outcome findings. The presence of conditions at discharge that clinicians agree should be corrected before discharge or monitored after discharge and that may result in poor outcomes if not corrected was found to be associated with an increase in instability at discharge, despite the fact that PPS was not found to be associated with an increase in either 30-day mortality or 6-month mortality. The authors make note of the possibility that other factors also changed in the period prior to and following the PPS's implementation.

10.1.6.2.2. Simultaneous Nonrandomized Design (Program–No Program)

Comparing two non-randomized populations simultaneously, one of which is served by the program and the other is not, is one way to get around the issue of changes that take place over time. This kind of design is essentially a cohort study where the "exposure" is the kind of healthcare that is being examined. The issue of how to choose exposed and nonexposed groups for research emerges, just like in any cohort study.

Many studies have been conducted on the topic of whether higher surgeon and hospital volumes are associated with better patient outcomes in recent years, which has attracted a lot of attention. The simultaneous, nonrandomized study of hospital volume that Jollis and colleagues reported is an example of that type of study. This study investigated the potential relationship between the volume of hospital procedures performed and variations in patient outcomes across hospitals. Hospitalizations following percutaneous transluminal coronary angioplasty were examined by the authors. They looked at the correlation between the number of angioplasties performed by the hospital and in-hospital mortality as well as the need for emergency bypass surgery during the index hospitalization. A dose-response relationship was discovered: hospitals with the lowest annual volume of angioplasties also had the highest rates of unplanned bypass surgery and in-hospital mortality. Regionalization of angioplasty services is supported by the finding that hospitals performing more angioplasties have lower short-term mortality. This finding has significant potential policy implications.

The correlation between improved patient outcomes and higher hospital volumes may be explained by the surgeons' higher volume of procedures rather than the total volume of procedures performed at these hospitals. This problem was addressed by Birkmeyer and associates. Utilizing Medicare claims data from 1998 and 1999, they looked at mortality rates for all 474,108 patients who had one of four procedures related to heart disease or four procedures related to cancer removal (Fig. 10.9). The study revealed that patients operated on by low-volume surgeons had a higher mortality rate than patients operated on by high-volume surgeons for the majority of procedures. Regardless of the hospital's surgical volume at the time of the procedure, this relationship persisted (Figure 10.7).

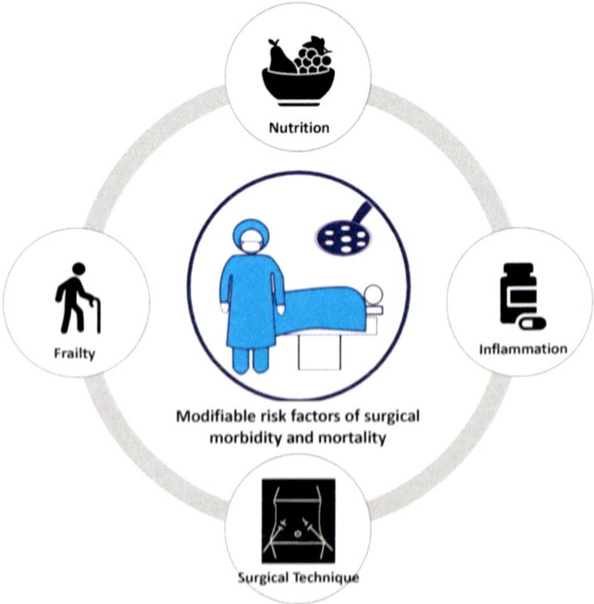

Figure 10.7. *modifiable risk factors influencing postoperative outcomes.*

Source: Lee B, Han H-S. Tackling surgical morbidity and mortality through modifiable risk factors in cancer patients. Nutrients. 2022; 14(15):3107. https://doi.org/10.3390/nu14153107.

10.1.6.2.3. Comparison of Utilizers and Non-utilizers

One approach for a simultaneous, nonrandomized study is to compare a group of people who use a health service with a group of people who do not (Figure 10.8).

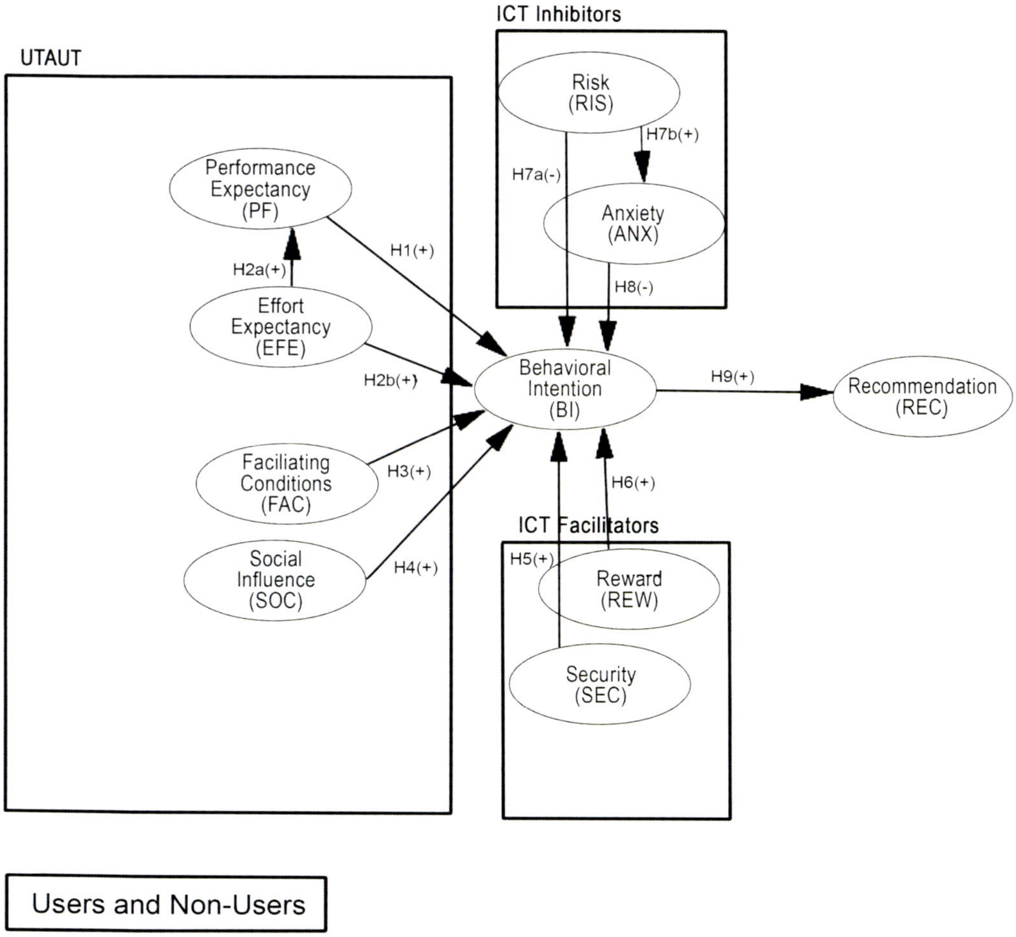

Figure 10.8. *Design of a nonrandomized cohort study comparing utilizers with non-utilizers of a program.*

Source: Saprikis V, Avlogiaris G, Katarachia A. A comparative study of users versus non-users' behavioral intention towards M-banking apps' Adoption. Information. 2022; 13(1):30. https://doi.org/10.3390/info13010030.

Long acknowledged are the self-selection issues this kind of design entails. Many years ago, Stine and colleagues published the findings of a study on prenatal care given to women who gave birth in Baltimore between 1960 and 1961 and were younger than 17 years old.

In this study, 1,397 young women received prenatal care and 315 did not. The neonatal death rate was 30.1 per 1,000 in those who received care and 88.9 per 1,000 in those who did not. The patients were not randomized, but decided themselves whether or not to seek care. As the authors pointed out, in the absence of randomization, we cannot conclude that the care reduced neonatal mortality. For we have the problem of selection: those who came in for care were probably more motivated regarding a broad array of health and prevention issues compared with those who did not.

Therefore, the observed difference in neonatal mortality could be as much a result of the traits shared by the two groups as it is of the care given. As long as the groups are not randomized, we can attempt to address the selection problem by describing the prognostic profiles of those who use and do not use care. However, this still leaves us with a persistent sense of uncertainty regarding whether some factors that could have distinguished between utilizers and non-utilizers and, consequently, impacted the health outcome were overlooked in the study.

10.1.6.2.4. Comparison of Eligible and Non-eligible Populations

Another method compares individuals who are eligible for the care being evaluated with a group of individuals who are not eligible due to the issue of potential selection biases in comparing groups of utilizers with non-utilizers (Fig. 10.9).

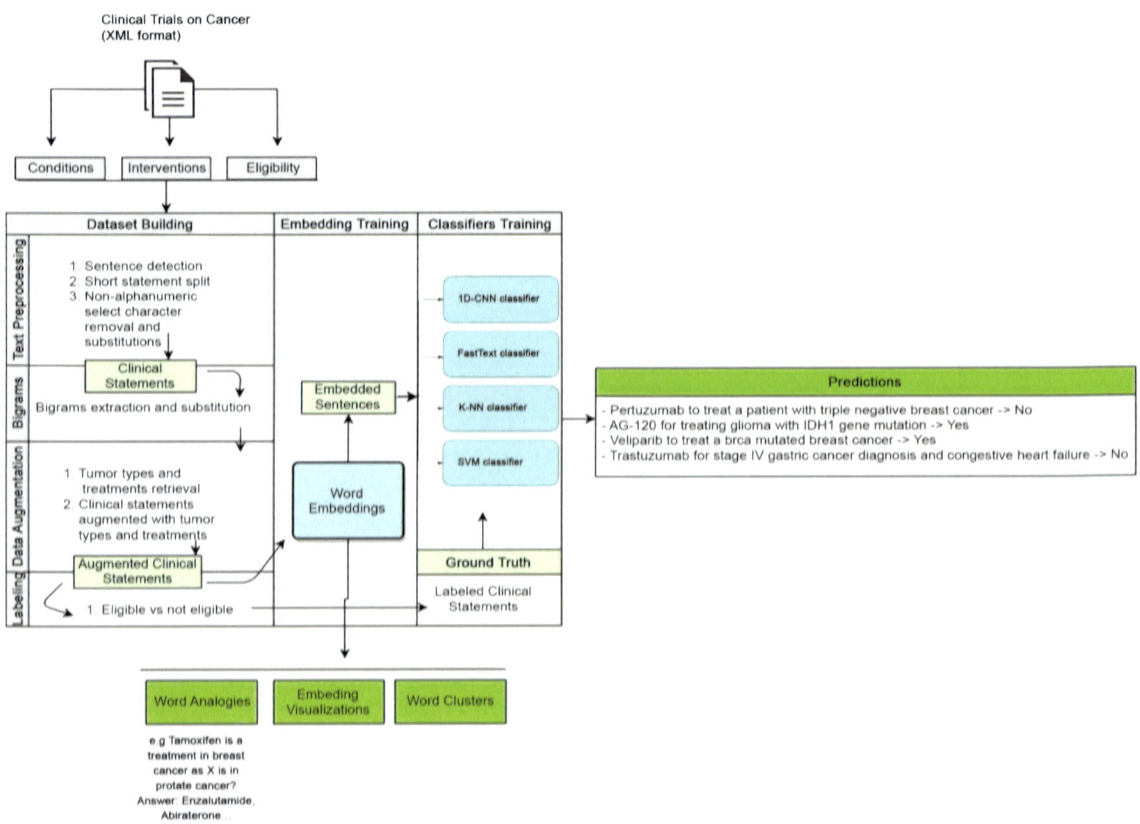

Figure 10.9. *Predicting whether or not short clinical statements concerning the type of tumor, including the molecular profile, the oncologic treatment, the medical history, or concomitant medication, were included in clinical trials.*

Source: Bustos A, Pertusa A. Learning Eligibility in Cancer clinical trials using deep neural networks. Applied Sciences. 2018; 8(7):1206. https://doi.org/10.3390/app8071206.

Since it is assumed that eligibility or non-eligibility has no bearing on the prognosis or outcome, selection bias is not introduced, which could have an impact on the study's conclusions. Examples of eligibility requirements are the kind of employment and the census tract in which one resides. Nevertheless, even with this design, one needs to be aware of potential sources of selection bias. For instance, it is evident that socioeconomic status may be related to a resident's census tract. Finding a suitable non-eligible population for comparison could be a crucial problem.

10.1.6.2.5. Combination Designs

A hypothetical outcome of a nonrandomized study comparing the morbidity level of a group that has not received healthcare (Group X) with a group that has (Group Y). We might be inclined to draw the conclusion that the health service lowers morbidity based on the fact that Group Y's observed level of morbidity is lower than Group X's. In order to arrive at this conclusion, we make the assumption that, prior to Group Y receiving care, the initial levels of morbidity in the two groups were comparable. We could interpret the finding of a lower level of morbidity in Group Y (Y_2) than in Group X (X_2) at a time after care has been administered as likely resulting from the care given if the morbidity levels for X_1 and Y_1 were similar.

It is plausible, nevertheless, that the groups were initially distinct and that their prognoses varied at that point, even in the absence of any care. Should that be the case, then any variations in morbidity noted following treatment (i.e., Y_2 being less than X_2) may simply represent the initial variations at the point prior to the delivery of care and may not provide insight into the efficacy of that care.

A combination design, which blends a before-and-after design with a program-no program design, is another method of program evaluation in light of this issue. The evaluation of outpatient treatment for children with sore throats serves as an illustration of this methodology.

The purpose of the study was to evaluate whether children who were eligible for outpatient treatment for sore throats had lower rates of rheumatic fever than did children who were not in order to determine the efficacy of this type of care for children. The reasoning was as follows: Children frequently get "strep" throats. Rheumatic fever can develop from "strep" throats if left untreated. It is possible to avoid rheumatic fever by treating "strep" throats appropriately. Therefore, fewer cases of rheumatic fever should arise in the children who received the treatment if these programs are successful in treating "strep" throats.

Comprehensive care programs for children and youth were started in many inner cities, including Baltimore, in the middle of the 1960s. The census tract in which the child lived determined their eligibility for care under this program. It was previously established that inner-city Baltimore was a hotspot for rheumatoid fever. It was feasible to determine and contrast a number of subgroups of Baltimore's youth and young adults, as well as compare their hospitalization rates for acute rheumatic fever episodes with those of the entire city. The groups comprised people living in census tracts that satisfied the requirements for comprehensive care eligibility as well as people living in census tracts that did not meet these requirements. The entire city of Baltimore was used to compare both.

A program versus no program comparison of black children's rheumatic fever rates is taken into account. The rate of rheumatic fever in children who qualified for comprehensive care was 10.6 per 100,000, while the rate in children who did not qualified was 14.9 per 100,000. In this simultaneous comparison, the eligible group's rate was lower, but the difference was not statistically significant (Figure 10.10).

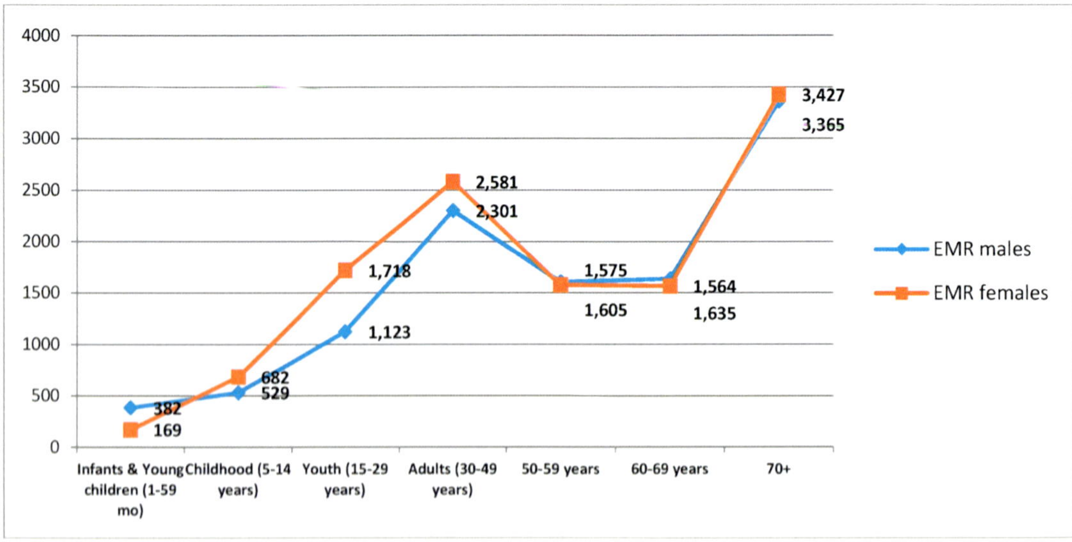

Figure 10.10. *Trends in total deaths (Y axis) from rheumatic heart disease by age and sex in the Eastern Mediterranean Region (EMR).*

Source: *Abul-Fadl AMAM, Mourad MM, Ghamrawy A, Sarhan AE. Trends in deaths from rheumatic heart disease in the eastern mediterranean region: Burden and challenges. Journal of Cardiovascular Development and Disease. 2018; 5(2):32. https://doi.org/10.3390/jcdd5020032.*

This combination design's subsequent analysis looked at how rates of rheumatic fever changed over time in both eligible and non-eligible groups. The incidence of rheumatic fever decreased by 60% in the qualifying census tracts between 1960–1964 (prior to the implementation of the programs) and 1968–1970 (during the program's run). The incidence of rheumatic fever remained essentially unchanged (+2%) in the non-eligible tracts. As a result, a decline in the quality of care offered is consistent with both components of the combination design.

It was unclear, though, if the programs' care was genuinely to blame for the drop in rheumatic fever because so much had changed in the inner city during this period. For that reason, another analysis was done. A streptococcal throat infection in a child can present with symptoms or not at all. It seems obvious that the only child who would have been brought to a clinic would have had a sore throat. We would expect the decline in incidence to be restricted to children with symptomatic clinical sore throats who would have sought care, rather than to have happened in asymptomatic children who had no clinically apparent infections, if our hypothesis about the clinic's care was to blame for the decrease in rheumatic fever incidence.

The entire decrease was restricted to kids who had previously had a clinically obvious infection; kids who had "strep" throat without any symptoms saw no change in the incidence of rheumatic fever. Thus, these results are in excellent agreement with the hypothesis that the decrease in the incidence of rheumatic fever was caused by medical care, or a factor closely related to it (Figure 10.11).

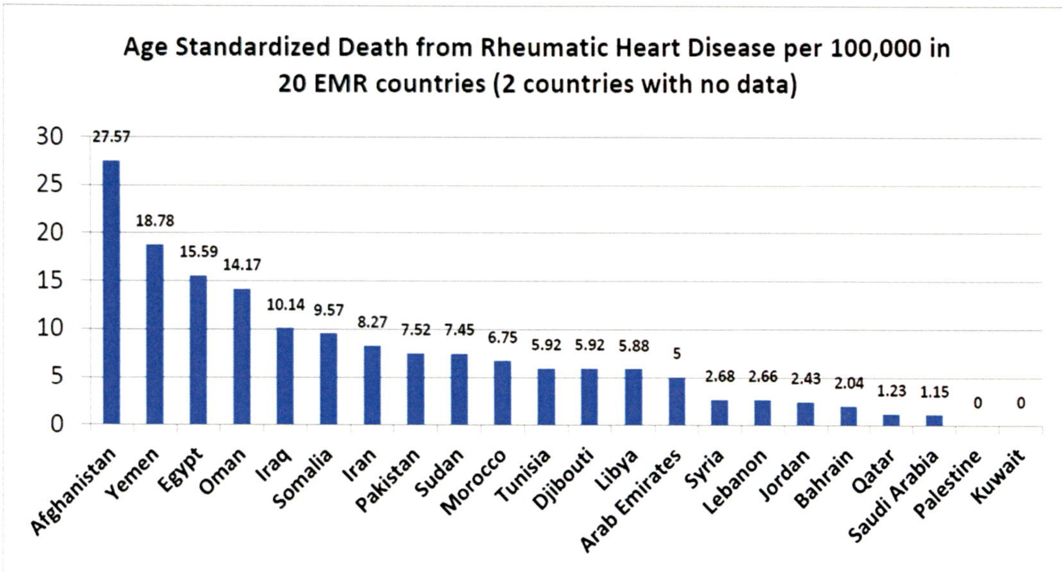

Figure 10.11. *Age standardized deaths per 100,000 from rheumatic heart disease for the 20 countries of the Eastern Mediterranean region.*

Source: (www.worldlifeexpectancy.com) Data source: published by WHO, 2014.

Source: Abul-Fadl AMAM, Mourad MM, Ghamrawy A, Sarhan AE. Trends in deaths from rheumatic heart disease in the eastern mediterranean region: burden and challenges. Journal of Cardiovascular Development and Disease. 2018; 5(2):32. https://doi.org/10.3390/jcdd5020032.

10.2. The Epidemiologic Approach to Evaluating Screening Programs

The methodical evaluation of the efficacy, efficiency, and impact of screening tests in identifying illnesses or conditions in a population is known as the epidemiologic approach to screening program evaluation. The natural history of diseases, the effectiveness of screening tests, and the results of screening programs are all studied using an approach based on epidemiological concepts and methodologies. Here are key components of the epidemiologic approach to evaluating screening programs:

10.2.1. The Natural History of Disease

Let's take a closer look at the natural history of disease before talking about the methodologic challenges associated with assessing the screening benefit. The disease's biological onset happens eventually. It is usually impossible to detect changes like this, which could be subcellular changes like a change in DNA. Later on, the illness develops symptoms or clinical signs; in other words, it enters the clinical phase. The patient seeks medical attention as a result of the clinical signs, and following a diagnosis and the start of the proper therapy, the patient may recover completely, experience reduced symptoms, become disabled, or pass away (Figure 10.12).

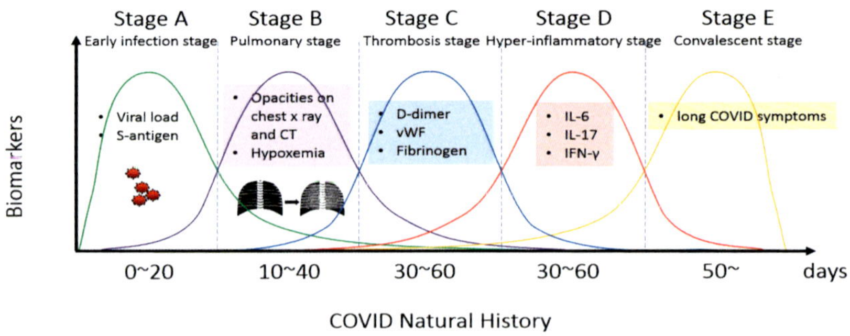

Figure 10.12. *The natural history of COVID-19 includes five stages. The first stage is the early infection stage, which is characterized by the elevation of the viral load and S-antigen levels in the serum. The second stage is the pulmonary stage, which is characterized by opacities on chest X-rays, glass opacities on computed tomography (CT), and hypoxemia. The third stage is the thrombosis stage which is characterized by elevated D-dimer, vWF, and fibrinogen levels. The fourth stage is the hyper-inflammatory stage which is characterized by the elevation of cytokines such as IL-6, IL-17, and interferons. The fifth stage is the convalescent stage where long COVID symptoms may be observed.*

Source: Liang KH, Teng YC, Liao YT, Yarmishyn AA, Chiang S-H, Hung WC, Hsiao CY, Tsai ET, Chang TJ, Yang DM, et al. The natural history of SARS-CoV-2-incurred disease: from infection to long COVID. International Journal of Translational Medicine. 2024; 4(1):72–86. https://doi.org/10.3390/ijtm4010004.

The appearance of symptoms indicates a critical stage in a disease's natural history, as shown in Figure 10.16B. The time when a disease is present can be split into two phases: the clinical phase of the disease is the time from the onset of signs and symptoms to the final result, which could be a cure, control of the disease, or death. The preclinical phase of the disease is the time interval between the biological onset of the illness and the emergence of symptoms. Primary prevention, as illustrated in Figures 10.16C and D, refers to intervention taken before a disease has manifested itself. This includes immunization and lowering exposure to agents that cause disease. Secondary prevention occurs during the preclinical phase of an illness, which is after the disease has developed but before clinical signs and symptoms have appeared. It involves detecting disease at an earlier stage than usual, such as through screening. Treating clinically ill people in order to stop illness-related complications, such as the patient's death, is known as tertiary prevention.

In order to encourage symptomatic individuals to seek medical attention sooner, we could implement health education programs with the goal of detecting disease earlier than usual. Finding asymptomatic patients with a disease, however, is a significant challenge.

Now, let's examine the disease's preclinical stage in more detail. The disease can eventually be identified during the preclinical stage using the tests that are currently accessible. The detectable preclinical phase of the disease is the time interval from this point to the emergence of signs and symptoms. When a disease is found through screening, the diagnosis process can occur sooner in the illness's natural course. The lead time is the difference between the typical time of diagnosis and the interval by which screening and early disease detection advance the time of diagnosis. The idea of screening and identifying a disease earlier than it would typically be discovered is intrinsic to the concept of lead time. The critical point in a disease's natural history is another key idea in screening. This is the point in the natural history where treatment is easier to administer and/or more effective before. If a disease has a chance of recovery, it might not be cured after this point but before. The point at which breast cancer spreads to the axillary lymph nodes, for instance, is crucial in women with this disease. The prognosis is significantly better if the disease is discovered and treated before that happens as opposed to after it has spread to the nodes.

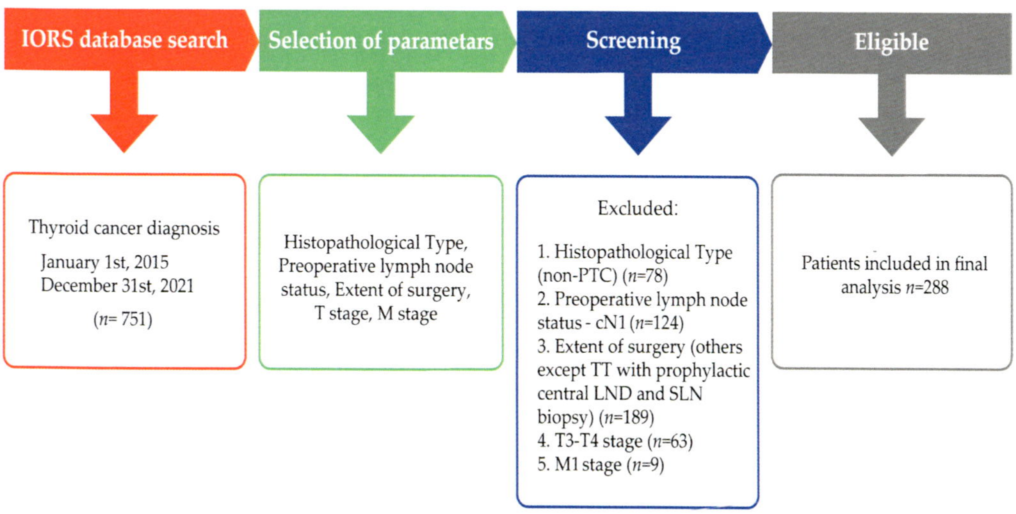

Figure 10.13. *An example of screening for lymph node spread.*

Source: Popović Krneta M, Šobić Šaranović D, Mijatović Teodorović L, Krajčinović N, Avramović N, Bojović Ž, Bukumirić Z, Marković I, Rajšić S, Djorović BB, et al. Prediction of cervical lymph node metastasis in clinically node-negative T1 and T2 papillary thyroid carcinoma using supervised machine learning approach. Journal of Clinical Medicine. 2023; 12(11):3641. https://doi.org/10.3390/jcm12113641.

A disease's natural history may contain several pivotal moments. For instance, the point at which the disease spreads from the axillary nodes to other body parts in a patient with breast cancer may be a second crucial point. Even in cases where the disease has not spread systemically, the prognosis is still better when it is limited to the axillary lymph nodes.

Since the critical point is a theoretical concept, we typically are unable to pinpoint the exact moment at which a given disease reaches its critical point. That is, nevertheless, a crucial concept in screening. It is evident that there is no justification for screening and early detection if we are unable to identify one or more pivotal moments in the disease's natural history. Early detection is predicated on the idea that a disease has a biologic point in its natural history, before which a patient will benefit more from treatment than from treatment after that point (Figure 10.13).

10.2.2. The Pattern of Disease Progression

We might expect to see a potential benefit from screening and early detection if the following two assumptions hold:

1. All or most clinical cases of a disease first go through a detectable preclinical phase.
2. In the absence of intervention, all or most cases in a preclinical phase progress to a clinical phase.

The two presumptions are fairly obvious. For instance, there's no need to run screening tests if none of the preclinical cases turn into clinical cases. On the other hand, there is no need to run screening tests if none of the clinical cases advance past the preclinical stage. Therefore, it's critical to consider both presumptions when evaluating any potential screening benefits.

Both presumptions, though, are debatable. Under some circumstances, the preclinical stage might be so brief that no program of periodic screening would likely find the disease. Furthermore, there is mounting evidence that certain diseases may experience spontaneous regression; as a result, not all preclinical cases inevitably develop into clinical disease.

The progression from a normal cervix to cervical cancer is taken here as an example. As more cases at the in situ (noninvasive) stage are found, we might anticipate a corresponding decline in the number of cases that progress to invasive disease.

The issue that some cases advance through the in-situ stage so quickly and the preclinical stage lasts for such a short time that, in actuality, there is no preclinical stage during which disease can be detected by screening makes assessing the benefits of cervical cancer screening more difficult. Furthermore, studies using nuclear DNA quantitation indicate that intraepithelial abnormalities in the cervical cavity may be an irreversible precursor to invasive cancer or a reversible state itself. Additionally, data imply that certain cases of cervical intraepithelial neoplasia identified by a Papanicolaou (Pap) smear spontaneously regress, both in the later stage (carcinoma in situ) and especially in the earlier stages.

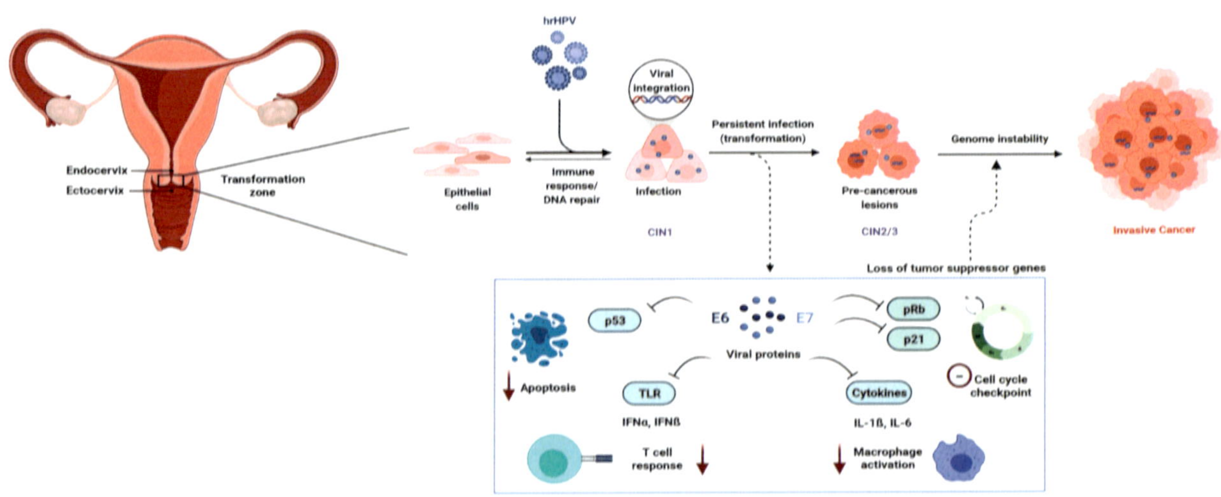

Figure 10.14. *A, Natural history of cervical cancer.*

Source: Ramachandran D, Dörk T. Genomic risk factors for cervical cancer. Cancers. 2021; 13(20):5137. https://doi.org/10.3390/cancers13205137

According to a study, 36% of women with abnormal Pap smears who declined treatment subsequently had normal Pap smears. Furthermore, current data indicate that various papillomavirus types may be linked to the majority, if not all, of in situ cervical neoplasias. As only neoplasia linked to specific papillomavirus types progresses to invasive cancer, we might be dealing with heterogeneity in the disease and the causative agent.

Therefore, early detection followed by effective intervention would be reflected by a commensurate reduction in the number of invasive lesions that subsequently develop. When evaluating the benefits of screening, it is important to consider the extent of both phenomena, spontaneous regression and extremely rapid progression, as this has a clear impact on the size of the decrease in invasive disease that may be anticipated as a result of early detection and intervention. These concerns are obviously pertinent to assessing the advantages of screening for a variety of diseases, even though they have been demonstrated in relation to cervical cancer (Figure 10.14).

10.2.3. Methodologic Issues

A few methodologic issues need to be considered in order to interpret the results of a study intended to assess the advantages of screening. Due to the challenges of randomly assigning a population for screening, the majority of research on screening programs that have been conducted have not been randomized trials. So, the question is, why can't we simply take a look at a group of individuals who have undergone screening and compare their mortality to that of a group who has not—that is, assess the efficacy of screening using a cohort design?

Assume for the moment that we are comparing a population of individuals who have undergone screening for a particular disease with a population that has not undergone screening. Let's further assume that individuals in whom disease is detected will receive treatment, if one is available. Let us turn to some of the methodologic issues involved. If we find a lower mortality from the disease in those in whom disease was identified through screening than in those in whom disease was not detected in this manner, can we not conclude that screening and early detection of disease has been beneficial?

10.2.3.1. Selection Biases

- **Referral Bias (Volunteer Bias):** The first thing we might look for when drawing a conclusion about the advantages of screening is if there was any bias in the process of choosing who was screened and who wasn't. It would be ideal if we could presume that people who were screened shared the same traits as people who weren't. The traits of people who take part in screening or other health programs and those who do not, however, differ greatly. Numerous studies have demonstrated that volunteers follow medical advice more frequently and are generally healthier than the general population. Even if early detection had no effect on improving prognosis, we might see lower mortality in the screened group if, for example, people whose disease had a better prognosis from the beginning were either referred for screening or self-selected. Of course, it's also possible that a large number of high-risk individuals who volunteer for screening do so because they experience anxiety due to favorable family history or lifestyle choices. The issue is that we are unsure of the direction in which selection bias may act or how it may impact the findings of the study.

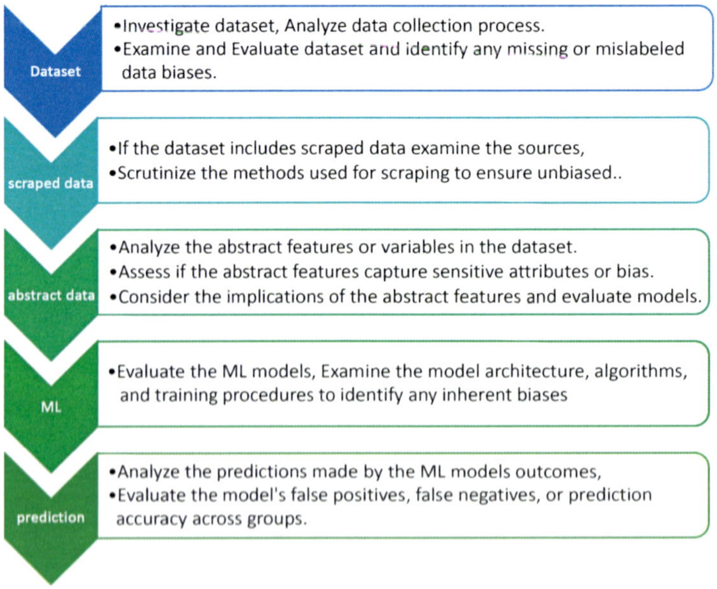

Figure 10.15. *Analyzes of bias in screening.*

Source: Siddique S, Haque MA, George R, Gupta KD, Gupta D, Faruk MJH. Survey on machine learning biases and mitigation techniques. Digital. 2024; 4(1):1–68. https://doi.org/10.3390/digital4010001.

It is best to conduct the comparison using a randomized experimental study, taking care to ensure that the two groups have similar initial prognostic profiles, in order to address the issue of selection bias that most significantly affects our interpretation of the results (Figure 10.15).

10.2.3.2. Length-Biased Sampling (Prognostic Selection)

The second category of selection issues that crop up when analyzing the data from a comparison between a screened and an unscreened group is potential selection bias; this has more to do with the kind of disease that the screening detects than with the individuals who come in for screening. If the outcome of those in whom disease is detected by screening is found to be better than the outcome of those who were not screened and in whom disease was identified during the usual course of clinical care, could the better outcome among those who are screened result from selective identification by screening of persons with a better prognosis? Could the better outcome be unrelated to the timing of diagnostic and treatment interventions? Does screening identify cases of the disease which have a better natural history?

Regarding these individuals, what is the preclinical phase? Preclinical and clinical phases are separated in the single continuous natural history of each patient's disease depending on when symptoms and indicators start to appear. Some have a short natural history, while others have a long natural history. This implies that the preclinical phase will likewise be lengthy if a person has a slowly progressing natural history and a lengthy clinical phase. On the other hand, a patient with a rapidly progressing illness and a brief natural history is likely to have a brief clinical phase, and it makes sense to assume that the preclinical phase will follow suit. The idea that a long clinical phase corresponds with a long preclinical phase and a short clinical phase corresponds with a short preclinical phase is supported by data, in fact.

Keep in mind that the goal of screening is to identify the illness in its preclinical stages, as during the clinical stages, patients are aware of the issue and, even in the absence of screening, will seek medical attention for symptoms. Which patient group is more likely to be identified by a one-time screening program in a community: those with a short preclinical phase or those with a long preclinical phase?

In order to address this query, let's look at a small sample that undergoes screening for a particular illness. Every case has a preclinical and a clinical phase, as demonstrated here. Every preclinical phase in the figure has the same duration as the corresponding clinical phase. The goal of the screening is to find cases in the preclinical, presymptomatic state because patients in the clinical phase will be identified in the normal course of medical care. Be aware that the preclinical stages of the cases shown here have varying durations. The greater the duration of the preclinical phase, the higher the probability that the screening program will identify the case in its preclinical stage. For instance, we will undoubtedly miss the majority of cases during the preclinical phase if we screen for a disease once a year for which the preclinical phase lasts only 24 hours. On the other hand, cases will be found if the preclinical phase lasts a year. Selective identification of cases with longer preclinical phases of illness is typically achieved through screening. Consequently, screening would continue to identify individuals with a long preclinical phase and, subsequently, a long clinical phase, even in the event that the subsequent therapy was ineffective (i.e., those whose prognosis is better). Even in the event that there was no screening program or no real benefits from screening, these individuals would still have a better prognosis.

There are various approaches to solving this issue. Using an experimental randomized design is one method, wherein efforts are made to maintain group comparability with respect to the duration of the detectable preclinical phase of illness. But that might not be so simple. Additionally, both the screened and the unscreened members of each group should have their survival examined. Survival in the screened group should be computed for both individuals whose disease is discovered through screening and for those whose disease is discovered in between screening exams, or "interval cases."

10.2.3.3. Lead Time Bias

A bias related to lead time also occurs when comparing the survival of those who undergo screening to the survival of those who do not; specifically, how much sooner can a diagnosis be made if the disease is discovered through screening as opposed to the typical timing of the diagnosis if screening is not done?

Examine four patients with a particular ailment. Each horizontal line's thicker portion indicates the apparent survival that is seen. The typical time of diagnosis and death are displayed in the first case (A). The second case (B) displays the same time of death but an earlier diagnosis. The patient is not any better off because death has not been postponed, even though survival appears better because the time between diagnosis and death is longer. The third case (C) indicates a delay in the disease's progression and an earlier diagnosis, both of which are obviously advantageous to the patient (presuming they have a good quality of life). The fourth case (D) concludes with an earlier diagnosis and subsequent prevention of the disease's death. Delay or prevention of death are the benefits we aim to achieve. While we have chosen to concentrate on death in this chapter, other valid outcome measures that we could have considered include morbidity, recurrences, quality of life, or patient satisfaction.

10.2.3.4. Lead Time and Five-Year Survival

Five-year survival is a frequently used measure of therapeutic success, particularly in cancer therapy. Let us examine the possible effect of lead time on apparent 5-year survival.

The natural history of colon cancer in a hypothetical patient diagnosed in the standard clinical setting without any screening is considered. The disease's biological onset occurred in 2000. After the patient's symptoms became apparent in 2008, a diagnostic evaluation revealed colon cancer. Despite having surgery in 2008, the patient passed away from colon cancer in 2010. This patient is obviously not a five-year survivor, having only lived for two years (from 2008 to 2010). This patient is considered a treatment failure if the 5-year survival rate is used as a measure of treatment success.

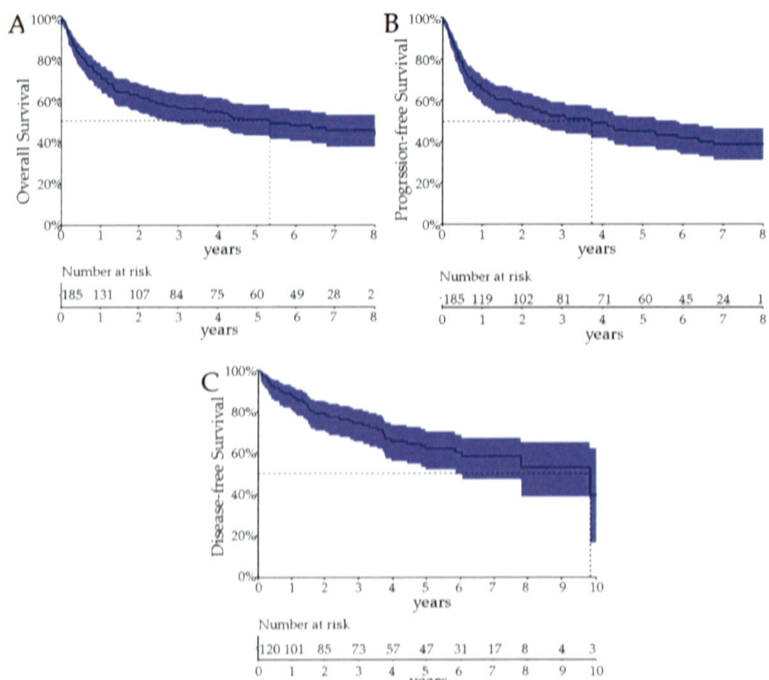

Figure 10.16. *Survival curves for 185 Brazilian patients with diffuse large B-cell lymphoma (DLBCL), NOS aged ≥ 70 years. (**A**) Overall survival, (**B**) progression-free survival, and (**C**) disease-free survival.*

Source: de Pádua Covas Lage LA, De Vita RN, de Oliveira Alves LB, Jacomassi MD, Culler HF, Reichert CO, de Freitas FA, Rocha V, Siqueira SAC, de Oliveira Costa R, et al. Predictors of survival, treatment modalities, and clinical outcomes of diffuse large B-cell lymphoma in patients older than 70 years still an unmet medical need in 2024 based on real-world evidence. Cancers. 2024; 16(8):1459. https://doi.org/10.3390/cancers16081459.

Think about the possible outcomes for this patient should he live in a community where a screening program is implemented (. Let's assume for the sake of this hypothetical example alone that there is actually no benefit to early detection, meaning that early intervention has no effect on the natural course of colon cancer. Although the patient in this instance has no symptoms, in 2005 they had a standard screening test, the results of which are positive. The patient underwent surgery in 2005 but passed away in 2010. The patient is now unquestionably a 5-year survivor having made it through five years.

He has survived for five years, though, not because death has come any later, but rather because the diagnosis was received sooner. Upon contrasting this screening scenario with the non-screened scenario, it is clear that the patient has not lived any longer as a result of the earlier detection. The patient may have suffered a reduction in life quality since the disease was discovered earlier through screening, which allowed him to receive additional medical care and postoperative care for an additional three years. Additionally, he may have lost out on three years of a normal life. This issue of an illusion of improved survival solely due to earlier detection is known as the lead time bias (Figure 10.16).

Because survival is measured from an earlier point of diagnosis, screening will appear to have a benefit even if there is no real benefit to early disease detection—even if death is not postponed. This is not to say that early detection has no benefits; rather, the lead time connected with early detection implies that benefits, such as increased survival, may manifest even in the absence of benefits. Therefore, when interpreting the findings of nonrandomized evaluations, lead time must be considered.

A scenario where no screening activity is being conducted is now considered. 30% of patients survive five years after diagnosis. The entire frame is moved to the left if we implement a screening program with a one-year lead time. Now, if we compute survival at five years following the updated diagnosis date, survival seems to be 50%, but this is only due to bias in lead time. The issue is that the ostensibly higher survival rate is not due to longer life expectancies for those who are screened; rather, it is the consequence of an early diagnosis made earlier in the disease's natural course.

Therefore, in order to detect any extension of survival beyond that caused by the lead time artifact, we must account for an estimated lead time in any comparison between screened and unscreened populations. In order for early detection to actually lead to better survival, the screened group's survival rate must exceed both the lead time and the control group's survival rate. As a result, we must estimate the lead time for the illness under investigation. An alternative approach is to contrast the overall screened group's mortality from the disease with that of the unscreened group, as opposed to solely focusing on the case fatality rate of individuals in whom the disease was identified through screening.

10.2.3.5. Overdiagnosis Bias

An additional possible bias is overdiagnosis. Sometimes those who start a screening program are incredibly passionate about it. Even pathologists who read Pap smears for cervical cancer can get overly excited about the test results and end up overinterpreting them, which can lead to false-positive readings. Should they overread, some average women will be added to the group of people who are believed to have positive Pap smears. As a result, women who are cancer-free will be added to the abnormal group. One could mistakenly believe that screening has increased the rate of early-stage cancer detection and diagnosis if normal individuals in the screened group are more likely than normal individuals in the unscreened group to receive an incorrect positive diagnosis—that is, to be diagnosed with cancer when they actually do not. Furthermore, the results would represent an inflated estimate of survival after screening in people thought to have cancer, leading to the incorrect conclusion that screening had been shown to improve survival from cancer in this population because many of the people in the screened group who were diagnosed with the disease would not actually have cancer and would therefore have good survival.

The possible quantitative impact of overdiagnosis resulting from screening is demonstrated in a hypothetical example shown in Figure 10.17. In Scenario 1, there is no screening. In this scenario, 1,000 patients with clinical lung cancer are followed for 10 years. At that point, 900 have died and 100 are alive. The 10-year survival for the 1,000 patients is therefore or 10%.

Consider Scenario 2, wherein overdiagnosis occurs due to screening. In this case, 4,000 individuals have positive lung cancer screening results. Of these, 3,000 are false positives—people who are not actually suffering from lung cancer but were mistakenly diagnosed as having it by the screening test—while the remaining 1,000 are the same patients with clinical lung cancer shown in Figure 10.17 A.

These three thousand people are still alive after ten years, as are the hundred individuals who had clinical lung cancer and survived. As a result, 3,100 of the 4,000 persons who initially tested positive have lived for ten years. In the original patient population of 1,000 with clinical lung cancer, 10-year survival in Scenario 2 is now 78%, compared with 10% in Scenario 1, as can be seen in the comparison of Scenarios 1 and 2. But Scenario 2's ostensibly "better" survival rate is solely attributable to the inclusion of 3,000 individuals who were over diagnosed by the screening but did not have lung cancer.

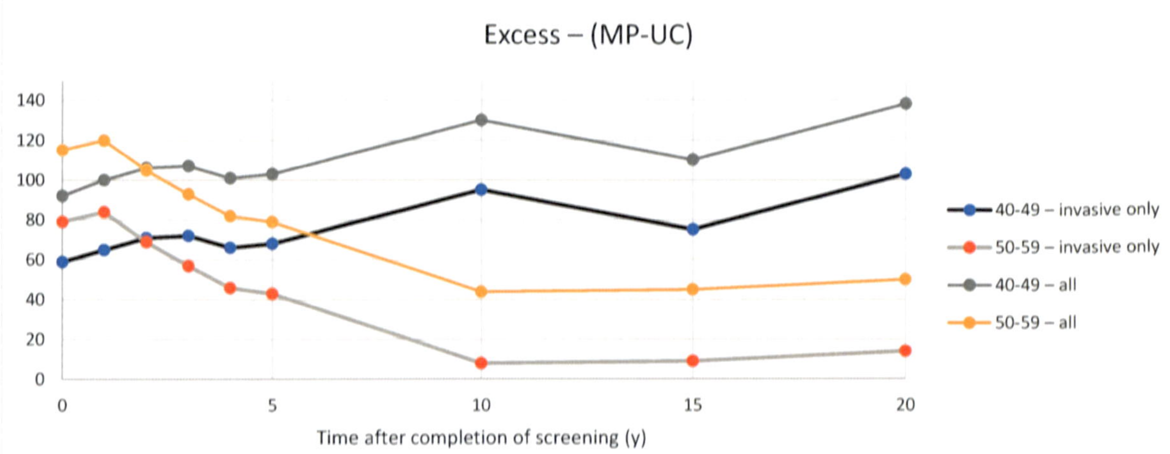

Figure 10.17. *Excess invasive cancers in the study group compared to the controls in the two CNBSS trials.*

Source: Yaffe MJ, Mainprize JG. Over detection of breast cancer. Current Oncology. 2022; 29(6):3894–3910. https://doi.org/10.3390/curroncol29060311.

10.2.4. Study Designs for Evaluating Screening: Nonrandomized and Randomized Studies

10.2.4.1. Nonrandomized Studies

We have essentially been discussing nonrandomized observational studies of screened and unscreened individuals—a cohort design—while talking about the methodologic challenges associated with nonrandomized screening studies.

As a means of evaluating the efficacy of screening, the case-control design has drawn more attention in recent years. People with advanced illnesses are the "cases" in this design; these are the kinds of diseases that screening is intended to prevent. Appropriate controls for this kind of research have been suggested on multiple occasions. It is obvious that they ought to be "non-cases," or individuals without severe illness. Many now feel that individuals chosen from the population from which the cases were derived make better controls, even though the "controls" used in early case-control studies for evaluating screening were people with disease in an early stage. To consider screening as a form of "exposure," we next ascertain the frequency of prior screening among the cases as well as the controls. An odds ratio can be computed, and if screening is successful, it will be less than 1 to 0. If this is the case, we would anticipate a higher prevalence of screening history among the controls than among those with advanced disease.

10.2.4.2. Randomized Studies

In a study of this kind, half of the population is randomly assigned to screening and the other half to no screening. Such a study is challenging to organize and conduct. The mammography-based breast cancer screening trial conducted by the Health Insurance Plan (HIP) of New York is arguably the most well-known randomized screening experiment.

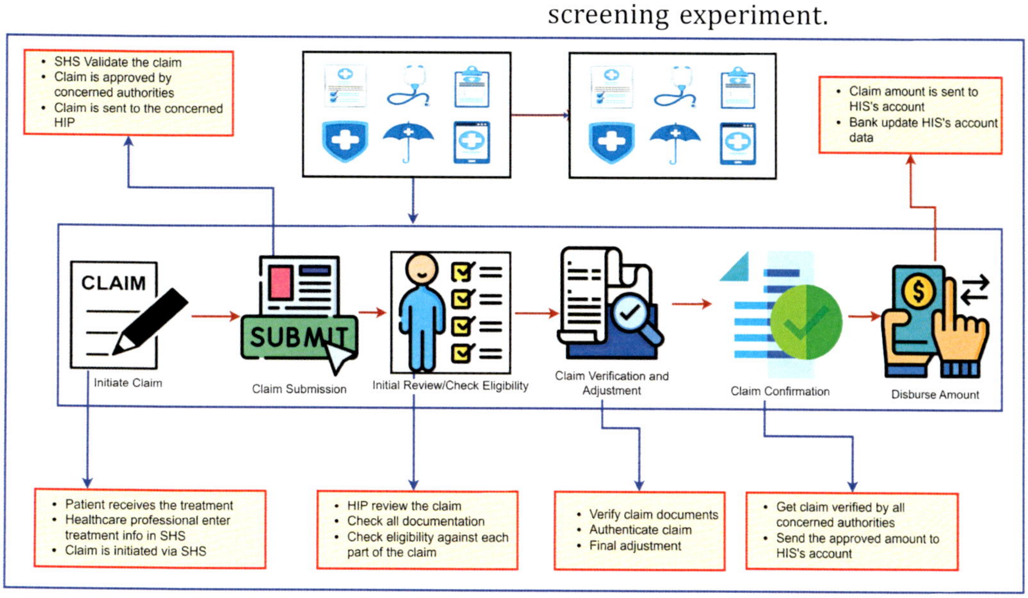

Figure 10.18. *Design of the health insurance claim (HIC).*

Source: Al-Quayed F, Humayun M, Tahir S. Towards a secure technology-driven architecture for Smart health insurance systems: An empirical study. Healthcare. 2023; 11(16):2257. https://doi.org/10.3390/healthcare11162257.

Women enrolled in the prepaid HIP program participated in a randomized trial carried out by Shapiro and associates. This study has established itself as a standard in the literature for reporting on the assessment of screening benefits using a randomized trial design, and it will be used as a template for similar studies in the future. In 1963, the study was started. Its goal was to ascertain whether routine screening for breast cancer using mammography and clinical examinations decreased the death rate from breast cancer in women between the ages of 40 and 64. A total of 62,000 women were randomized into two groups: 31,000 each for the study and the control. Screening exams were provided to the study group; 65% of participants took the first exam and were then offered yearly follow-up exams. The majority of these women underwent one of the three available yearly screening exams. The screening process included an interview, a mammography, and a physical examination. Under the prepayment program, control women got the standard medical care (Figure 10.18).

The figure below shows the number of breast cancer deaths and the mortality rates in the world (Figure 10.19).

The 5-year case-fatality for the women in both groups who developed breast cancer is displayed in Figure 10.31. In the control group, case fatalities accounted for 40% of cases. The case-fatality rate for the entire study group—that is, women who were randomly assigned to undergo mammography, regardless of whether they were screened or not—was 29%. This group was then split into those who were screened and those who declined screening by Shapiro and colleagues. 35% of those who declined screening became fatal cases. The case-fatality rate among those who underwent screening was 23%.

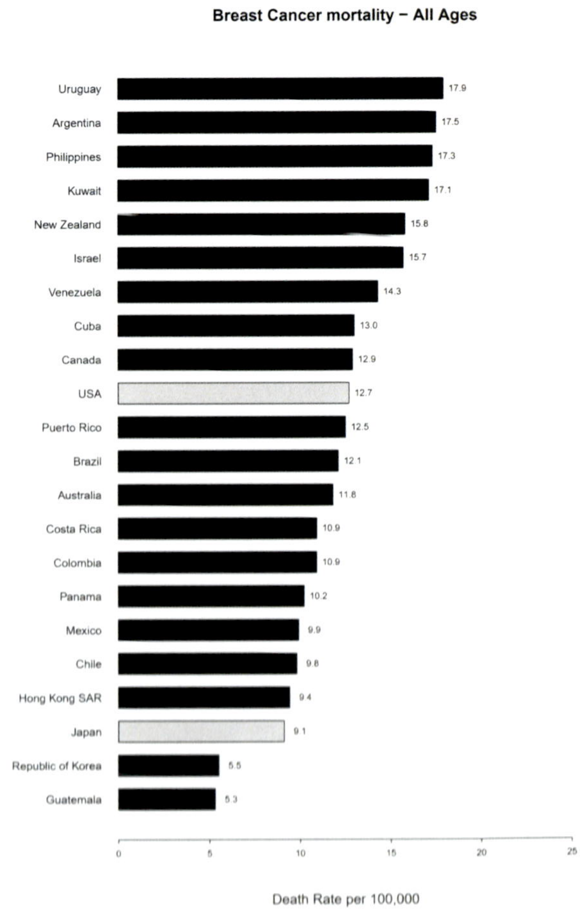

Figure 10.19. *Bar plot of the age-standardized (world population) rates for breast cancer registered in 2017 (or 2015 for Kuwait), ordered from the highest to the lowest rate.*

Source: Wojtyla C, Bertuccio P, Ciebiera M, La Vecchia C. Breast cancer mortality in the Americas and Australasia over the period 1980–2017 with predictions for 2025. Biology. 2021; 10(8):814. https://doi.org/10.3390/biology10080814.

The survival rates of women whose breast cancer was discovered during the screening exam and those of women whose breast cancer was discovered in between screening exams—that is, in cases where no breast cancer was found during screening but the women developed symptoms prior to the next examination, which took place a year later—were then compared by Shapiro and colleagues. The case-fatality rate would have been only 13% if the cancer had been identified through mammography. On the other hand, the case-fatality was 38% if the breast cancer was an interval case, meaning it was discovered in between exams. The likely explanation for this variation in case-fatality is that the disease was rapidly progressive when it was discovered between routine mammograms. Because it was so aggressive, it was found before the next regularly scheduled examination, which was scheduled a year later, even though it was not visible during the routine mammography examination (Figure 10.20).

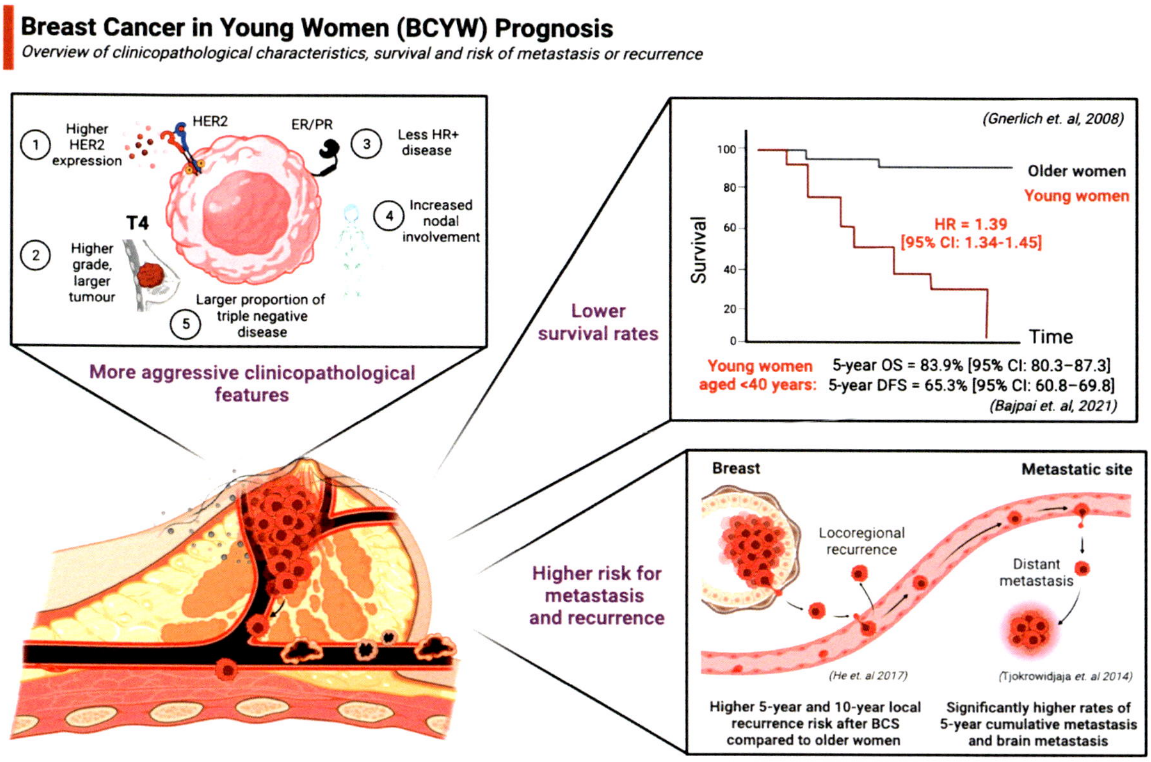

Figure 10.20. *Understanding fatality among patients with breast cancer.*

Source: Zhu JW, Charkhchi P, Adekunte S, Akbari MR. What Is known about breast cancer in young women? Cancers. 2023; 15(6):1917. https://doi.org/10.3390/cancers15061917.

The long preclinical phase and low case-fatality of 13% in women whose cancer findings were discovered during screening suggested a long clinical phase as well. Given the high case fatality of the group, the women with normal mammograms and whose disease manifested clinically prior to the subsequent examination experienced a brief preclinical phase and a brief clinical phase.

Those who did not show up for screening had a far higher mortality rate over five years than those who did. The answer is obvious: volunteer bias, the well-documented finding that people who participate in health programs differ from those who do not in many ways, including health status, attitudes, educational and socioeconomic levels, and other factors. Since the screening was limited to breast cancer, why should those who came for screening and those who did not manifest different mortality rates for causes other than breast cancer? This serves as further evidence that comparing program participants to non-participants is an invalid method of program evaluation.

We might stray from our topic of the HIP study to discuss an intriguing use of these data that Shapiro and colleagues conducted. In the United States, whites have a higher 5-year relative survival rate from breast cancer than blacks.

There has been discussion about whether this is because black patients may take longer to receive a diagnosis and treatment for their disease than white patients do. It has also been suggested that there may be differences in the biology of the disease between black and white populations. Shapiro and associates realized that the mammography randomized trial presented a unique chance to investigate this query. First, let's focus only on the survival curves for the black and white control group.

The data show that the prognosis was worse for Blacks and Hispanics than for Whites. Now, let's take a closer look at the curves for Whites and Blacks in the study group of women who underwent screening; since screening was done according to a set schedule, there was no difference in their access to care or use of it. There is almost no difference between the two curves, which show significant overlap. This strongly implies that the racial disparity in survivability had been eliminated by the screening and that the typically noted racial disparity in breast cancer prognosis is actually the consequence of black people's lower utilization of or access to care, which has delayed diagnosis and treatment (Figure 10.21).

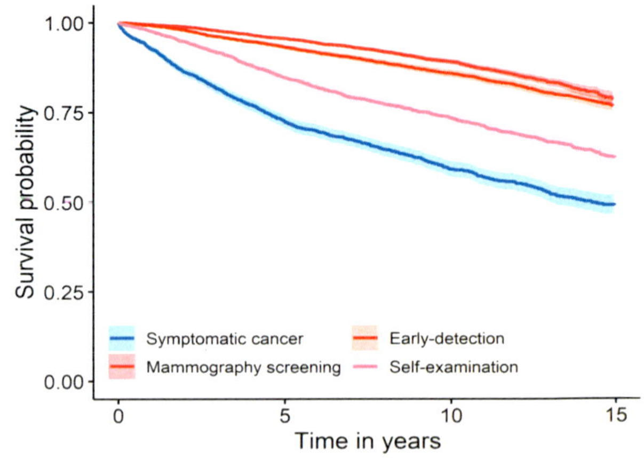

Figure 10.21. *Survival of breast cancer for different modes of detection with the pointwise 95% confidence interval in shaded bands.*

Source: Schumann L, Hadwiger M, Eisemann N, Katalinic A. Lead-time corrected effect on breast cancer survival in Germany by mode of detection. Cancers. 2024; 16(7):1326. https://doi.org/10.3390/cancers16071326.

10.2.4.3. Examples of Studies Evaluating Screening

10.2.4.3.1. Mammography for Women 40 to 49 Years of Age

The question of whether mammography should be routinely advised for women in their 40s has been at the center of a significant controversy in recent years. The benefits of routine mammography exams for women 50 years of age and above were demonstrated by the data from Shapiro's study and other studies. For women in their 40s, the information is less clear. The results of randomized trials conducted in various populations can be difficult to interpret. While it has been estimated that women in their 40s who undergo annual mammograms will experience a 17% reduction in mortality, the majority of the data that are currently available come from studies that were not intended to evaluate potential benefits in this age group. Furthermore, a considerable number of the trials included women in their late 40s, raising the possibility that, despite any benefits that may have been noted, they may have come from mammograms done on women 50 years of age or older.

A similar problem is considered. When 50-year-old women who were 50 years of age or older and were either screened or not, the mortality curves split approximately 4 years after enrollment, with the mammography group exhibiting longer-lasting lower mortality. But when 40-year-old women who were screened and those who weren't, the mortality curves show no discernible variations in mortality for a minimum of 11–12 years following enrollment. To find out if the divergence in the mortality curves will continue and genuinely benefit women who had mammograms in their 40s, more observation is required. The women in these studies who have been followed for ten years or longer have passed the age of fifty, making it difficult to interpret these curves. Consequently, any benefit observed may be attributable to mammograms performed after age 50 rather than mammograms performed in their 40s, even if mortality in screened women declines after 11 years. Clarification of these issues may be aided by additional follow-up with women enrolled in many of these studies as well as in newly started studies enrolling women in their early 40s.

The National Institutes of Health established a Consensus Panel in 1997 to examine the scientific data supporting the advantages of mammography for women between the ages of 40 and 49. The panel came to the conclusion that there was insufficient evidence to support recommending mammography to all women in their 40s. The Panel suggested that each woman make her own decisions about whether to get a mammogram. Her choice may be influenced by her personal medical history, an objective assessment of the available scientific data, her perception of and assessment of each possible risk and benefit, her values associated with each, and her approach to dealing with uncertainty. A woman should have access to the most up-to-date, pertinent information on the advantages and risks of the treatment, presented in an intelligible and practical manner, considering the significance and complexity of the issues involved in evaluating the evidence.

The majority of women will rely significantly on the expertise and understanding of their doctors; one significant issue in this context is that many doctors lack the knowledge of cancer screening statistics necessary to offer women and their families the support they require to carefully review the findings and recommendations, as well as the validity, of mammography studies for women in their 40s. In a recent study, Wegwarth and colleagues reported the findings of a nationwide survey of primary care doctors in the U.S and discovered that the majority of these doctors mistook higher detection and improved survival rates with screening for proof that screening saves lives. Few people appropriately noted that decreased mortality in a randomized trial is proof positive screening is beneficial. The Consensus Panel further stated that in order to prevent financial barriers from influencing a woman's decision to undergo a mammogram, third-party payors or health maintenance organizations should cover the costs of the exams for women in their 40s who choose to have them performed. The National Cancer Institute, which had initiated the panel's formation, along with other organizations, declined the panel's recommendations. Strong political forces were obviously in favor of mammography for women in their 40s at the time, based on the available evidence.

The 2001 publication of a review by Olsen and Gøtzsche of the data supporting mammography at any age broadened the debate surrounding the procedure. The investigators brought up a number of concerns, including the potential insufficiency of the randomization process and the potential unreliability of the assessment of the cause of death. They also noted that in certain trials, women with preexisting cancer were excluded from the studies only after they had been screened, and they concluded that the two best trials did not find any benefit.

The review was published in an issue of the Lancet that included an accompanying editorial that stated, in part, that there was currently insufficient evidence from large randomized trials to support screening mammography programs. An article published in 2004 refuted the claims made by Olsen and Gøtzsche, concluding that the previous consensus regarding mammography was accurate.

Nonetheless, the dispute is still going strong. In the year 2002, the U. S. After reviewing the available data, the Preventive Services Task Force advised women 40 years of age and above to undergo screening mammography every one to two years. This Task Force reexamined the issue of mammography for women in their 40s in 2009 and proposed that screening mammograms be performed every two years for women between the ages of 50 and 74. However, they also came to the following conclusion: "There is moderate certainty that the net benefit is small for biennial screening mammography in women aged 40 to 49 years." The Task Force rated its recommendation a "C," emphasizing that it advises against routinely screening women between the ages of 40 and 49. The Task Force advocates for informed and personalized decision-making regarding the appropriate age to begin mammography screening, they continued."

New guidelines regarding mammography for women in their 40s were released by the American College of Physicians in 2007. These guidelines were based on a comprehensive systematic review that looked at both potential benefits and risks. The group came to the conclusion that mammography carries significant risks and that the evidence for net benefit is less clear for women in their 40s than for women in their 50s. They said that the evidence did not support a blanket recommendation. The National Health Service of the United Kingdom released guidelines in 2011 suggesting that women between the ages of 47 and 73 should have a mammogram every three years.

Thus, the debate between supporters and detractors is far from over and is unlikely to be resolved to everyone's satisfaction with the opinions of experts. More extensive trials are unlikely to address the intricate issues with methodology and interpretation. These studies are time-consuming, costly, and difficult to start and finish. They are also constrained in that the results frequently do not take into account the most recent advancements in mammography technology. But since there is so much conflicting information in the data, it is likely that new technologies for breast cancer detection will lead to advancements in the field. Meanwhile, because of the significant uncertainties in the available data, women are left to make difficult decisions about their own mammography options.

10.2.4.3.2. Screening for Cervical Cancer

The Pap smear is arguably the most widely used cancer screening test. It follows that there must be copious evidence supporting its efficacy in lowering the death rate from invasive cervical cancer. Regretfully, no well-designed randomized, controlled trial has been conducted on cervical cancer screening, and it is unlikely that one will be conducted in the future as cervical cancer screening has been deemed effective by the public and health authorities alike. Considering the enormous resources that have been used globally to screen for cervical cancer, this situation is astounding.

Despite the lack of concrete proof of Pap smears' efficacy, it would be unethical to conduct a randomized trial of the procedure. Many other methods have been employed in the absence of randomized trials. Comparing incidence and mortality rates across populations with varying screening rates has probably been the most common evaluation design. An alternative method has involved tracking variations in the rates of carcinoma in situ diagnosis over time. A third strategy has involved conducting case-control studies, wherein women diagnosed with invasive cervical cancer are compared to control groups, and the frequency of prior Pap smears is investigated in each cohort.

Notwithstanding these misgivings, the evidence suggests that the majority of carcinomas in situ most likely do progress to invasive cancer; as a result, early detection of cervical cancer in the in situ stage would considerably save lives, albeit at a rate that may be less than many optimistic estimates. The lack of an initial well-designed randomized trial contributes significantly to the uncertainty surrounding cervical cancer screening. This observation highlights the fact that new pharmaceutical agents in the U.S must meet certain requirements before they are licensed for use in humans, but new technologies and health initiatives are subject to a different, less strict set of requirements. In the U.S, no medication would be approved without evaluation through randomized, controlled trials; sadly, however, prior to the introduction of screening or other programs and procedures, no such evaluation is necessary.

10.2.4.3.3. Screening for Neuroblastoma

Some of the issues just discussed are encountered in screening for neuroblastoma, which is a tumor that occurs in young children. The rationale for screening for neuroblastoma was outlined by Tuchman and colleagues: (1) Outcome has improved little in the past several decades. (2) Prognosis is known to be better in children who manifest the disease before the age of 1 year. (3) At any age, children in advanced stages of disease have worse prognoses than those in early stages. (4) More than 90% of children presenting with clinical symptoms of neuroblastoma excrete higher than normal amounts of catecholamines in their urine. (5) These metabolites can easily be measured in urine samples obtained from diapers.

These data provide compelling justification for neuroblastoma screening. Data from Japan, where a significant neuroblastoma screening initiative was implemented, are considered here. The percentages of children under one year old with neuroblastoma were compared in Sapporo, Hokkaido, before and after screening was implemented. These data were then cross-checked with birth data from the remaining parts of Hokkaido, where screening programs were not implemented. Following the start of screening, Sapporo had a higher percentage of cases of neuroblastoma in children under the age of one year than the rest of Hokkaido (Figure 10.22).

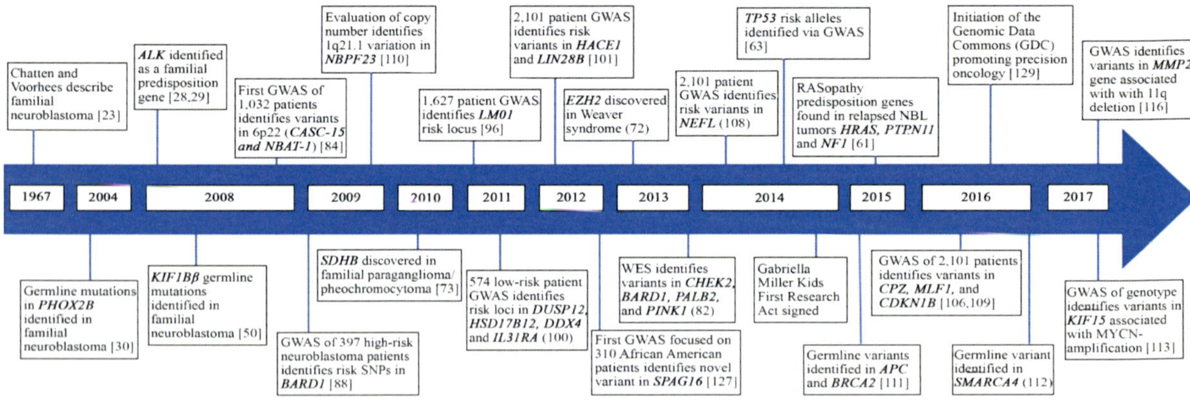

Figure 10.22. *Timeline of identified genetic variation predisposing to neuroblastoma. GWAS, genome-wide association studies.*

Source: Barr EK, Applebaum MA. Genetic predisposition to neuroblastoma. Children. 2018; 5(9):119. https://doi.org/10.3390/children5090119.

Nevertheless, evaluating the advantages of neuroblastoma screening presents a number of significant issues. We now know that neuroblastoma is a biologically heterogeneous disease, with some cases obviously having a better prognosis from the outset than others. Many tumors have a good prognosis because, even in the absence of therapy, they spontaneously regress. Furthermore, aggressive, quickly growing tumors are less likely to be detected by screening than slow-growing, less malignant tumors.

10.3. Epidemiology and Public Policy

One of epidemiology's main functions is to provide a foundation for the creation of policies pertaining to human health, such as illness prevention and control. Epidemiologic study results may have bearing on problems pertaining to clinical practice, community health, and population-based strategies for illness prevention and health promotion.

10.3.1. Epidemiology and Prevention

Understanding fundamental epidemiologic concepts and the potential interpretation of epidemiologic study results is necessary for identifying populations at increased risk, determining the cause of their increased risk, and weighing the costs and benefits of removing or reducing exposure to the causal factor or factors. Furthermore, it is crucial to evaluate the quality of the evidence and note any restrictions on the conclusions that can be drawn or the extent to which the results can be applied. As a result, epidemiology is regarded as the "fundamental science" of prevention. The question of what level of epidemiologic evidence is necessary to support a preventive effort is obviously difficult to answer. Depending on whether primary or secondary prevention is being considered, different issues are involved. When it comes to primary prevention, the answer relies on a number of factors, including the severity of the ailment, the costs (both monetary and in terms of human suffering and loss of quality of life), the strength of the evidence linking a particular causative factor or factors to the disease in question, and the difficulty of minimizing or completely removing exposure to that factor.

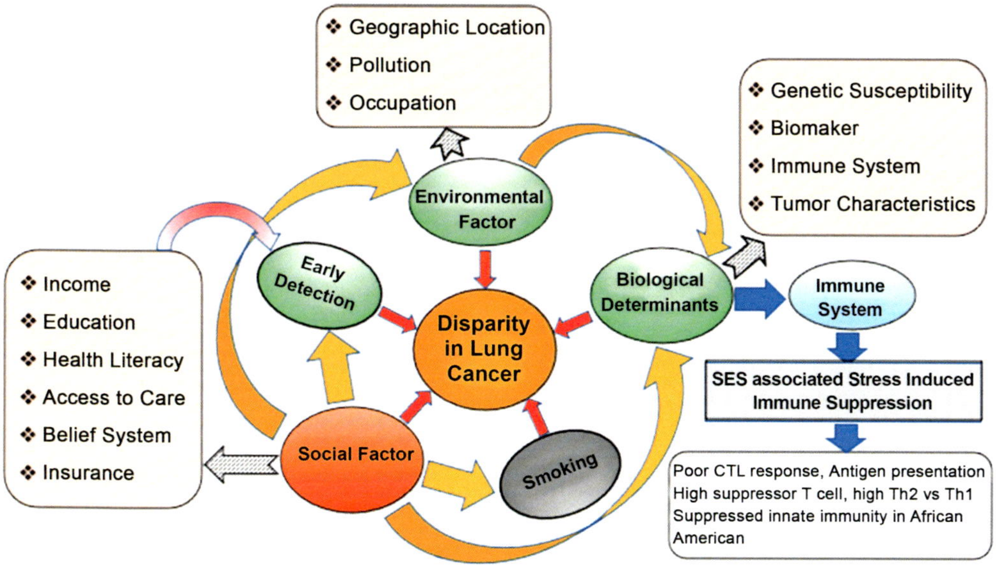

Figure 10.23. *Social and biological determinants of lung cancer. The diagram shows an association of social factors such as income, education, health literacy, access to care, belief system, and insurance status with racial differences in lung cancer incidence and outcome. Low socioeconomic status negatively impacts education, income, health awareness, and access to insurance, leading to lower screening rates, unhealthy geographical location, forced choice of occupation, and frequent proneness to exposure to hazards. Low SES also induces chronic stress, impacting the biology of lung cancer and favoring an immunosuppressive environment in African Americans.*

Source: Brock BA, Mir H, Flenaugh EL, Oprea-Ilies G, Singh R, Singh S. Social and biological determinants in lung cancer disparity. Cancers. 2024; 16(3):612. https://doi.org/10.3390/cancers16030612.

Extending the so-called traditional risk factor model of epidemiology, which examines the relationship between an independent factor like exposure and a dependent factor like the outcome of a disease, has received a lot of attention in recent years.

The problems differ slightly with secondary prevention. We still need to take into account how serious the illness is. It is also necessary to consider whether screening can identify the disease earlier than usual, how costly and invasive this kind of detection would be, whether treating a patient earlier than usual will benefit them, and whether screening has any negative side effects. It is evident that epidemiology is a very useful method for addressing a lot of these problems.

It has been proposed that this approach should be broadened in two ways. Firstly, it should measure not only the negative outcome, or the disease itself, but also the effects the disease has on the individual, his or her family, and the community in terms of the economy, society, and psychology. Secondly, it is evident that a population's exposure to a putative causal agent is typically not distributed evenly. Therefore, if prevention is to be achieved by lowering the exposure, the factors that determine whether an individual becomes exposed must be investigated (Figure 10.23).

The relationship is influenced by determinants of susceptibility of the individual to the exposure, which include genetic factors along with environmental and social influences. The full model is even more complex. While an expanded approach like this makes sense intuitively and offers a great framework for analyzing public health issues, it still needs to be shown whether specific exposures or other independent variables are linked to higher risks of particular diseases.

In any case, societal factors, such as a society's values and priorities, will determine the quantity and kind of data we need for prevention. Along with other fields, epidemiology can supply a large portion of the scientific data required to address questions related to risk and prevention.

However, societal values, political factors, and economic factors will ultimately determine whether or not to start a preventative program. Simultaneously, it is envisaged that these determinations will also rest on a solid basis of scientific data furnished by epidemiology and other pertinent fields.

Making the distinction between exposures to the macro- and microenvironments is crucial. Exposures that impact populations or entire communities, like air pollution, are referred to as macroenvironmental exposures. Microenvironmental exposures include things like food, smoking, and alcohol use that have an impact on a particular person. From the perspective of prevention, macroenvironmental factors are more easily controlled and modified because this can be achieved through laws and regulations (e.g., establishing pollution-related environmental standards). On the other hand, changing personal habits and lifestyles is necessary to alter microenvironmental factors, and this can often be a much more difficult task.

When it comes to microenvironmental factors, it is often insufficient to merely present risk estimates and scientific proof to persuade people to change their lifestyles in order to prevent harm. The degree to which people are willing to take risks in various areas of their lives, including their health, varies widely. Furthermore, a person's actions may vary based on whether they are exposed to the "risk" of a favorable event or the possibility of a negative outcome. Furthermore, people frequently shift the blame for lifestyle-related health issues elsewhere.

Therefore, the previously mentioned concept of risk communication needs to go beyond just providing policymakers with risk data. In order to encourage people to take accountability and take the best possible care of their own health, it must also address how to communicate with the public in a way that is clear and relevant given how each person perceives their own level of risk. Therefore, epidemiologists and health educators should collaborate to appropriately educate the public about risk factors.

10.3.2. Population Approaches Versus High-Risk Approaches to Prevention

Whether our strategy should focus on individuals who are known to be at high risk or whether it should expand primary prevention efforts to the general public is a crucial question in the field of prevention. Rose brought up this topic in 1985, and Whelton expanded on it in 1994 during a talk about preventing hypertension and heart disease deaths (CHD).

There is no known threshold for the risk of death from CHD, according to epidemiologic studies, which show that it increases steadily with increases in both systolic and diastolic blood pressure. The systolic blood pressure distribution of 347,978 men who underwent screening for the Multiple Risk Factor Intervention Trial (MRFIT) is considered here. The risk rises gradually as blood pressure rises. People who had a blood pressure of 180 mm Hg or greater had a 5.65 times greater chance of dying from CHD than people whose blood pressure was less than 110 mm Hg.

A person is considered to have no excess deaths if their blood pressure is less than 110 mm Hg. More than two thirds of the excess CHD deaths were caused by people with hypertension, even though less than one-fourth of all people had the condition. Given that these individuals have the highest relative risk, it makes sense to focus our preventive efforts on preventing high systolic blood pressure.

Nonetheless, blood pressure in the 140–159 mm Hg range (stage 1) was present in nearly 80% of the hypertensive individuals. About 43% of the excess risk of dying from coronary heart disease (CHD) in the general population and roughly 64% of the excess risk of CHD death in hypertensive subjects were related to stage 1 hypertension.

Therefore, focusing preventive efforts on individuals with the highest blood pressure extremes is insufficient to address the overall burden of CHD deaths linked to elevated blood pressure. If we are to stop the majority of excess deaths linked to elevated blood pressure, we also need to concentrate on those with less noticeable elevations in blood pressure.

It therefore seems reasonable to combine a high risk with a population approach: one set of preventive measures addressed to those at particularly high risk and another designed for primary prevention of hypertension and addressed to the population in general.

Preventive programs may be significantly impacted by these analyzes. Preventive measures that are appropriate for the general population are not the same as those that may be used for high-risk individuals. High-risk patients are more likely to put up with more costly, uncomfortable, and intrusive procedures if they are aware of their increased risk.

But, in order for a preventive measure to be widely accepted, it must be inexpensive and only minimally invasive; if it is to cause the majority of people any pain or discomfort, it must also be reasonably minor.

The aim of a population-based strategy, as illustrated in Figure 10.24, is to shift the entire blood pressure distribution curve downward when a community-wide blood pressure-lowering intervention is implemented.

Given that the majority of people in the population have blood pressure that is higher than the very lowest levels that are thought to be ideal, even a slight downward (or leftward) shift in the curve is probably going to have a significant positive impact on public health.

In actuality, a change of this kind would stop more strokes in the general population than effective treatment restricted to "high-risk" patients. In addition, Rose3 made the point that the "high-risk" strategy is a temporary fix required to safeguard vulnerable people.

In the end, though, we want to identify the fundamental reasons why the condition occurs—in this case, high blood pressure—and create and put into practice the appropriate strategies for its (primary) prevention.

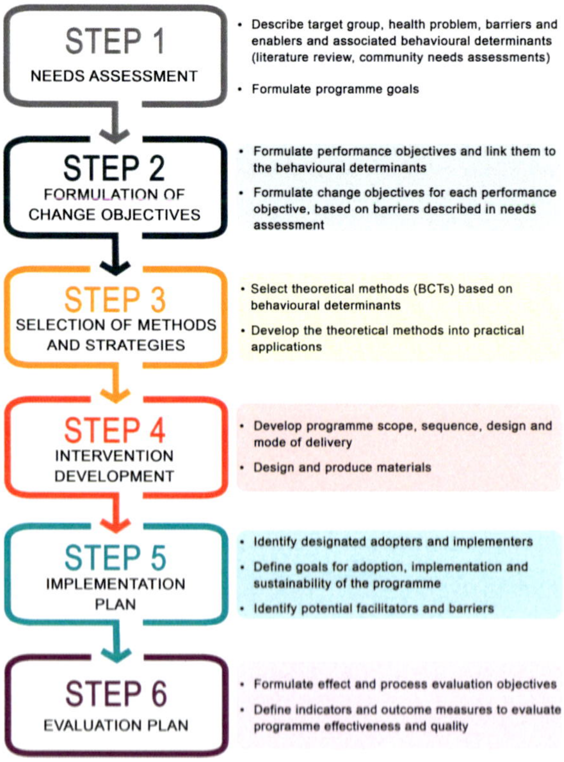

Figure 10.24. *An example of intervention mapping.*

Source: N Dieberger AM, van Poppel MNM, Watson ED. Baby steps: Using intervention mapping to develop a sustainable perinatal physical activity healthcare intervention. International Journal of Environmental Research and Public Health. 2021; 18(11):5869. https://doi.org/10.3390/ijerph18115869.

10.3.3. Epidemiology and Clinical Medicine: Hormone Replacement Therapy in Postmenopausal Women

The foundational science of clinical research is epidemiology. In many cases, clinical decision-making requires the use of data from epidemiologic studies. A thorough understanding of epidemiology is essential to the process of creating significant research on the efficacy of clinical interventions, the quality of various diagnostic techniques, and the natural history of disease. Numerous ambiguities and conundrums in clinical policy, many of which are difficult to solve, can be addressed with great relevance by epidemiology.

Subsequently, several nonrandomized observational studies were published that reported additional health benefits, including decreased incidence of hip fractures, osteoporosis, and heart attacks and strokes. When taking into account the total amount of available data, it seemed clear and generally consistent that estrogen shielded women from heart disease. It was recommended that women should consult their doctors about starting hormone replacement therapy (HRT) once they turned 50 years old in order to guard against heart disease and other aging-related ailments.

Two randomized trials were started, the Heart and Estrogen/Progestin Replacement Study (HERS) and the Women's Health Initiative (WHI), after it was determined that there was insufficient evidence to support the use of hard disease endpoints in these trials, such as the risk of myocardial infarction. 2,763 women with documented coronary heart disease (CHD) were included in the HERS study. It was discovered that contrary to popular belief, combination hormone replacement therapy elevated women's risk of myocardial infarctions in the first few years following initiation of therapy. The study's nearly seven-year follow-up period yielded no proof that HRT provided protection (Figure 10.25).

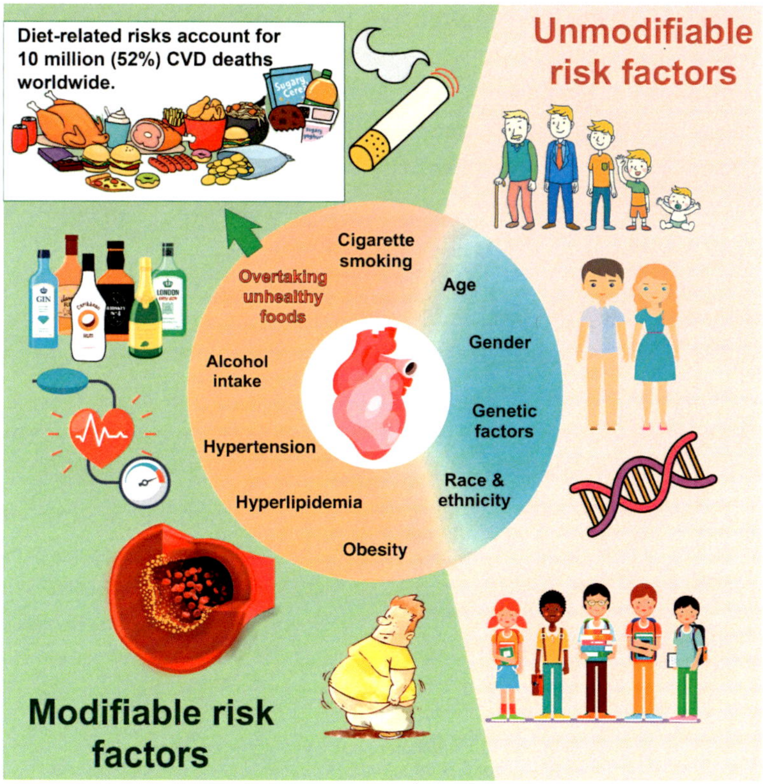

Figure 10.25. *The factors of incidence of coronary heart disease events.*

Source: Chen W, Zhang S, Hu X, Chen F, Li D. a review of healthy dietary choices for cardiovascular disease: from individual nutrients and foods to dietary patterns. Nutrients. 2023; 15(23):4898. https://doi.org/10.3390/nu15234898.

In order to assess HRT as primary prevention for heart disease and other disorders common in the elderly, 16,608 women participated in the WHI, a randomized, placebo-controlled trial that was conducted in 1991 and 1992. The trial was scheduled to run for 8.5 years. An estrogen plus progestin randomized, placebo-controlled trial was conducted as one of the study's arms on postmenopausal women with an intact uterus. Due to results showing increased risks of blood clots, breast cancer, heart attacks, and strokes by the time this component of the study was stopped three years early. The risks associated with HRT exceeded these advantages overall, even though the study indicated lower incidence of osteoporosis, bone fractures, and colorectal cancer.

Adverse events occurred in only 2.5 percent of the enrolled women. Based on the study findings, an estimate has been made that, in a year, there should be 7 more heart attacks (37 women taking estrogen plus progestin experienced heart attacks compared to 30 women taking a placebo), 8 more strokes, 8 more cases of breast cancer, and 18 more blood clots for every 10,000 women taking estrogen plus progestin. Five fewer hip fractures and six fewer cases of colorectal cancer would be anticipated at the same time.

The WHI results shocked a lot of women who had been taking HRT. The results clearly suggest that the risks of cardiovascular endpoints are actually increased in women who take estrogen plus progestin to prevent heart disease. These women were left wondering if they should look for other options or keep using HRT. Many also felt that the medical community had misled them because, despite the lack of conclusive evidence from placebo-controlled randomized trials, their doctors had for years reassured them about the safety and efficacy of HRT. The WHI did not address the issue that many women face when deciding whether to take combination hormone replacement therapy (HRT) for short periods of time in order to prevent or relieve postmenopausal symptoms like hot flashes, which complicates the decision-making process for women going through menopause.

The reason for the significant disparity between the outcomes of the placebo-controlled randomized WHI study and the results of numerous nonrandomized observational studies that had previously suggested that combination hormone replacement therapy (HRT) provided protection against heart disease is a significant methodologic question. This is a crucial topic because, in many fields of medicine and public health, our knowledge is based on the results of nonrandomized observational studies rather than randomized trials due to cost concerns or other impediments.

Numerous justifications have been put forth. The women who received HRT prescriptions in the observational studies were frequently healthier individuals with lower cardiovascular risk profiles. Compared to women who do not use HRT, those who do frequently have higher socioeconomic status, are leaner, more educated, more physically active, are less likely to smoke, and are more health conscious. Women who were prescribed HRT were frequently perceived as compliant, and compliant people frequently exhibit other positive behavioral patterns. Therefore, in the observational studies, confounding by lifestyle and other factors might have occurred. Furthermore, it's possible that the periodic cross-sectional measurements employed in the observational studies did not always detect early adverse effects that resulted in HRT discontinuation. It is obvious that when nonrandomized, observational studies are the foundation for clinical and public health policy in the future, these issues must be addressed.

10.3.4. Risk Assessment

Risk assessment is one of the main uses of epidemiology in relation to public policy. The characterization of possible harmful health effects of human exposure to environmental hazards is known as risk assessment. As illustrated in Figure 10.26, risk assessment is seen as a component of a larger process that starts with research, moves through risk assessment, and ends with risk management.

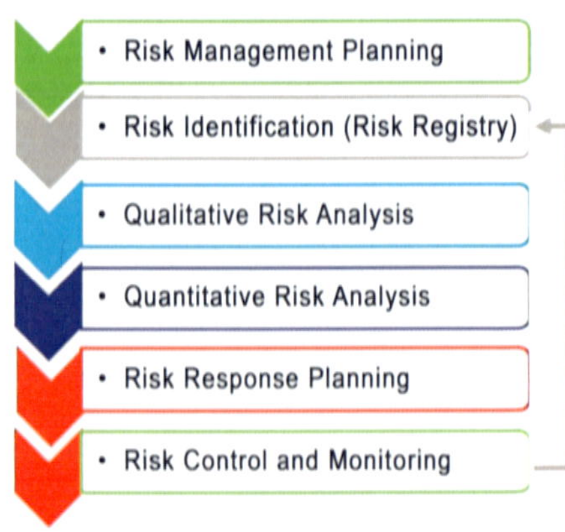

• Risk Management Planning
• Risk Identification (Risk Registry)
• Qualitative Risk Analysis
• Quantitative Risk Analysis
• Risk Response Planning
• Risk Control and Monitoring

Figure 10.26. *Risk assessment and management workflow diagram*

Source: Lee SY, Hnottavange-Telleen K, Jia W, Xiao T, Viswanathan H, Chu S, Dai Z, Pan F, McPherson B, Balch R. Risk Assessment and management workflow—an example of the southwest regional partnership. Energies. 2021; 14(7):1908. https://doi.org/10.3390/en14071908.

Samet et al. examined the connection between epidemiology and risk assessment and defined risk management as a process that includes choosing the best course of action and weighing the pros and cons of potential regulatory actions. Risk communication, which is the dissemination of risk assessment results to individuals who require them in order to engage in policy formation and implement suitable risk management measures, comes after risk management.

The National Research Council (1983) listed four steps in the process of risk assessment:

1. **Hazard Identification:** Determination of whether a particular chemical is causally linked to particular health effects.
2. **Dose-Response Assessment:** Determination of the relationship between the magnitude of exposure and the probability of occurrence of the health effects in question.
3. **Exposure Assessment:** Determination of the extent of human exposure before or after application of regulatory controls.
4. **Risk Characterization:** Description of the nature—and often the magnitude—of human risk, including attendant uncertainty.

Although epidemiology is not the only pertinent scientific field in the risk assessment process, epidemiologic data are unquestionably crucial in each of these steps. Toxicology in particular plays a significant role, and when results from the two fields disagree, it can be difficult to reconcile epidemiologic and toxicologic data.

A multitude of significant methodological issues impact the application of epidemiology in risk assessment. Thorough evaluation of every variable is essential because epidemiologic studies typically focus on the connection between an environmental exposure and the chance of contracting a disease.

10.3.4.1. Assessment of Exposure

Exposure data typically originate from multiple sources. There are benefits and drawbacks to every kind of source; the latter include incompleteness and reporting biases. Investigators often consult multiple sources when gathering information about exposure, but when disparate sources produce contradicting data, issues frequently arise.

Macroenvironmental factors typically affect many people at once, making it challenging to measure individual exposures. This presents another challenge for exposure assessment. Consequently, aggregate measurements are frequently used in ecological approaches rather than individual ones, and the aggregation is frequently done over wide areas. Individuals living in a community are therefore attributed with its characteristics; however, it is frequently debatable whether characterizing an individual exposure through this process is valid. Moreover, obtaining personal exposure histories is challenging from both a prospective and retrospective standpoint. Furthermore, it is necessary to determine long-past exposures, which is particularly difficult, due to the lengthy latent or induction period between exposure and development of disease.

A related set of issues arises when attempting to describe a worker's occupational exposures and establish a connection between a work-related exposure and a negative health consequence. In an industrial setting, workers are likely to be exposed to a variety of agents, making it challenging to isolate the risk associated with a single specific exposure. Second, studies of the exposure-disease relationship may be challenging because there is frequently a lengthy latent period between the exposure and the subsequent development of disease; for instance, recall may be poor and exposure records may have been lost. Third, people who live close to an industrial plant may be more susceptible to disease, making it challenging to determine how much of a worker's risk comes from living there and how much is related to occupational exposure at work.

All of the sources and measures that have been discussed thus far are indirect, which may be the most fundamental issue when it comes to measuring exposures in epidemiologic studies. For instance, there has been a lot of interest in the potential health effects of electromagnetic fields (EMF) in recent years. The 1979 study by Wertheimer and Leeper, which found that children who lived close to high-voltage transmission lines had higher incidences of leukemia, sparked this interest. Many methodological concerns have since been brought up, and it is still unclear whether these fields have a negative impact on people's health.

Numerous methods are employed in the study of EMF to quantify exposure, such as self-reports of electrical appliance use, spot or 24-hour measurements of the fields, and home wiring configurations. However, depending on the kind of exposure measurement that was employed, the findings of various studies regarding the risk of disease vary. In actuality, compared to wire configuration codes, actual magnetic field measurements—even 24-hour measurements—produce weaker associations with childhood leukemia. This finding begs the question of whether there is any possible cause-and-effect relationship between disease incidence and magnetic field exposure. Most of the time, important questions remain unanswered even with the best indirect measure of exposure. Firstly, exposure is rarely binary, so information on exposure dose is required to investigate potential dose-response relationships. Finding out if the exposure was continuous or sporadic is crucial, too. For instance, in the pathophysiology of cancer, periodic exposure alternating between periods of exposure and nonexposure may permit DNA repair during the nonexposure periods; continuous exposure would prevent such repair from occurring. Last but not least, latency information is crucial: How long is the latent period and what is its range? Knowing this will help us concentrate our efforts on identifying exposure during a window of time that appears to be one in which a causal exposure may have very well happened. Because of these problems in measuring exposure using indirect approaches, much interest has focused on the use of biological markers of exposures. The use of such biomarkers has been termed biochemical epidemiology or molecular epidemiology. The advantage of using biomarkers is that such use can overcome the problem of limited recall or lack of awareness of an exposure. In addition, biomarkers can overcome errors resulting from variations in individual absorption or metabolism by focusing on a later step in the causal chain.

Biomarkers can be defined as indicators of exposure, indicators of changes in the body brought on by exposures, or indicators of vulnerability or risk. The figure below shows their types (Figure 10.27).

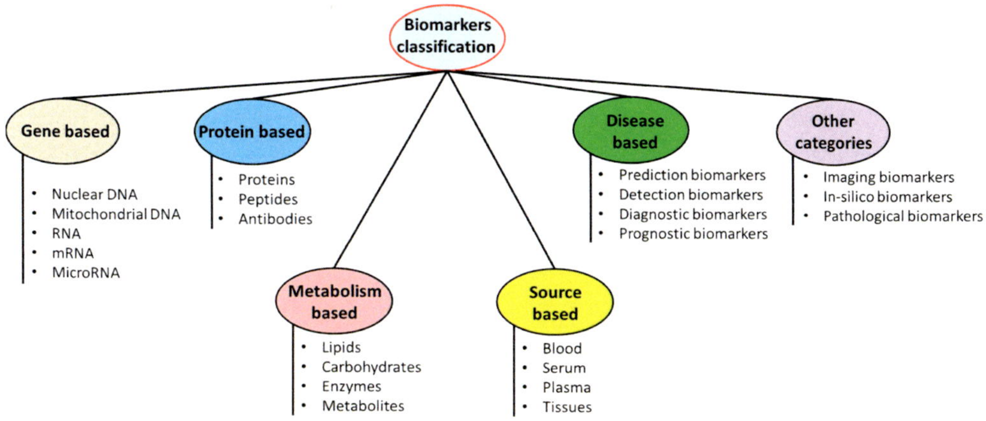

Figure 10.27. *What are biomarkers?*

Source: Ahmad A, Imran M, Ahsan H. Biomarkers as Biomedical bioindicators: Approaches and techniques for the detection, analysis, and validation of novel biomarkers of diseases. Pharmaceutics. 2023; 15(6):1630. https://doi.org/10.3390/pharmaceutics15061630.

The amount of potentially harmful substances in the general environment, the amounts to which a particular person is exposed, the amount absorbed, or the amount of the absorbed substance or its metabolite that reaches the target tissue are all possible metrics to measure. We are getting closer to measuring an exposure at a particular point in the process where an exposure is connected to a disease in humans thanks to biomarkers. For instance, we can quantify DNA adducts, which represent the impact of a material on biological processes in the body following absorption, in addition to environmental concentrations of the substance.

10.3.5. Meta-Analysis

Several scientific questions arise when epidemiologic data are used for formulating public policy:

1. Can epidemiologic methods detect small increases in risk?
2. How can we reconcile inconsistencies between animal and human data?
3. How can we use incomplete or equivocal epidemiologic data?
4. How can results be interpreted when the findings of epidemiologic studies disagree?

Many of the risks we are dealing with may be very small, but given the large number of individuals exposed and the potential for many of them to experience adverse health effects, they may potentially be very important for public health. However, bias or other methodologic limitations could easily be the cause of an observed slight increase in relative risk above 1.0; as a result, such results should be interpreted extremely cautiously until the results have been replicated and additional supporting data has been gathered.

Systematizing the process of reviewing the epidemiologic literature on a given topic has been attempted, owing to the possibility of inconsistent and occasionally dramatically conflicting results from different epidemiologic studies. "The statistical analysis of a large collection of analysis results from individual studies for the purpose of integrating the findings" is the definition of a related procedure known as meta-analysis. In contrast to a systematic review, a meta-analysis enables the results of several studies to be combined, appropriately weighting each study according to the number of subjects it samples and other factors. When study results are conflicting, providing a broad overview of the problem can be helpful.

However, there are a lot of issues and concerns surrounding meta-analysis. First, should all available studies be included in the analysis, or should it only include published studies? Secondly, how can the quality of the reviewed and aggregated studies be addressed? Lastly, when relative risks or odds ratios from different studies differ, a meta-analysis may obscure significant differences among individual studies. Therefore, a meta-analysis mustn't take the place of a thorough assessment of each study that is part of the analysis, including a close look at each study's methodologic limitations and results. Fourth, it's not always possible for other analysts to replicate the findings of meta-analyzes. An example is depicted in Figure 10.28.

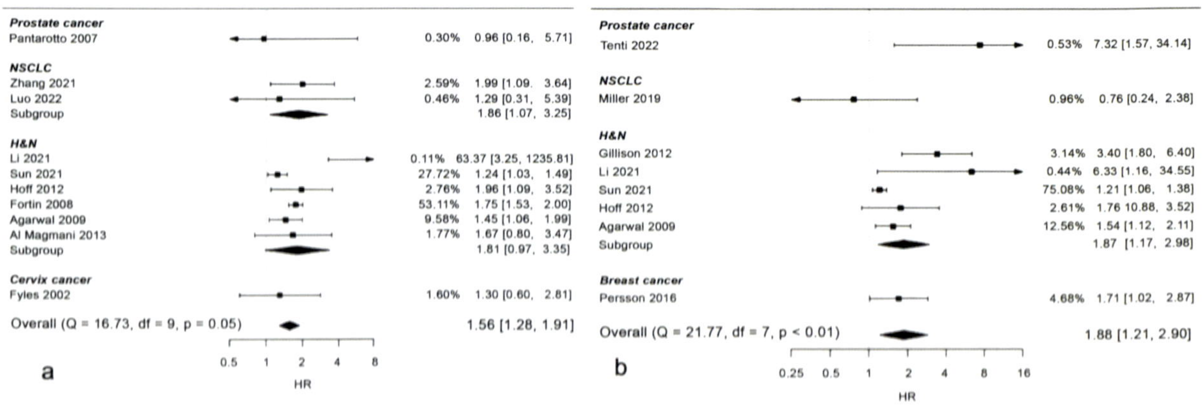

Figure 10.28. *Forest plots on pooled Hazard Ratios (HRs) on smoking during radiotherapy and efficacy. (**a**) Smoking during radiotherapy and locoregional recurrence free survival; (**b**) smoking during radiotherapy and disease-free survival. HR > 1 indicates worse outcome for smokers during radiation treatment, whereas HR < 1 indicates better outcome. Comparison group is non-smoker (former or never). Abbreviations: NSCLC, non-small-cell lung cancer; H&N, head and neck cancer.*

Source: Bergman M, Fountoukidis G, Smith D, Ahlgren J, Lambe M, Valachis A. Effect of smoking on treatment efficacy and toxicity in patients with cancer: A systematic review and meta-analysis. Cancers. 2022; 14(17):4117. https://doi.org/10.3390/cancers14174117.

Although meta-analysis is typically utilized in conjunction with randomized trials, it is also increasingly being applied to nonrandomized observational studies, such as case-control and cohort studies. In these cases, there may not be a common research design among the studies. Therefore, the question of how similar these studies must be for them to be included in a meta-analysis makes sense. Furthermore, biases (like selection and misclassification bias) must be appropriately controlled. However, this can be a very difficult task in meta-analyzes. Given the aforementioned considerations, there is still a great deal of disagreement regarding meta-analysis.

Putting a quantitative stamp on the estimation of a single relative risk or odds ratio from all the studies may give rise to a false sense of certainty regarding the risk's magnitude, which brings us to our final issue with meta-analysis: in light of all the challenges raised. When a number is attached to a finding, people frequently have an excessive amount of faith in its validity. As a result, many of the challenges that arise in meta-analysis may occasionally go unnoticed.

A Closer Look

Epidemiology And Public Policy

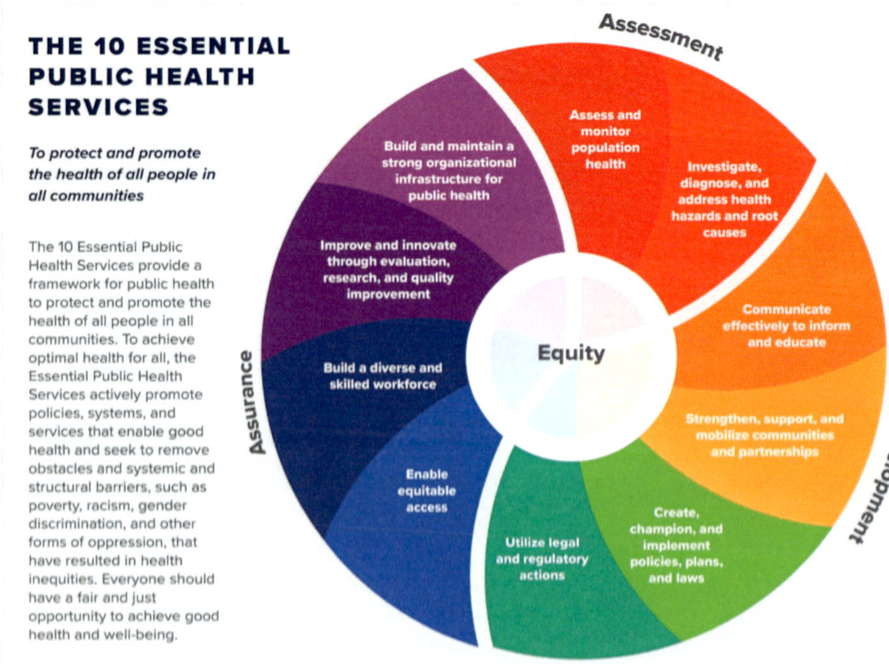

Epidemiology, as the study of the patterns, causes, and effects of health and disease conditions in populations, plays a crucial role in informing public policy decisions. By closely examining the distribution and determinants of health and disease, epidemiologists provide valuable insights that guide the development and implementation of effective public health policies.

Through rigorous data collection, analysis, and interpretation, epidemiologists identify trends and risk factors associated with various health outcomes. They investigate the spread of diseases, assess the impact of interventions, and evaluate the effectiveness of preventive measures. This evidence-based approach helps policymakers understand the burden of different health conditions within communities and prioritize resources accordingly.

Moreover, epidemiological research often uncovers disparities in health outcomes among different demographic groups, highlighting areas where targeted interventions are needed to address inequities. By identifying social, economic, and environmental factors that contribute to health disparities, epidemiologists inform policy efforts aimed at promoting health equity and reducing inequalities in access to care. Public policy decisions informed by epidemiological evidence can range from implementing vaccination programs and smoking bans to enacting regulations on food safety and environmental pollution. Epidemiologists collaborate with policymakers to design policies that are not only based on scientific evidence but also feasible and acceptable to the affected populations.

In essence, the close relationship between epidemiology and public policy underscores the importance of using scientific research to inform decision-making processes aimed at improving population health and well-being. By leveraging epidemiological insights, policymakers can develop strategies that effectively address public health challenges and promote healthier communities.

SUMMARY

- Epidemiology serves as a foundational tool in shaping public health policy through its rigorous approach to studying disease patterns, risk factors, and the effectiveness of interventions. Epidemiological research provides essential evidence that informs the evaluation of health policies and guides decision-making processes at local, national, and global levels.
- Epidemiology plays a crucial role in evaluating the impact of existing health policies and interventions. Through observational studies, randomized controlled trials (RCTs), and other study designs, epidemiologists assess whether specific policies or interventions have achieved their intended outcomes. For example, they might evaluate the effectiveness of vaccination programs in reducing disease incidence or analyze the impact of smoking bans on public health outcomes like cardiovascular disease rates.
- Randomization eliminates the problem of selection bias that results from either self-selection by the patient or selection of the patient by the health care provider. Usually, study participants are assigned to receive one type of care versus another rather than to receive care versus no care. For many reasons, both ethical and practical, randomizing patients to receive no care usually is not considered.
- All health care interventions cannot be subjected to randomized trials for several reasons. First, such trials are often logistically complex and extremely expensive. Because so many different health care measures are in use at any time, it is not feasible to subject all of them to randomized evaluations.
- The epidemiologic approach to evaluating screening programs involves systematically assessing the effectiveness, efficiency, and impact of screening tests in detecting diseases or conditions in a population. This approach relies on epidemiological principles and methods to study the natural history of diseases, the performance of screening tests, and the outcomes of screening programs.
- A major role of epidemiology is to serve as a basis for developing policies that affect human health, including the prevention and control of disease. As seen in previous chapters, the findings from epidemiologic studies may be relevant both to issues in clinical practice and community health, and to population approaches to disease prevention and health promotion.
- Identifying populations at increased risk, ascertaining the cause of their increased risk, and analyzing the costs and benefits of eliminating or reducing exposure to the causal factor or factors all require an understanding of basic epidemiologic concepts and of the possible interpretation of the findings of epidemiologic studies.

References

1. Birkmeyer, J. D., Stukel, T. A., Siewers, A. E., et al. (2003). Surgeon volume and operative mortality in the United States. *New England Journal of Medicine, 349*(22), 2117–2127.
2. Drummond, A. E., Pearson, B., Lincoln, N. B., et al. (2005). Ten-year follow-up of a randomized controlled trial of care in a stroke rehabilitation unit. *BMJ, 331*(7515), 491, 492.

3. Gordis, L. (1973). Effectiveness of comprehensive-care programs in preventing rheumatic fever. *New England Journal of Medicine, 289*(7), 331–335.
4. Gornick, M. E., Eggers, P. W., Reilly, T. W., et al. (1996). Effects of race and income on mortality and use of services among Medicare beneficiaries. *New England Journal of Medicine, 335*(11), 791–799.
5. Grady, D., Herrington, D., Bittner, V., et al., for the HERS Research Group. (2002). Cardiovascular disease outcomes during 6.8 years of hormone therapy: Heart and estrogen/progestin replacement study follow-up (HERS II). *JAMA, 288*(1), 49–57.
6. Grodstein, F., Clarkson, T. B., & Manson, J. E. (2003). Understanding the divergent data on postmenopausal hormone therapy. *New England Journal of Medicine, 348*(7), 645–650.
7. Jollis, J. G., Peterson, E. D., DeLong, E. R., et al. (1994). The relation between the volume of coronary angioplasty procedures at hospitals treating Medicare beneficiaries and short-term mortality. *New England Journal of Medicine, 331*(24), 1625–1629.
8. Kahn, K. L., Rubenstein, L. V., Draper, D., et al. (1990). The effects of DRG-based prospective payment system on quality of care for hospitalized Medicare patients: An introduction to the series. *JAMA, 264*(15), 1953–1955.
9. Kalra, L., Evans, A., Perez, I., et al. (2000). Alternative strategies for stroke care: A prospective randomized controlled trial. *Lancet, 356*(9233), 894–899.
10. Kosecoff, J., Kahn, K. L., Rogers, W. H., et al. (1990). Prospective payment system and impairment at discharge: The "quicker and sicker" story revisited. *JAMA, 264*(15), 1980–1983.
11. Michels, K. B. (2003). Hormone replacement therapy in epidemiologic studies and randomized clinical trials—Are we checkmate? *Epidemiology, 14*(1), 3–5.
12. Samet, J. M., Schnatter, R., & Gibb, H. (1998). Epidemiology and risk assessment. *American Journal of Epidemiology, 148*(10), 929–936.
13. Stine, O. C., Rider, R. V., & Sweeney, I. (1964). School leaving due to pregnancy in an urban adolescent population. *Journal of Public Health, 54*(1), 1–6.
14. The Women's Health Initiative. (2002). Risks and benefits of estrogen plus progestin in healthy postmenopausal women: Principal results. The Women's Health Initiative randomized controlled trial. *JAMA, 288*(3), 321–333.
15. Wertheimer, N., & Leeper, E. (1979). Electrical wiring configurations and childhood cancer. *American Journal of Epidemiology, 109*(3), 273–284.
16. Whittemore, A. S., & McGuire, V. (2003). Observational studies and randomized trials of hormone replacement therapy: What can we learn from them? *Epidemiology, 14*(1), 8–10.

INDEX

G

H

I

L

M

N

S

T

FSC
www.fsc.org
MIX
Papier | Fördert gute Waldnutzung
FSC® C083411

Kolibri 360 GmbH
Ferdinand-Jühlke-Straße 7
99095 Erfurt, Deutschland
produktsicherheit@kolibri360.de